D0154390

The A–Z of Death and Dying

The A–Z of Death and Dying

Social, Medical, and Cultural Aspects

MICHAEL BRENNAN, EDITOR

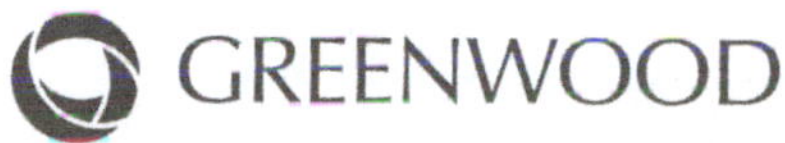

AN IMPRINT OF ABC-CLIO, LLC
Santa Barbara, California • Denver, Colorado • Oxford, England

Library of Congress Cataloging-in-Publication Data

The A–Z of death and dying : social, medical, and cultural aspects / Michael Brennan, editor.

pages cm

Includes index.

ISBN 978-1-4408-0343-7 (hardback : alk. paper) — ISBN 978-1-4408-0344-4 (ebook)

1. Thanatology—Encyclopedias. 2. Death—Encyclopedias. I. Brennan, Michael, 1973 April 17–

HQ1073.A22 2014

306.9—dc23 2013033528

ISBN: 978-1-4408-0343-7

EISBN: 978-1-4408-0344-4

18 17 16 15 14 1 2 3 4 5

This book is also available on the World Wide Web as an eBook.
Visit www.abc-clio.com for details.

Greenwood
An Imprint of ABC-CLIO, LLC

ABC-CLIO, LLC
130 Cremona Drive, P.O. Box 1911
Santa Barbara, California 93116-1911

This book is printed on acid-free paper ∞

Manufactured in the United States of America

Contents

Acknowledgments

Any undertaking of this sort relies inevitably upon the help and support of others, without whom it would not have been possible. There are therefore many people to whom I owe a debt of gratitude. Thanks are due to the editorial staff at ABC-CLIO, especially Mike Nobel, who commissioned this project, and Maxine Taylor, who helped see the manuscript through to completion. My thanks are due too to Allison Nadeau, media editor at ABC-CLIO, for her work in helping to select and obtain images for the book. Thanks are also due to the many contributors, especially those who delivered their manuscripts on time and in the form requested, and whose knowledge and expertise have helped ensure the final product resembles that as it was first envisioned. I am also grateful to my colleagues in the Department of Sociology and Archaeology at the University of Wisconsin–La Crosse for their friendship and collegiality; to my friends and colleagues involved in the annual International Conference on Death, Grief and Bereavement at the University of Wisconsin–La Crosse for their warmth and humility; and to my colleagues at Plymouth University, UK, for helping to stimulate my thinking on all things sociological. Special mention and thanks are owed to my wife, Lilach, for her continued support throughout this project (including help with copyediting and proofreading the final manuscript, as well as in helping to organize and process my voluminous file of e-mail correspondence with contributors), and to my little girl, Amelie, for her joyous laughter and for always helping to put a smile on my face.

Introduction

When, in the 1950s, Geoffrey Gorer first raised the possibility that death in modern society had been reduced to a crude form of entertainment akin to a kind of "pornography," he could not quite have anticipated the future possibilities by which this purported trend could at once be accelerated but also reversed in a range of representations, encounters, and activities related to mortality that are often sensitive, enriching, and deeply meaningful. This popular interest in mortality (from the renaissance in public mourning and *memento mori* practices such as RIP tattoos and postmortem photography, to Facebook grieving and the informal philosophical discussion of mortality in so-called death cafés) is mirrored in the academic interest in death, dying, and bereavement, often in ways that are increasingly suggestive of, and dependent upon, reciprocal relations between popular and scholarly domains.

Since the 1950s, what was once a fledgling scholarly interest in death and dying has grown exponentially into a well-established and interdisciplinary field of death studies (or thanatology) that traverses a wide variety of disciplines (sociology, psychology, history, anthropology, theology, and religious studies) and domains (clinical medicine, palliative care, social work, and tourism). After several decades of continual expansion, the field of death studies has now reached a stage of maturity reflective of an apparent shift in public attitudes, whereby death and dying, once closeted, are now very much part of public life. Witness, for example, the 35 million visitors worldwide to the "Body Worlds" exhibition of human cadavers since it first opened in 1996, or the seeming public appetite for the consumption of "pathographies" by celebrities and public figures who have chosen, often in a very public way, to narrate their intimate experiences of dying. In light of these developments, the second decade of the 21st century is therefore an extremely timely moment at which to consolidate the accumulated body of knowledge about death and dying by providing an accessible and up-to-date reference work that captures the longer trajectory of historical change as well as recent developments and innovations, both within the field of death studies as well as in society at large.

Drawing upon the expertise of international scholars and practitioners from across the interdisciplinary field of thanatology, the approximately 180 entries contained within this A–Z compendium are as capacious and wide-ranging as life itself; of which death and dying are themselves an intrinsic and inescapable part. Indeed, a guiding principle and philosophical assumption underpinning the work of early pioneers within the field of death education, as well as many contributors to this volume, is that a fuller understanding of death can help enhance our appreciation of life; that thanatology can help one live better by reminding us of our own fragile and finite existence.

In putting together this encyclopedia (and reflected in its subtitle), particular emphasis has been given to the social, cultural, and medical aspects of death and dying in ways that serve as a reminder that while death is an immutable and biological certainty, all other practices, attitudes, and beliefs surrounding it are mutable: group specific and subject to historical variation and change. In light of this, we can see how our attitudes and practices regarding death and dying (including the ways we grieve) are often, without us necessarily realizing it, influenced by others. So too, our social interactions and beliefs in relation to death and dying take place *within* a given culture and are thereby subject to variation by gender, age, race/ethnicity, social class, and so on. In a narrower sense, culture in the shape of art and literature, film, television, and interactive digital technologies provide a specific focus for the conveyance (or avoidance) of death and dying in ways that serve as a cultural barometer of continuity and change. That modern medicine provides another dimension and focus of the entries contained in this volume should come as little surprise given that today, in contrast to a century ago (when almost the exact opposite was the case), the overwhelming majority of people (some 80 percent) die in hospitals, hospices, and residential care facilities rather than at home.

This transformation in the place of death speaks volumes about the medicalization of death in modern societies, as well as the ability provided by modern medical technology to sustain life (and also potentially prolong suffering), in ways that have been of profound and ongoing concern to campaigners advocating dignity in death and those working within the hospice and palliative care movement. That much of our understanding of death (including the definition and point at which a person is said to have died) and grief is underscored by prevailing medical and scientific discourses can be seen in recent discussion surrounding the eagerly awaited revision to the *Diagnostic and Statistical Manual of Mental Disorders* (*DSM-5*). The redefinition of grief by the American Psychiatric Association (by which bereavement was traditionally excluded as the basis for providing a psychiatric diagnosis, such as depression, in the immediate aftermath of a personal loss) has raised concerns among some who fear that the release of the newest edition of the *DSM-5* will inevitably lead to the unnecessary medication of individuals who have experienced a recent bereavement. While loss is a distressing and universal experience involving significant psychosocial transition, it does not however, in most cases, require medical intervention.

The entries contained within *The A–Z of Death and Dying* both reflect and span a wide array of areas and themes, not least the social, historical, demographic, and epidemiological aspects of death and dying in ways that correlate closely with the benchmarking standards of health education in the United States. In this vein, death provides a useful social indicator that reveals much, not only about the way life is lived in a particular society at a particular moment in time, but can also (especially when placed in comparative context) throw much-needed light on the social progress and overall health of a nation. Death rates, infant mortality, and life expectancy, for example, all tell us a great deal about how our society has changed, as well as about how our own society differs from others, by providing a focus for cross-cultural comparison. The reduction in mortality rates and growth in average life expectancy (which, as data from the U.S. Census Bureau indicate, has increased from 47 to 78 years in the United States since 1900) have had the effect of raising our expectations about life and living, death and dying, often to the extent that people behave as if they were immortal, failing to make adequate preparations—whether financial, psychological, or social—for their own and deaths of others whom they love.

In reading Abraham Verghese's 2009 novel *Cutting for Stone,* I was reminded of the differing expectations about death and dying within a global cultural context when the book's protagonist and narrator, Dr. Marion Stone, has to deliver the news of a fatal condition to a patient for the first time in America. The narrator tells us how it felt as if he had just delivered news of a fatal condition for the very first time and how, in Ethiopia or Nairobi, "people assumed that all illness—even a trivial or imagined one—was fatal; they expected death." In contrast, the narrator describes how in America "death or the possibility of it always seemed to come as a surprise, as if we took it for granted that we were immortal, and that death was just an option."

The timeless significance of loss, together with the renewed public (and academic) interest in death and dying, suggests a need to consolidate the accumulated corpus of work within a growing and expansive field in a convenient and easily accessible A–Z reference work. *The A–Z of Death and Dying* attempts to do just that, bringing together, in a single volume, a wide variety of entries reflective of the latest cutting-edge theory and research that would otherwise remain spread across a range of disparate, and sometimes difficult-to-access, sources (specialist journals, books, and academic colloquia). These concise yet comprehensive entries are intended to have wide appeal, providing an essential entry point for those new to the topic, as well as for those with a long-standing interest in death and dying. In keeping with *The Chicago Manual of Style*, 16th edition, and per the publisher's style guidelines, whereby the use of plural pronouns ("they", "their") to avoid gender generalization is discouraged, I have alternated between male and female pronouns to avoid the implication of stereotypic gender roles; I have done so randomly unless circumstances demand gender-specific language.

The A–Z of Death and Dying will also help support health curricula by demonstrating, for example, ways in which health inequalities and differences in health behaviors during life have been used as an explanation and predictor of differential rates of premature death between social groups. Extensively cross-referenced and containing a comprehensive index in order to facilitate easy navigation of the text, as well as to encourage reading across a range of interrelated topics and themes, it has been my intention to provide a book that will serve as an invaluable resource for high-school and undergraduate studies in universities and four-year colleges; researchers looking for information on a particular topic; as well as the wider public and those working with the dying, dead, and bereaved. The pace of change, whether to legislation around the world regarding assisted dying; technologies used for the enhancement of bodily disposal; or to facilitate as well as communicate grieving and dying, means that it is almost impossible to provide a text that is fully conversant and abreast of the very latest developments. I have, nevertheless, striven to provide a resource that will serve as an accessible and trusted source of knowledge and hope that readers will find something valuable in it.

The Contributors

Ahmed M. Abdel-Khalek
University of Alexandria, Egypt

David A. Anderson
University of Wisconsin–La Crosse, USA

Michael Ashby
University of Tasmania, Australia

David E. Balk
City University New York at Brooklyn College, USA

Christopher Bartley
University of Liverpool, UK

Sandra L. Bertman
Mount Ida College, USA

Jason Bertrand
University of Wisconsin–La Crosse, USA

Regina A. Boisclair
Alaska Pacific University, USA

Lucy Bregman
Temple University, USA

Michael Brennan
Plymouth University, UK

Andrea Malkin Brenner
American University, USA

Inge B. Corless
Massachusetts General Hospital, USA

Gerry R. Cox
University of Wisconsin–La Crosse, USA

Illene Cupit
University of Wisconsin–Green Bay, USA

Priscilla Dass-Brailsford
Georgetown University, USA

Douglas J. Davies
University of Durham, UK

Dixie Dennis
Austin Peay State University, USA

Michael Robert Dennis
Emporia State University, USA

Erin Dermody
Brunel University, UK

Kenneth J. Doka
College of New Rochelle, USA

James Claude Upshaw Downs
Georgia State Regional Medical Examiner's Office, USA

Demetrea Nicole Farris
University of West Alabama, USA

Christopher J. Ferguson
Texas A&M University, USA

Scott Gelfand
Oklahoma State University, USA

Richard B. Gilbert
Mercy College, USA

Ann Gleig
University of Central Florida, USA

Richard Greene
Weber State University, USA

Rabbi Earl A. Grollman
Beth El temple Center, USA

Harry Hamilton
University of Alabama at Birmingham, USA

Darcy Harris
King's University College, Ontario, Canada

Bert Hayslip Jr.
University of North Texas, USA

Laurel Hilliker
Park University, USA

Christine Hippert
University of Wisconsin–La Crosse, USA

Jason M. Holland
University of Nevada, USA

Glennys Howarth
Plymouth University, UK

Asa Kasher
Tel-Aviv University, Israel

Michael C. Kearl
Trinity University, USA

Karen A. Kehl
University of Wisconsin–Madison, USA

Karin T. Kirchhoff
University of Wisconsin–Madison, USA

Dennis Klass
Webster University, USA

Jody LaCourt
University of Minnesota, USA

Michael R. Leming
St. Olaf College, USA

Lynn Letukas
University of Wisconsin–La Crosse, USA

Michael LuBrant
University of Minnesota, USA

Una MacConville
University of Bath, UK

Michael Matthews
University of Minnesota, USA

Charles Maynard
University of Washington, USA

Vanessa McGann
Co-Chair Clinician-Survivor Task Force, Clinical Psychologist, Private Practice, New York City, USA

Jane Moore
King's University College, Ontario, Canada

Harold Mytum
University of Liverpool, UK

Robert A. Neimeyer
University of Memphis, USA

Dudley L. Poston Jr.
Texas A&M University, USA

Irene Renzenbrink
Lakeside Expressive Arts, Melbourne, Australia

Leigh Rich
Armstrong Atlantic State University, USA

Rachel Robison-Greene
University of Massachusetts at Amherst, USA

Melissa Sandefur
Middle Tennessee State University, USA

Neil Small
University of Bradford, UK

Harold Ivan Smith
St. Luke's Hospital, Kansas City, USA

Carla Sofka
Siena College, USA

Silke Steidinger
Inform (The Information Network on Religious Movements) London School of Economics and Political Science, UK

Robert G. Stevenson
Mercy College, USA

Albert Lee Strickland
Pacific Publishing Services, USA

Neil Thompson
Avenue Consulting, UK

Tim Thornton
University of Wisconsin–La Crosse, USA

John Troyer
University of Bath, UK

Gail A. Van Norman
University of Washington, USA

Claire Villarreal
Rice University, USA

Kate Woodthorpe
University of Bath, UK

Qian Xiong
Texas A&M University, USA

A

ABORTION

Abortion describes the end of a pregnancy before the embryo or fetus is able to survive outside the womb. Abortion may be *spontaneous*—where it is more typically referred to as "miscarriage"—resulting from natural causes or an accident; or *induced*, where a pregnancy is terminated intentionally. In many societies, the termination of a pregnancy may produce a grief reaction in women that varies in onset and intensity. Some women may experience little or no grief, while others may experience a grief that is not only severe but is also complicated by feelings of guilt. The onset of grief may be delayed by weeks, months, and sometimes even years. In societies where abortion is surrounded with social stigma, the grief that many women experience may not be validated or supported by others, rendering it "disenfranchised."

Since 1973—the year of the landmark *Roe v. Wade* Supreme Court decision that legalized abortion—the number of legal abortions in the United States has exceeded 50 million, which is more than the combined populations of New York, Florida, and Illinois. Instead of a population of 311 million, without abortion, the population of the country could have been 17 percent larger. According to a 2011 report by the Guttmacher Institute, more than one in five American women will have had an abortion in her lifetime. Abortion remains the most common surgical procedure for women in America.

Rates of Abortion across Social Groups

Minority women are significantly more likely to have abortions than non-Hispanic white women. In 2004, 11 of 1,000 white women had abortions, compared to 28 for Hispanic women and 50 for black women. Such discrepancies have led some minority leaders to claim that the procedure constitutes racial genocide. Writing in the *Quarterly Journal of Economics*, John Donahue and Steven Levitt have linked states' legalization of abortions in the late 1960s and early 1970s with the decline in crime rates between 1985 and 1997.

However, rates of abortion have been in decline. The number of abortions in the United States declined from 1.6 to 1.2 million between 1990 and 2005, and the proportion occurring during the first trimester increased from 38 to 61 percent between 1973 and 2002. At the end of the first decade of the 21st century, approximately 23 of every 100 pregnancies ended in abortion—slightly more than it was in 1974 and considerably less than its peak of 30. Worldwide, between one-quarter and one-fifth of all pregnancies are terminated by abortion. In

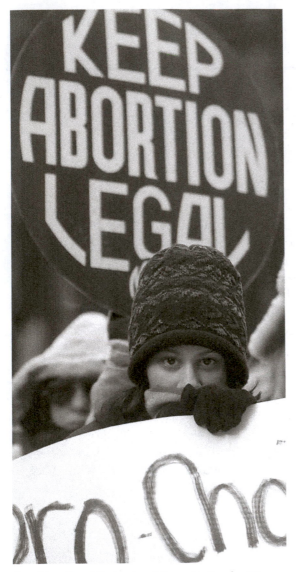

Amy Votteler of the National Organization for Women at a Chicago, Illinois, rally on January 22, 2003, marking the 30th anniversary of the Supreme Court's *Roe v. Wade* decision legalizing abortion. (AP/Wide World Photos)

Russia, 44.7 percent of all pregnancies ended in legal abortion in 2008, whereas in Chile and Panama, less than 0.02 percent ended in legal abortion (Johnston, 2010).

The Abortion Debate

Norma McCorvey did not celebrate the 30th anniversary of the historic *Roe v. Wade* decision that legalized abortion. McCorvey had used the pseudonym Jane Roe to remain anonymous as the lead plaintiff in the 1973 *Roe v. Wade* decision, wherein the U.S. Supreme Court legalized first-trimester abortions and overturned the statutes of two-thirds of the states that prohibited the procedure. No longer agreeing with the court's argument that fetuses within the womb are not full-fledged citizens with rights protected under the Constitution, McCorvey had "switched sides." Her change in position is indicative of the nation's ambivalence toward what Sheldon Ekland-Olson has described as "the knotty problem of whether all human life, all moments in life are equally worthy of living, protecting, and prolonging."

Few moral issues have so divided Americans since the time of slavery than the issue of abortion. As a moral issue, in which emotions have run especially high, the debate surrounding abortion has often exceeded the bounds of rational discourse, spilling over into violence. "Pro-life" activists have murdered abortion providers—or, from their perspective, have committed the "justifiable homicides" of those who kill babies in the midst of a national "holocaust"—and have, between 1977 and 1993, been complicit in 36 bombings, 81 arsons, 131 death threats, 84 assaults, 2 kidnappings, 327 clinic invasions, 71 chemical attacks, and more than 6,000 facility blockades (Ekland-Olson, 2012).

The abortion debate is also a moral issue that has been heavily politicized in a way that political (and religious) affiliation can often be correlated with opposing "pro-life" and "pro-choice" positions. Historically, the ideologies underlying both the "pro-choice" and "pro-life" advocates have shifted considerably, as have their political alignments. In the late 1970s, for instance, strong Republicans were more likely to support abortion than were strong Democrats; four decades later, the latter were twice as likely to be supporters.

By 2009, for the first time, more Americans considered themselves to be "pro-life" than "pro-choice." Attitudes are strongly nuanced in terms of the context of mothers' pregnancies. According to the 2008 and 2010 National Opinion Research Center (NORC) General Social Surveys, which include random samples of noninstitutionalized Americans 18 years of age and older, a large majority—some 87 percent—approve of a women's right to a legal abortion if her health is seriously endangered. Further, some 74 percent support the right of a woman to have a legal abortion if there is a strong chance of a serious birth defect or if the pregnancy was the result of rape (77 percent). Support for a woman's right to a legal abortion diminishes considerably if the woman is married and does not want any more children (46 percent), is poor and cannot afford any more children (44 percent), is not married (41 percent), or if she simply wants an abortion "for whatever reason" (42 percent).

Beliefs are also influenced by understandings of where the line between existence and nonexistence is drawn. The Catholic Church, for instance, holds that life begins at conception. When an aspiring mother's fertilized egg was mistakenly discarded by a fertility clinic, a Cook County judge ruled in 2005 that it was legally a "human being," clearing the way for a Chicago couple to file a wrongful-death suit. In the waning months of the George W. Bush administration, Health and Human Services officials in 2008 considered a regulation that would classify most birth control pills and intrauterine devices as forms of abortion because they prevented the development of fertilized eggs into fetuses. Three years later, a Georgia state legislator introduced a bill criminalizing miscarriages which, along with abortion, constitute "prenatal murder." Such attempts to create moral certainty will invariably fail given new scientific insights and advances in medical science.

Michael C. Kearl

Further Reading

Boven, Luc. "The Rhythm Method and Embryonic Death." *Journal of Medical Ethics,* 32 (2006): 355–56.

Doka, K.J. (ed.). *Disenfranchised Grief: Recognizing Hidden Sorrow.* Lexington, MA: Lexington Books, 1989.

Donahue, John J. III, and Steven D. Levitt. "The Impact of Legalized Abortion on Crime." *The Quarterly Journal of Economics,* 116(2) (2001): 379–420.

Ekland-Olson, Sheldon. *Who Lives, Who Dies, Who Decides? Abortion, Neonatal Care, Assisted Dying, and Capital Punishment.* New York: Routledge, 2012.

Johnston, William Robert. 2010. http://www.johnstonsarchive.net/policy/abortion/wrjp334pd.html

Kearl, M. C. "The Abortion Issue in the United States." In *Handbook of Death and Dying, Volume 1: The Presence of Death,* edited by Clifton D. Bryant (pp. 386–96). Thousand Oaks, CA: Sage, 2003.

Padawer, R. "The Two-Minus-One Pregnancy." *New York Times,* August 10, 2011. http://www.nytimes.com/2011/08/14/magazine/the-two-minus-one-pregnancy.html?pagewanted=all

Schroedel, Jean Reith. *Is the Fetus a Person? A Comparison of the Policies across the Fifty States.* Ithaca, NY: Cornell University Press, 2000.

ACCIDENTAL DEATH

Accidents were the fifth leading cause of death in the United States in 2011, accounting for 122,777 deaths. More than a quarter of these were due to motor vehicle accidents, which remain the largest cause of accidental deaths, accounting for 33,687 deaths in 2010. In children and adolescents aged 1–19 years, accidents are the single leading cause of death, with the vast majority of these resulting from motor vehicle accidents. More than 9,000 young people die annually in the United States from injuries sustained in motor vehicle accidents, with other leading accidental causes of death being falls, fires, drownings, poisoning, and exposure to noxious substances. The Centers for Disease Control and Prevention (CDC) reported a sharp decline in accidental deaths to children and adolescents between 2000 and 2009, falling 30 percent, due largely to a decline in deaths resulting from motor vehicle accidents.

While the rate of fatalities from motor vehicle accidents remains alarmingly high, it has fallen since its peak in the 1960s due largely to advances in car safety and technology, such as antilock brakes, front and side impact airbags, and seat belt restraints. Fatalities from motor vehicle accidents are highest among young people, especially adolescent males aged 16–19, for whom the rate of death is almost twice that of their female counterparts. In 2010 alone, seven teenagers aged 16–19 died in the United States every day from injuries incurred in motor vehicle accidents. When combined with data reporting that teenage drivers are more likely to engage in risk-taking behaviors (such as speeding, texting while driving, driving under the influence of alcohol, and without a seat belt), the higher incidence of fatalities from motor vehicle accidents among young people suggests that accidents are less likely the result of "bad luck" or "fate" than they are of reckless choices and poor decision making.

Accidents more generally may, of course, be the result of simple misfortune but can also, as we have seen, be caused by reckless or risky behavior; they may sometimes occur as the result of negligence on the part of an individual, a company, or some other organization and would therefore constitute *wrongful death.* While human life is inherently full of risks, many societies attempt to minimize the opportunities for accidental death through public information campaigns warning the public of, for example, the dangers of drinking and driving or of walking on frozen lakes and ponds, which may become unsafe due to melting ice. Most contemporary Western societies go further still by enacting legislation and implementing measures aimed at ensuring public health and safety. In the United Kingdom, *The Black Report* into inequalities in health between different socioeconomic groups indicated that children of families in the lowest social classes were at greater likelihood of dying accidentally than their peers in higher social classes and that this could be linked to the greater environmental hazards affecting communities in poorer socioeconomic neighborhoods. The report indicated that deaths caused by fire, falls, and drowning for boys in social class V (the lowest socioeconomic group) were 10 times greater than those for boys in social class I (the highest socioeconomic group). This is a powerful reminder that while accidents *do* happen, they are often not simply a chance occurrence, nor is their distribution within the population necessarily random.

Michael Brennan

See also: Adolescents; Children; Health Promotion.

Further Reading

Centers for Disease Control and Prevention. http://www.cdc.gov/motorvehiclesafety/

"Leading Causes of Death," Centers for Disease Control and Prevention. National Vital Statistics System, 2010. http://www.cdc.gov/nchs/data/dvs/LCWK1_2010.pdf

Vigilant, Lee Garth. "Accidental Death." In *Encyclopedia of Death and the Human Experience*, edited by Clifton D. Bryant and Dennis L. Peck (pp. 5–8). Thousand Oaks, CA: Sage.

ACTIVE DYING

Active dying is the final phase in a patient's life when death is imminent and likely to occur within a matter of hours or days. Just as the term "active labor" marks the onset of birth and the beginning of the life cycle, so "active dying" signals the end of the life course. The term is best understood within the wider context of a *dying trajectory* (see **Dying Trajectory**). It is usually reserved for situations in which a person has been severely ill for a prolonged period of time, in which death is both anticipated and expected, and is characterized by discernible physical changes such as decreased appetite and thirst, incontinence, nausea, and vomiting. During this natural process, in which dying accelerates and the body begins to shut down, other physical signs indicating the nearing of death include heightened agitation and restlessness, disorientation and confusion, and diminished consciousness. Active dying may also be manifested by disturbances in breathing (which may be labored, irregular, or short), changes in vital signs (including blood pressure, temperature, and pulse), and the cooling of extremities, which may take on a mottled bluish or purplish complexion. This is especially pertinent to nursing staff working with the elderly and terminally ill in hospices and residential care facilities, whose role is to provide comfort care in a patient's last few remaining hours, as well as to reassure relatives by explaining the bodily changes occurring when a person is actively dying. This is particularly the case when secretions in the throat or the relaxing of muscles in the throat may lead to noisy breathing, sometimes referred to as the "death rattle," which can be alleviated by medication or repositioning the patient. Just before death occurs, a person may experience a brief and momentary sense of mental clarity, known as "terminal alertness," after which the chest may heave as if to breathe.

Michael Brennan

ADEC (ASSOCIATION FOR DEATH EDUCATION AND COUNSELING)

The Association for Death Education and Counseling (ADEC) was founded in 1976 and is the single largest professional organization within the field of thanatology (see **Thanatology**). Based in the United States, ADEC is an international and interdisciplinary organization whose chief goal is the promotion of excellence and recognition of diversity in death education, care of the dying, grief counseling, and research in thanatology. In addition to providing information, support, and resources to the general public, ADEC organizes an annual international conference and offers continuing education accreditation and professional certification in thanatology through workshops, webinars (online seminars), and self-study programs. Its membership consists primarily of educators and counselors and includes a wide variety of human service providers and practitioners—from social workers, funeral directors, and clergy to nurses and psychologists—whose work brings them into contact with the dead, dying, and the bereaved. In the early days, and against the backdrop of denial and repression of death and dying in American society in the first half of the 20th century (see **Death Denial**), ADEC provided a professional meeting place for those who felt isolated in their work. Today, in ways reflective of the growth of thanatology since the 1970s, ADEC provides ample opportunities for professional networking and the development and sharing of professional knowledge and skills. In addition to maintaining a comprehensive database of specialists in thanatology, ADEC publishes the *Forum*, a hybrid publication between a professional newsletter and scientific journal that provides opportunities for sharing research, experience, and clinical practice, encompassing an overarching mission of ADEC by serving as a bridge between research and practice. ADEC is also affiliated with a number of key publications in the fields of death, dying, and bereavement, including *Death Studies, Omega: Journal of Death and Dying,* and *Grief Matters: The Australian Journal of Grief and Bereavement.*

Michael Brennan

See also: Death Awareness Movement; Death Education.

Further Reading

http://www.adec.org

ADOLESCENTS

Adolescence is a period of time from as early as age 10 through 21. While younger children have difficulties understanding death cognitively, by the time they reach adolescence, they can think abstractly and critically and can understand that death is permanent and universal (see also **Children**). Cognitively, adolescents know that death is the cessation of physical functioning. While they may recognize that death will happen to them, adolescents often act as if "it won't happen to me."

Adolescence is a difficult time for a child in the best of circumstances. The period of adolescence is fraught with daunting tasks—developing identity, achieving peer acceptance, and separating from parents. These tasks complicate the adolescent's response to death. It is a time when children pull back from family and adults and seek the support of their peers. It is a time when withdrawal and experimentation are often the norm. It is a time for finding oneself and sorting through questions. Adolescents frequently have the same cognitive understanding of death as do adults, but they may express their grief in different ways.

Adolescents often feel that they are invulnerable. They practice risk-taking behaviors on a regular basis—driving too fast, not being cautious, drug and sexual experimentation, and so on. While they may cognitively know that they will one day die, their behaviors do not support that belief. These risk-taking behaviors can proliferate when adolescents experience the death of someone close to them. The adolescent may feel that there is nothing to live for or may find that the "rush" of risk-taking behaviors momentarily takes them away from

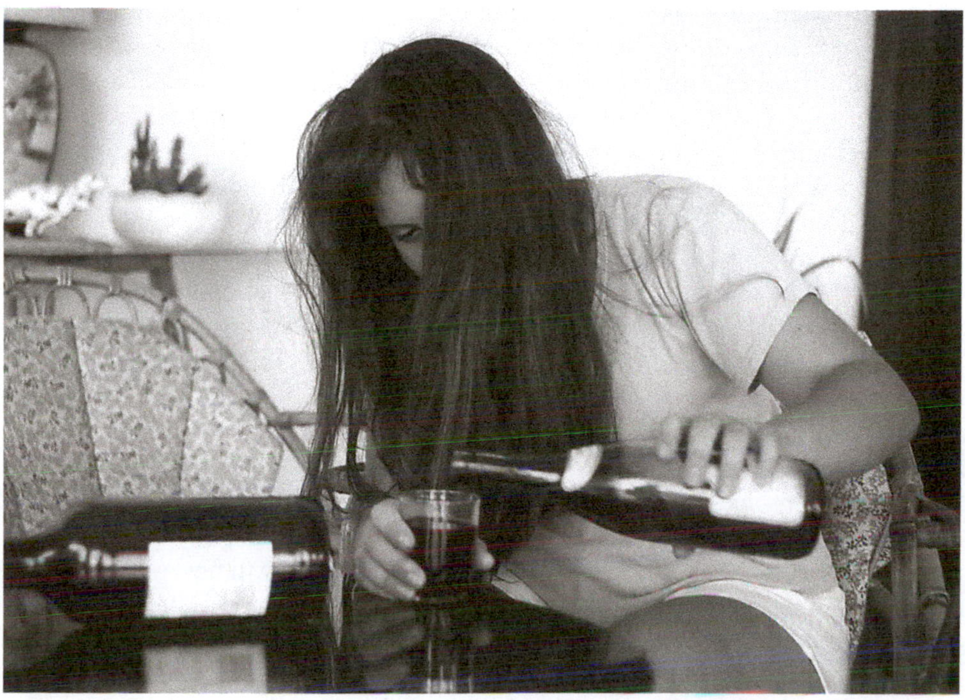

Risk-taking behaviors, such as alcohol consumption, can increase when an adolescent is experiencing grief. The longer children delay alcohol use, the less likely they are to develop any problems associated with it. (PhotoDisc, Inc.)

their grief. Engaging in promiscuous sexual activity may be seeking to fill a void that a death has created inside the adolescent, but it cannot be filled that way, and unrestrained, unprotected sexual activity can result in sexually transmitted diseases and further emotional upheaval, as well as strained relationships with adults and caregivers.

Adolescents are looking within themselves and sorting through their identity, so they are frequently preoccupied with this internal struggle. In addition, adolescents are often trying to "fit it" with their peers. Experiencing the death of a family member or close friend makes them different. As a result, they may withdraw from peers, losing interest in activities in which they had consistently participated, like sports or the arts. They may go out of their way to avoid places or situations that remind them of the deceased and in doing so, further remove themselves from support systems that are already in place for them.

When the person who died is a parental figure or caregiver, the adolescent may seek to live up to that person's expectations. In the extreme, this may give rise to perfectionism, where the adolescent expectations for themselves are unrealistic and the cause of frustration and greater turmoil.

Supporting Adolescents Who Are Grieving

Adolescents who are grieving need monitoring by caring adults. Indicators that the adolescent may need support include changes in eating habits, sexual activity, drinking, drug use, cutting or branding, the loss of friends and interest in activities, and a substantial drop in school grades. Emotionally "uncharged" conversations and acceptance of the adolescent's feelings provide the adolescent with the opportunity to share and question his or her experiences. At this age level, peer support groups may provide help. In such a group, the adolescent is not alone in his or her grief and finds peers that have also experienced the loss of a loved one.

One of the things that is most confounding when dealing with grieving adolescents is the fact that they re-grieve their losses as they reach new developmental understandings. This is often something that catches adults by surprise. They expect that the children in their lives have "dealt" with a death and then find that the child is experiencing new, raw feelings and emotions. When a child experiences the death of a loved one as a preschooler, they might ask questions that indicate that they are waiting for the person to return. There may not be a reoccurrence of the questions and concern for many years. As a child reaches adolescence, and develops an understanding of what "forever" means, there may come a whole new period of grief as the adolescent realizes that the loved one will never return. In the school setting, this can translate to a student who suffered a death in kindergarten entering middle school and exhibiting some of the behaviors associated with grief that are age appropriate. This makes the cause of those behaviors difficult to recognize when the death occurred so long ago. It is sometimes difficult to tell what behaviors result from a death and which are typically adolescent behaviors.

Re-grieving is a key concept for all people working or living with bereaved children and adolescents. It is a normal part of the grieving process and can affect adolescents' lives on an ongoing basis, being more intense at some times than others.

Death Rates among Adolescents in the United States

The U.S. Department of Health and Human Services reports deaths of adolescents (aged 15–19 years) at the rate of 64.4 deaths per 100,000. The death rate for males is notably higher than that for females (90.7 vs. 36.8 per 100,000). Unintentional injury is the leading cause of death in this age group, with the second and third leading causes of death being homicide and suicide. Homicide and suicide are followed by deaths due to cancer and diseases of the heart.

Deaths due to unintentional injury include those that are the result of motor vehicle accidents. Nearly a third of those accidents involved an adolescent driver under the influence of alcohol. Firearms are the second leading cause of fatal injury, followed by poisoning, suffocation, and drowning.

Homicide and Suicide

It is noteworthy that homicide is the leading cause of death for 15- to 24-year-old African American males in the United States—the highest incidence of firearm-related deaths in this age group in the world.

Male youth die by suicide five times more often than do female adolescents. Yet, females are more likely to make suicide attempts. Forty-five percent of suicides by adolescents used firearms. Risk factors for suicide include mental illness, substance abuse, life-limiting illnesses, recent stressful events, presence of firearms in the household, self-injury, suicidal attempts, and low self-esteem. Demographics figure significantly in predicting suicide. Risks increase if the adolescent is male, white, and/or gay or bisexual. (NCIPC, 2003)

Factors that protect adolescents from completing suicide include family and school connections, lack of access to firearms, academic achievement, and self-esteem. Schools have developed suicide-prevention programs, yet there is controversy as to whether these programs help prevent suicide or make students more aware of suicide as a possible solution to seemingly insurmountable problems.

Adolescents with Life-Limiting Illnesses

Adolescents are often fully aware of the implications of a life-limiting diagnosis. They want medical personnel to talk *with* them rather than *to* them or to their parents. During treatment phases, adolescents are particularly sensitive to physical changes to their body when, developmentally (and societally), appearance means a great deal. Adolescents with life-limiting illnesses may be isolated from peers because of constraints imposed by the illness (communicability) or those imposed by treatments (low resistance to infection). Adolescents frequently want to learn as much as possible about their illness and make decisions regarding their care. This can cause conflict, as parents may wish to try any means to prolong the life of their child, while the adolescent may want to decide the trajectory of his or her illness and its treatment (including the cessation of treatment).

As in the case of young children with life-limiting illnesses, siblings of adolescents who are dying can experience struggles with concerns about being affected by the same condition, jealousy over the attention received by the ill adolescent, and guilt over these feelings.

Dying adolescents, like adults, are concerned that they will be comfortable and safe during the dying process. The death process for adolescents is often complicated by the fact that they are not legally able to make medical decisions, yet can be at odds with their parents in terms of treatment, cessation of treatment, and extraordinary measures of life sustainment. Open communication between family members and health care providers, as well as a growing number of hospices that work with children and adolescents, can provide a less stressful dying experience for all concerned.

Jane Moore

Further Reading

American Association of Suicidology: http://www.suicidology.org/c/document_library/get_file?folderId=248&name=DLFE-484.pdf

Doka, K.J. and A.S. Tucci. *Living with Grief: Children and Adolescents.* Washington, DC: Hospice Foundation of America, 2008.

Mitchell, G., J. Murray, and J. Hynson. "Understanding the Whole Person: Life-Limiting Illness across the Life Cycle." In *Palliative Care: A Patient-Centered Approach,* edited by G. Mitchell (pp. 79–107). London: Radcliffe, 2008.

National Center for Injury Prevention and Control (NCIPC). *Fatal Injuries: Leading Causes of Death Reports.* Atlanta, GA: Centers for Disease Control and Prevention, 2003.

U.S. Department of Health and Human Services, Child Health USA 2008–2009. http://mchb.hrsa.gov/chusa08/hstat/hsa/pages/225am.html

ADVANCE DIRECTIVES

Advance directives are legal documents that permit adults to state their preferences for future care in the event of an emergency or other life-threatening situation. Advance directives are state specific; those that live in more than one state would need to have documents meeting each state's requirements. "Five Wishes" is a form that that meets requirements in 42 states. Advance care planning is the process of discussion of burdens and benefits of treatment that would result in completion of an advance directive. The document(s) may be in two forms: a living will and a health care power of attorney (HCPOA), or a single document combining both.

A living will states the person's preferences for life-sustaining treatments and comes into effect when the patient becomes terminally ill. An HCPOA designates a decision maker for medical affairs when the person cannot communicate. These documents may be changed and should be reviewed or updated as needed, especially with changes in health status.

In medical decision making there is an order of priority. When patients are able, they continue to make decisions. If the patient is unable to communicate, then the advanced directives are used. If there are no documents, health care providers are left to discern a direction, asking family members about past conversations (or statements). If none were had (or made), they will ask about the personality and activities of the person before the event causing hospital admission. The presence of advance directives has been shown to lessen the stress families experience when asked to make decisions about withdrawing life support.

In 1991, The U.S. Congress passed The Patient Self-Determination Act, requiring health care institutions to inquire whether patients had completed advance directives and, if not, to provide information about them upon the patient's admission to the health care facility. The intent was to prevent the prolongation of dying in cases where interventions might not have been desired and, once instituted, were difficult or impossible to reverse without information from the patient.

However, the flaws of the legislation were numerous. In a death-denying society, the likelihood of discussions about impending death, or preparing for it, is low. No incentive was provided to encourage the completion of the forms, nor was professional help provided to assist patients to do so. Patients were responsible to find the forms and complete them, and so completion rates have been consistently low. Advance directives, when present, may not cover a particular situation in terms of interventions desired (or undesired), or the time lapse since completion of the advance directive may cause the health professional to question its relevance. If the patient is not deemed to be terminally ill, the living will may be thought not to be relevant. The HCPOA may not have been notified of a change in the patient's status or may not have a copy of the document.

In order to optimize advance directives, the patients' preferences about their future health care should be elicited during an advance care planning discussion in a less stressful setting and time than during hospital admission. Choices about interventions that patients make may vary depending upon differing circumstances. For example, a patient may not wish to be sustained by mechanical ventilation if she suffered severe brain trauma, but might be willing to be ventilated for a short time if she were in a car accident.

The HCPOA overcomes some of these limitations because surrogates make decisions in real time with the information available to them. The surrogate's role is to make decisions that the patient would want and not what the surrogate wants. A surrogate who knows the role of a substitute decision maker and is informed about the patient's preferences will be the best person to speak for the patient.

Copies of advance directives should be provided to the primary care provider, the HCPOA, and family likely to be available in an emergency. Hopefully, there will be greater accord and no attempts to override the HCPOA at the time of decision making.

When a patient is chronically ill, completion of advance directives, with consideration of the use of resuscitation, becomes more critical. Explanations about the likelihood of surviving a respiratory or cardiac arrest should be part of the decision making on whether to accept cardiopulmonary resuscitation (CPR). This is the only medical treatment that is given *without* consent and needs to have a medical order Do Not Resuscitate (DNR) written, or a patient's refusal to accept it, in order to prevent resuscitation. Rates for returning to previous levels of function following resuscitation are quite low (below 12%) and drop further still if the event is not witnessed or the patient has cancer or some other serious comorbidity.

In the home, a "vial of life," a baggie that is taped to the refrigerator, gives instructions to first responders if 911 is called. The baggie would contain the advance directive, a recent electrocardiogram (EKG), a picture (if helpful), and any DNR documentation. First responders have been told to search for this baggie for guidance in approaching the patient's treatment.

Another complication of locating paper documents is that they might reside in one setting but not where the patient is sent for care in an emergency. In a health care system, advance directives given to the primary care provider may be stored in the database. Across unrelated settings, for example, from hospital to nursing home, Physician Orders for Life-Sustaining Treatment (POLST) are medical orders indicating life-sustaining treatment wishes for seriously ill patients. These orders enhance advance directives by changing the preferences for treatment into actionable medical orders signed by a health care provider. These orders have been followed more consistently than advance directives. Some individual states have endorsed the program; others are developing alternative programs, while some have no program at all.

Attempts to promote the implementation of advance directives have been numerous. Educating the public and making forms more readily available will help increase the prevalence of advance directives. "Respecting Choices" is a comprehensive program to help educate health care professionals on how best to honor patients' end-of-life choices.

Karin T. Kirchhoff

See also: Good Death; Terminal Illness and Care.

Further Reading

Advance Care Planning: http://www.ahrq.gov/research/endliferia/endria.htm
Five Wishes: http://www.agingwithdignity.org/five-wishes-states.php
POLST: http://www.ohsu.edu/polst/
Respecting Choices: http://respectingchoices.org/

AFRICAN AMERICANS

African American culture has played a significant role in shaping African Americans' beliefs surrounding death and dying. Due to the historical and structural factors that have led to a mistrust of the health care system, such as racial discrimination and a denial of equitable access to health care, African Americans are less likely to rely upon the medical community for end-of-life care such as hospice and palliative services, compared to other racial and ethnic groups. Most African American families tend to care for sick family members in their private homes. In addition, they are less likely to support discontinuing life-support treatment once it is started, or organ donation, for fear of having an external source take control of their health care decision making or bodies. Similarly, African Americans do not typically support other methods of terminating life, such as physician-assisted suicide. They are also much more likely to focus on prolonging life and taking advantage of life-sustaining measures than whites.

Traditions Related to Death and Bereavement

Spirituality plays a central role in African American tradition surrounding grief, bereavement, death, and dying. Death is not seen as the end of life or a final act, but rather a continuation or passage of life from earth to another place. According to John Mbiti, African Americans typically refer to the process of death as

> returning home, going away, being called away, becoming God's property, and so on. All these words show the belief that death is not a complete destruction of the individual. Life goes on beyond the grave. Therefore, people combine their sorrow over the death of someone with the belief that that is not the end and that the departed continue to live in the hereafter. (Mbiti, 1970, 119)

Thus, the word "death" is rarely used to refer to deceased members of the African American community, rather "transition" is used to imply that the individual is not gone, but has moved on or "passed" into the next life. This view of death is rooted in traditional African culture, where deceased family members and relatives are still considered part of the family circle as the "living dead," who are always present among them in spirit. African Americans often believe that during times of emotional distress, crisis, and joy, their deceased loved ones are spiritually with them and watching over them. This allows individuals to keep deceased family members in their memories and cope with their loss. Thus, African Americans tend to have a circular view of life and death and spirituality, which is often depicted in African drawings and art with the image of the circle. In contrast, traditional Western views of life and death follow a much more linear model, since there is little to no emphasis placed on spiritual presence in the afterlife.

African American Church and Funerals

The African American church plays an important role in assisting grieving family members who have recently lost a loved one and during end-of-life discussions. The church generally serves as a central gathering place for friends and family members, even if the individual did not regularly attend church and is not a member of the particular church congregation. As long as the immediate or extended family of the individual regularly attends church, there is a strong enough tie to hold services at the given location.

Community is also a very important part of dealing with death and illness, especially end-of-life decisions. It is not uncommon for members of the immediate and extended family to visit loved ones in the hospital for extended time periods. In addition, medical decisions are often made as part of a collective group, rather than by one individual in the immediate family. When an individual is about to die, family and friends are expected to immediately gather at the person's bedside for a prayer vigil to comfort him and help him transition to the next life.

Prior to the funeral, the mourning period lasts for roughly seven days and includes a ceremony, called a wake, where friends and family can view the body of the deceased individual and pay their respects. In addition, family members often gather together over food and drink and reflect on fond memories of their loved one. While the wake can take place in a funeral home, it is not uncommon for it to take place in the church or the deceased individual's home.

Beyond cultural and grieving practices, there are also differences between the white and African American communities surrounding funeral practices, namely the eulogy and music selection. Generally, black funerals tend to be more emotive than funerals of other racial and ethnic groups.

Since African Americans often experience prejudice and discrimination during their lifetime in the United States, funerals are a posthumous attempt to praise deceased individuals and achieve a high level of esteem. To this end, the eulogy and music selection are all centered on generating a positive sense of self-identity and remembrance. In addition, grief is not suppressed, but rather encouraged. Black funerals rely heavily upon the eulogy. The purpose of a eulogy is to verbally remember the deceased individual by openly discussing her attributes and achievements throughout her life. During white funerals, the eulogy tends to focus on the individual accomplishments of the deceased person. Then, the pastor asks God to have mercy on the deceased for any sins they may have committed during their life on earth. In contrast, during African American funerals, the focus is on enhancing the personal or social image of the deceased, often playing up their accomplishments, in order to leave the most favorable imagery in the minds of grieving family and friends at the ceremony. Thus, the minister's eulogy does not need to ask for God's forgiveness since the image portrayed of the dead individual is so positive and hopeful (see also **Eulogy**).

In the African American community, music and dance have often been an outlet for cultural and individual expression that is not typically accepted in mainstream white society. According to Masamba and Kalish (1976), the music at black funerals essentially serves the dual purposes of remembering the relationship that the audience has had with the deceased individual, and bringing back specific memories that one had with the deceased individual during prior church ceremonies. A central aspect of African American funerals focuses on emotions and unscripted singing from audience members. In contrast, during white funerals, music is often provided by either an individual performer with a violin or piano, or a group of choir members who sing in a somewhat choreographed manner, and the audience expresses very little personal emotion.

Jazz Funerals and Second Lines

Among Africans Americans in New Orleans, music has played a key role in burial rituals since the early 20th century. Jazz bands and parades called "second lines" are frequently featured at funerals and represent the history of New Orleans as having a distinct regional culture. These music or jazz funerals are typically spiritual celebrations that are performed for musicians or individuals who are part of the music industry, as well as other members of society.

Their origin dates back to two traditions in the colonial era when (1) brass band members played in procession to honor deceased politicians and generals, and (2) African slaves formed circles to properly honor the spirits of their ancestors. Out of these two traditions, came burial ceremonies with jazz bands and marching processions to remember and celebrate the dead. Often, when the time for mourning is over, these second line parades take the form of a "massive moving street festival" with choreographed street dancers. Parades typically draw between 3,000 and 5,000 people on any given Sunday (Regis, 1999, 427).

These rituals and ceremonies at African American funerals are illustrative of regular ceremonies that take place within the black church, which is a central institution within the black community. Typically, church masses consist of high levels of emotion, energy, singing, and praise.

African American Health Disparities

According to the CDC, the top 10 leading causes of death among non-Hispanic African Americans across both sexes and all ages in 2010 included (1) heart disease, (2) cancer, (3) cerebrovascular disease (such as hypertension and stroke), (4) diabetes, (5) unintentional accidents, (6) kidney disease, (7) chronic lower respiratory disease, (8) homicide, (9) septicemia, and (10) Alzheimer's disease.

Throughout U.S. history, race has been a consistent predictor of morbidity and mortality rates, regardless of geographic region. There are sharp contrasts between health disparities among African Americans and other racial groups across life expectancy, obesity, heart disease, death rates, infant mortality, and other measures of health. For example, while the average life expectancy of a white American is 78.4 years, the average African American could only expect to live 73.6 years. Moreover, the infant mortality rate for African Americans is 2.4 times that for non-Hispanic white Americans (see also **Infant Mortality**).

According to the CDC, a variety of factors contribute to disparities in health outcomes among African Americans, including cultural barriers, lack of access to health care, and racial discrimination. One such cultural factor has been African American mistrust of the predominantly white medical community and doctors due to their history of maltreatment and deception of African Americans, and their refusal to treat black patients. In particular, beginning in 1932, the white physicians at the Tuskegee Institute in Macon County, Alabama, received funding from the National Public Health Service to examine the long-term effects of syphilis on African American men without use of informed consent. Participants in the study were told they were being treated for "bad blood," a local term used to describe much of the ailments associated with syphilis; however, they did not receive proper treatment for their disease. While penicillin became the drug of choice for syphilis by 1947, researchers did not offer it to their subjects. The study continued until 1972, when media coverage of the study generated national outrage surrounding the unethical treatment of participants.

Lynn Letukas

Further Reading

Barrett, Ronald and Helen Keller. "Death and Dying in the Black Experience." *Journal of Palliative Medicine,* 5 (2001): 793–99.

Bolling, John L. "Guinea across the Water: The African American Approach to Death and Dying." In *A Cross-Cultural Look at Death, Dying and Religion,* edited by Joan Parry and Angela Ryan (pp. 145–59). Chicago: Nelson-Hall Publishers, 1995.

Centers for Disease Control and Prevention, Minority Health. http://www.cdc.gov/minorityhealth/populations/REMP/black.html#10

Dancy, Joseph and Willie Davis. "Family and Psycho-Social Dimensions of Death and Dying in African Americans." Institute on Care at the End of Life, Duke Divinity School, 2004.

Heron, Melonie. "Deaths: Leading Causes for 2009." *National Vital Statistics Report,* 61 (October 26, 2012).

Masamba, Jean, and Richard Kalish. "Death and Bereavement: The Role of the Black Church." *Omega,* 7 (1976): 23–24.

Mbiti, John. *African Religions and Philosophy.* New York: Anchor Books, 1970.

Moore, James and Clifton Bryant. "Black Funeralization and Culturally Grounded Services." In *Handbook of Death and Dying, Vol. 1,* edited by Clifton D. Bryant (pp. 598–603). Thousand Oaks, CA: Sage, 2003.

"QuickStats: Infant Mortality Rates, by Mother's Place of Birth and Race/Ethnicity—United States." *Morbidity and Mortality Weekly Report.* Centers for Disease Control and Prevention, 2007.

Regis, Helen. "Second Lines, Minstrelsy, and the Contested Landscapes of New Orleans Afro-Creole Festivals." *Cultural Anthropology,* 14 (1990): 472–504.

Sullivan, Martha Adams. "May the Circle Be Unbroken: The African American Experience of Death, Dying and Spirituality." In *A Cross-Cultural Look at Death, Dying and Religion,* edited by Joan Parry and Angela Ryan (pp. 160–72). Chicago: Nelson-Hall Publishers, 1995.

AFTERLIFE BELIEFS

All living creatures are part of a cycle of life and death. Across cultures and throughout history, humans have constructed belief systems that explain death in cosmological, spiritual, and/or religious terms. These explanatory systems, even though widely diverse, usually deal with death in some way because, like no other social event or situation, death inherently challenges the taken-for-granted meanings of all societies. Cross-cultural studies of death reveal that most societies seem to have a concept of a soul and immortality. For some, a belief in the concept of a soul explains what happens during sleep and after death. For others, a belief in souls explains how the supernatural world becomes populated.

All of the world's five major religious traditions provide perspectives on death and views of the afterlife. These five religious traditions are Judaism, Christianity, Islam, Hinduism, and Buddhism.

Judaism

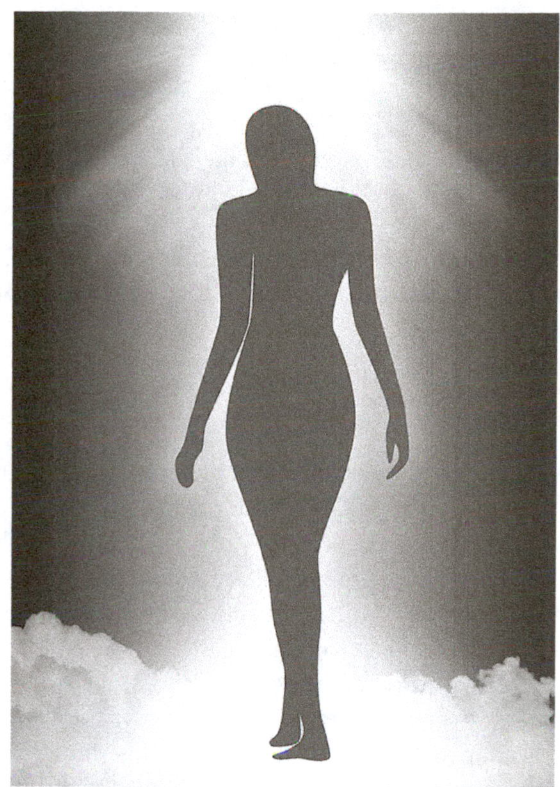

The possibility of an afterlife is addressed by the five major religions: Christianity, Judaism, Buddhism, Hinduism, and Islam. (Dreamstime)

Death in the Jewish tradition came into being as a result of Adam and Eve's sin, which caused them to be expelled from the Garden of Eden. When Adam and Eve ate the fruit from the "Tree of Knowledge," they received the curse of pain in childbirth, the burden of work, and the loss of physical immortality. According to the Biblical account in Genesis (2:4–3:24), although death was a punishment, it also brought the ability to distinguish between good and evil, as well as the power and responsibility to make decisions that have a future consequence.

Among contemporary Jews, including those who consider themselves religious, opinion differs regarding personal immortality. Some contend that there is no *afterlife,* only an *afterdeath*—the dead go to *Sheol,* where nothing happens, and the soul eventually slides into oblivion. Other Jews believe in a resurrection of the soul, when individuals are brought to a final judgment. Regardless of the content of Jewish beliefs regarding the immortality of the soul, Jewish funeral customs and rituals emphasize that God does not save us—as individuals—from death, but saves Israel for history, regardless of death (see also **Judaism**).

Christianity

Although Christianity shares much of the historical and mythical foundations of Judaism, there are many distinct differences in the Christian approach to death and afterlife beliefs. For the Christian, death is viewed as the entrance to eternal life and, therefore, is preferable to physical life. There is a strong belief in the immortality of the soul, the resurrection of the body, and a divine judgment of one's earthly life after death, resulting in the eternal rewards of heaven or the punishments of hell. For the Roman Catholic, there are four potential dispositions of the soul after death—heaven, hell, limbo, and purgatory (see also **Catholicism; Heaven; Hell; Purgatory**).

For the Christian, the teachings of Jesus and the Apostle Paul are the most important sources in arriving at a theology of life after death. Jesus declares to his followers:

> I am the Resurrection and the Life, he who believes in Me, though he die, yet shall he live, and whoever lives and believes in Me shall never die. (John 11:25, RSV)

Therefore, from the Christian perspective, faith in Jesus Christ provides for the individual Christian victory *over* death and eternal life with God (see also **Christianity**).

Islam

As in Christianity, life after death is also an important focus within the Islamic tradition. Earthly life and the realm of the dead are separated by a bridge that souls must cross on the Day of Judgment. After death, all people face a divine judgment. Then they are assigned eternal dwelling places where they will receive either eternal rewards or punishments, determined by the strengths of their faith in God and the moral quality of their earthly lives. According to the Qur'an, there are seven layers of heaven and seven layers of *alnar* ("Fire of Hell"), and each layer is separated from the layer above by receiving fewer rewards or greater punishments. The fundamental reason that individuals might be condemned to a life of torment in the Fire of Hell is a lack of belief in God and in the message of his prophet Muhammad. Other reasons include lying, being corrupt, committing blasphemy, denying the advent of Judgment Day and the reality of the Fire of Hell, lacking charity, and leading a life of luxury.

Like Jews and Christians, followers of Islam believe that God is fundamentally compassionate and place a similar emphasis on God as just. Therefore, individuals are held accountable for moral integrity at the time of their death. The primary expression of the Islamic concern for justice and accountability is found in the belief in the assignment to paradise or damnation. Accordingly, the Qur'an provides very vivid sketches of both paradise and hell. However, many Islamic theologians also stress that God's judgment is tempered with mercy, that the angel Gabriel will intercede on behalf of those condemned to punishment, and that they will eventually be pardoned (see also **Islam**).

Hinduism

Three concepts are central to an understanding of Hinduism—*karma, dharma,* and *moksha. Karma* refers to a moral law of causation; it suggests that an individual's actions produce results for which the individual is responsible. *Karma* also refers to the balance of good and bad deeds performed in previous existences. *Dharma* is religious duties, requirements, and/or prescriptions. The extent to which one fulfills one's *dharma* determines one's *karma.* In turn, *moksha* is the reward for living a saintly life. The main ways of achieving *moksha* are overcoming spiritual ignorance by acquiring true knowledge, performing good deeds, and living a life of love and devotion to God.

The central doctrine affecting death-related attitudes and behavior in the Hindu religion is reincarnation and the transmigration of souls (*samsara*). For the Hindu, one's present life is determined by one's actions in a previous life. Furthermore, one's present behavior will shape the future.

By way of contrast, whereas Jews, Christians, and Muslims believe in the immortality of the soul and hope for an afterlife, Hindus hope that their soul will be absorbed at death. For the Hindu, the goal is not to experience life after death, but rather to have one's soul united with the Oversoul. Punishment for the devout Hindu might be to have "everlasting spiritual rebirth."

Buddhism

Like the Hindu, for the Buddhist the goal is not to experience life after death, but rather to experience *nirvana*—which has the property of neither existence nor nonexistence. According to Margaret Ayer (1964: 52), nirvana is the "state of peace and freedom from the miseries of the constantly changing illusion which is existence."

The location of nirvana is to be found in the image of the flame when a candle is "blown out"—it is in a place beyond human understanding. According to Ayer (1964: 53), whenever people achieve nirvana "they 'will be seen no more.' It is through loss of desire, selfishness, evil, and illusion that this state of wisdom, holiness, and peace is reached." Buddhism contends that whereas physical death causes one to experience life again in a transmigrated form, "death to this world" (via *nirvana*) provides the gateway for ultimate happiness, peace, and fulfillment. Unlike Hinduism and the other religious traditions considered above, the ultimate goal of Buddhism is a state of consciousness, and not a symbolic location for the disembodied soul.

Michael R. Leming

Further Reading

Ayer, M. *Made in Thailand.* New York: Alfred A. Knopf, 1964.
Moreman, C. M. *Beyond the Threshold: Afterlife Beliefs and Experiences in World Religions.* Lanham, MD: Rowman and Littlefield, 2010.

AGING

In a century or so since 1900, the United States has undergone a profound shift in its demographic profile; namely, the proportion of the population who are aged 65 and older. During that time, the percentage of Americans aged 65 or above has trebled from 4 percent in 1900, to almost 13 percent in 2009. The increase in the number of elderly residents in the United States has been most acute since the 1950s, when the population overall was relatively "young," due to high fertility, declining rates of infant and childhood mortality, and high rates of immigration by young workers and their families in search of employment. Since 1950, when the proportion of Americans aged 65 and over stood at 8.1 percent, the percentage of Americans aged 65 and older has increased dramatically, to 12.8 percent in 2009, and is projected to reach 20.2 percent by 2050. Put another way, this means that by 2050, one in five of the U.S. population will be aged 65 and upward.

This dramatic increase in the proportion of elderly Americans presents serious policy challenges, not least in terms of the expanded need for retirement and health care systems to accommodate them, but also because of the simultaneous shrinkage in the number of people of working age to support them. While today's aged (and increasingly aging) population is due in part to improvements in public health, nutrition and lifestyle that have extended life expectancy beyond what could be reasonably expected several generations ago, many of those who live into old age experience a radically diminished quality of life due not only to the loss of faculties (such as hearing, memory, and sight), but also the loss of close and long-established relationships. To survive one's spouse, friends, and even one's own children, can be a lonely experience, one in which many elderly residents of nursing and care homes are left alone waiting to die (see also **Social Death**). This is in sharp contrast to the distant past, as Michel de Montaigne, a contemporary of William Shakespeare, observed in 1575, "To die of old age is a death rare, extraordinary, and singular . . . a privilege rarely seen."

The Old as the Cultural Shock Absorbers of Death

For most of human history (and remaining the case today in the least developed societies), death was largely the province of children. In Puritan New England, when a young couple married, they did so with the expectation that two or three of their children would die before the age of 10. Centuries later in the antebellum United States, between one-fifth and one-third of all children died before age 10. As late as the 19th century, if one survived childhood, it seemed that people tended to die at the peak of their social engagements.

During the 20th century, owing to medical successes against lethal microbes, creations of safer technologies, reductions in pollution, and healthier lifestyles, we have witnessed a largely successful "war" against most forms of premature death. Most of those who die "before their time" increasingly perish because of man-made (hence theoretically avoidable) causes: suicide, homicide, and accidents. Nowadays in the developed world, it is the old who are the cultural death lepers. Nearly 8 in 10 deaths in America occur among those who are "old." For the non-old, the prospects of death have largely been removed from conscious consideration when making plans. For example, those planning to enlarge their families rarely consider the possibility of a spouse dying during pregnancy.

Although such developments would seem to be the cause for collective celebration, old age has become understood as a cultural and social "problem." As societies at earlier periods of history viewed children as "quasi-persons" owing to their high rates of mortality, nowadays it is the elderly whose status is marginalized because of their association with death. As colonial Puritan parents usually sent their children away to the home of relatives or friends as a method of discipline and a way to prevent the parents from becoming too emotionally attached to their children, so now the elderly are disengaged from their roles in work and the community, sent to retirement communities, and often to assisted-care nursing homes to be cared for by others.

Given the basic confinement of death to the elderly, the cultural meanings of death shape the meaning and status of old age. And, within contemporary American society, where dying and death have been largely removed from the public sphere to institutionalized settings, death has become a cultural taboo. Perhaps all of the attention given to the longest lived of our species, to the *quantity* as opposed to the *quality* of life, is evidence of a reduction in the influence of religion and philosophy in mitigating fears of and about death. Nevertheless, the broad cultural fears surrounding death have shifted from concerns over postmortem judgment to concerns over aging and dying. To delay and obscure our aging (and our inevitable deaths), there has arisen a multibillion dollar antiaging industry featuring hair dyes, antiwrinkle creams, vitamin supplements, exercise regimens, and cosmetic surgery. Another strategy, one employed by celebrities and former leaders (such as Margaret Thatcher and Ronald Reagan), is simply to become invisible from public life, perhaps not wanting to diminish public memories of when in their prime.

How the Old Die

> I have observed, as a matter of fact, that it is only people who exceed the age of ninety who attain *euthanasia*—who die, that is to say, of no disease, apoplexy or convulsion, and pass away without agony of any sort; nay, who sometimes even show no pallor, but expire generally in a sitting attitude, and often after a meal—or, I may say, simply cease to live rather than die. (Bauman, 1992)

Accompanying changes in "who" dies (i.e., the elderly at the end of a long life, rather than the young) are basic changes in "how" people die; in the quality of death. Sociologically, the old die a number of mini-deaths before actually physiologically expiring. These include the death of one's working self (with "retirement" becoming a cultural consolation for those who must die), civic self (where individuals are placed within an emeritus status, a "roleless role"), spousal status with widowhood, and, if and when finally institutionalized, one's autonomous self (see also **Social Death**).

When Thomas Jefferson was asked if he would choose to live life over again, he responded affirmatively, but only between the ages of 25 and 60. Thereafter, he wrote, "the powers of life are sensibly on the wane, sight becomes dim, hearing dull, memory constantly enlarging its frightful blank and parting with all we have ever seen or known, spirits evaporate, bodily debility creeps on palsying every limb, and so faculty after faculty quits us, and where then is life?" The major causes of death have shifted since Jefferson's time, from relatively quick deaths owing to infectious disease and accidents, to slow-motion deaths resulting from such chronic maladies as heart disease, cancer, cerebrovascular disease (stroke), chronic obstructive lung disease (COPD), and diabetes (see also

Cardiovascular Disease; Disease; Dying Trajectory). These deaths often follow long periods of debilitation and debasement, such as from Parkinson's disease and late-stage Alzheimer's. The number of people with the latter doubles every five years after age 65, afflicting at least one-half of those 85 and older. Because of the aging revolution, Alzheimer's is projected to be *the* disease of the 21st century (see also **Alzheimer's Disease**). Fears of being robbed of all memories and mechanisms of self-control, of losing personal autonomy and becoming a burden on others, have largely replaced concerns over personal salvation. Fewer than 2 in 10 people who live to age 65 or beyond are fully functional in their last years of life.

The Commodification and Politics of the End of Life

The Great Recession made it clear that the United States can no longer afford to spend 17 percent of its GDP on health care, a sizable proportion of which is expended on older people. In 2008, Medicare paid $50 billion just for doctor and hospital bills during the last two months of patients' lives—more than the budget of the Department of Homeland Security or the Department of Education.

In capitalist economies, dying has, like so many other aspects of life (e.g., courtship, marriage, parenting, etc.), become highly commodified. There is more profit to be made from illness and pain than from preventative medicine. There is much profit to be made from terminal disease and the final few months of life. A 2011 study that analyzed data for the nearly 2 million Medicare recipients 65 and older who had died in 2008 found that nearly one recipient in three had surgery in the last year of life. Almost 1 in 5 had surgery in the last month of life; nearly 1 in 10 had surgery during the last week of life.

The inevitable cutbacks in federal expenditures toward Social Security, Medicare, Medicaid, and pensions for both public sector workers and military veterans, will likely be disproportionately shouldered by the old, reinforcing the negative connotations of the final stage of life.

The Griefs and Bereavements of the Old

In age-graded societies such as our own—where individuals are accompanied and tracked through and over a lifetime by their age-mates: as fellow students, spouses, coworkers, and friends—the griefs occasioned by death experienced outside of a family context are nowadays largely confined to older individuals. Retirement and the loss of a spouse, family members, and friends rank among life's most stressful experiences—and it is the old, those with the least psychic reserves, who largely must deal emotionally with such losses. With death largely reserved for the elderly, it is also largely the old who must deal with the stigmas associated with the proximity of those who die and who occupy the bereavement statuses of widow and widower.

Michael C. Kearl

See also: Alzheimer's Disease.

Further Reading

Bauman, Zygmunt. *Mortality, Immortality, and Other Life Strategies.* Stanford, CA: Stanford University Press, 1992.

Cohen, Eric, and Leon R. Kass. "Cast Me Not Off in Old Age." *Commentary,* 121(1) (2006): 32–39.

"Cost of Dying," *CBS 60 Minutes,* November 22, 2009. http://www.cbsnews.com/video/watch/?id=5725483n

Hochschild, Arlie. *The Unexpected Community: Portrait of an Old Age Subculture.* Berkeley, CA: University of California Press, 1978.

Kwok, Alvin, Marcus E. Semel, Stuart R. Lipsitz, Angela M. Bader, Amber E. Barnato, Atul A. Gawande, and Ashish K. Jha. "The Intensity and Variation of Surgical Care at the End of Life: A Retrospective Cohort Study." *The Lancet,* 378(9800) (2011): 1408–13.

ALCOHOL

Ethyl alcohol, or ethanol, is the intoxicating ingredient found in beer, wine, and liquor. Alcohol is produced by the fermentation of yeast, sugars, and starches.

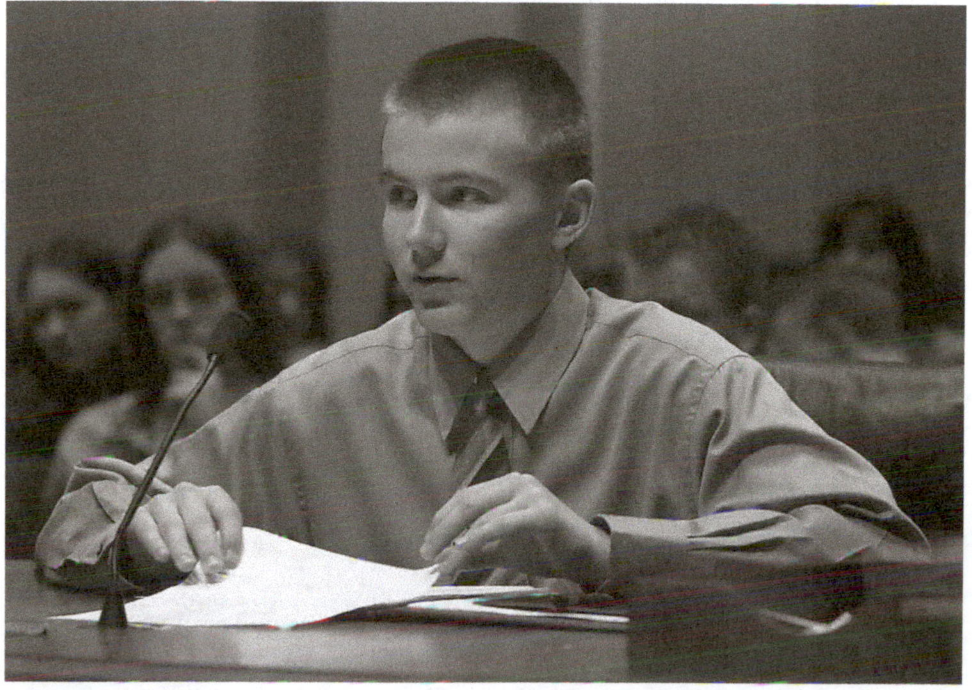

High school junior Curt Reha testifies before the General Affairs Committee in Lincoln, Nebraska, in February, 2001, in favor of bills that would make consumption of alcohol by a minor illegal. Reha told the committee of his 16-year-old cousin and another girl who had been killed in a car accident where there was evidence that the driver of the car, who survived, had been drinking. (AP Photo/Nati Harnik)

How Is Alcohol Consumed?

There are various ways to consume alcohol, but drinking the substance is by far the most popular. Another popular method includes mixing alcohol with food and eating the alcohol-infused food. "Eyeballing," the process of pouring alcohol in your eye sockets, has become popular in the past few years among college students around the world. Research shows that the majority of people that are experimenting with eyeballing are doing it because they are already under the influence of alcohol, not solely to get intoxicated. Another method of alcohol consumption is by soaking a tampon in alcohol and then inserting the tampon into the rectum or vagina. This method delivers the alcohol directly into the bloodstream through the membrane walls for a quicker and more intense effect.

Effective Dose/Lethal Dose

Each drug has an effective dose and a lethal dose. Effective dose is the amount of the drug that needs to be taken to reach the desired effect. Lethal dose is the amount of the drug that needs to be taken to prove fatal in the majority of the population. A drug's effective/lethal dose ratio shows how dangerous a drug is in terms of potential for overdose. Alcohol has an effective/lethal dose ratio of 1:10, which shows that if it takes 40 ounces of alcohol to get the desired "high," it will take 400 ounces to kill the average person. In comparison, heroin has an effective/lethal dose ratio of 1:5, cocaine's effective/lethal dose is 1:15, and marijuana has an effective/lethal dose of 1:>1,000.

Alcohol-Related Deaths

Alcohol is the third largest risk factor for disease in the world. It is the leading risk factor in the Americas. Nearly 4 percent of all deaths in the world are related to alcohol. Most alcohol-related deaths are caused by disease or injury, including cancer, liver cirrhosis, and cardiovascular disease. Alcohol has been proven to weaken the immune system and effect judgment, thereby increasing the risk for HIV/AIDS and sexually transmitted diseases.

Other Considerations

The National Institute on Alcohol Abuse and Alcoholism defines binge drinking as a pattern of drinking that brings a person's blood alcohol concentration (BAC) to 0.08 grams percent or above. This typically happens when men consume five or more drinks, and women consume four or more drinks, in about two hours. Many people associate binge drinking with kegs of beer and college aged students, when in fact, people over the age of 65 binge drink the most. Binge drinking may lead to health problems, such as cardiovascular disease. Binge drinking is also noted as causing mental health issues, social harm, and high economic costs.

Withdrawal

After chronic or prolonged ingestion of alcohol, the body gets used to the drug and has a difficulty functioning without it. Once the drug is no longer introduced into the body, withdrawal symptoms may occur. Symptoms can be light, mild, or severe ranging from anxiety, headaches, and even convulsions. There are specific treatments for each of these withdrawal symptoms.

Public Health Policy

Proactive measures are being taken through policy implementation to fight the high number of alcohol-related deaths. One example of proactive alcohol policy is limited alcohol licenses in each city or county. The lower the number of liquor licenses available in each area, the less likely underage youth will have access to alcohol. Limiting liquor licenses has also proved to lower alcohol-related crimes. Restrictions placed on the age of alcohol consumption are a simple way to attempt to monitor and safeguard against drinking. In the United States, a person must be 21 years of age to consume or purchase alcohol. Limiting the amount of alcohol that a person can consume while operating a motor vehicle is yet another public policy that is beneficial.

Jason Bertrand

Further Reading

Bennet, P. "Preventing Alcohol Problems Using Healthy Public Policy." *Health Promotion International,* 7 (1992): 297–306. http://pubs.niaaa.nih.gov/publications/Newsletter/winter2004/Newsletter_Number3.pdf

Hingson, R., T. Heeren, A. Jamanka, and J. Howland. "Age of Onset and Unintentional Injury Involvement after Drinking." *Journal of American Medical Association,* 12 (2000): 1527–33.

Hingson, R., T. Heeren, M. Winter, and H. Wechsler. "Magnitude of Alcohol-Related Mortality and Morbidity among U.S. College Students Ages 18–24: Changes from 1998 to 2001." *Annual Review of Public Health,* 26 (2005): 259–79.

Levy, D. and S. Mallonee. "Alcohol Involvement in Burn, Submersion, Spinal Cord, and Brain Injuries." *Medical Science Monitor,* 10 (2004): 17–24.

Miller J. and T. Naimi. "Binge Drinking and Associated Health Risk Behaviors among High School Students." *Pediatrics,* 119 (2007): 76–85.

National Institute of Alcohol Abuse and Alcoholism (NIAAA). "National Institute of Alcohol Abuse and Alcoholism Council Approves Definition of Binge Drinking." *NIAAA Newsletter,* 3 (2004): 3.

ALZHEIMER'S DISEASE

Alzheimer's is an age-related type of dementia involving the gradual wasting of brain tissue that results in severe cognitive impairment, including memory loss. The disease takes its name from Alois Alzheimer, the German psychiatrist who, in 1906, first described the anatomical characteristics of the condition. As the most common form of dementia, Alzheimer's was the sixth leading cause of death in America in 2010, affecting 5.4 million people, and one in eight seniors in the United States. Although Alzheimer's can only be definitively diagnosed with autopsy, the hallmarks of the disease—aside from a decline in memory—include impairment to at least one of the following abilities: the execution of motor skills; the aptitude for generating and comprehending language (either written or spoken); and the capacity to recognize or identify objects. Even though Alzheimer's begins to attack the brain well before symptoms are first manifested, onset of the disease typically occurs between the ages of 45–65, but is most common among the population of those aged 65 and over. As a degenerative condition that progressively worsens over time, four distinct phases can be discerned, characterized chiefly by the following:

1. A reduction in energy, difficulty in remembering things, and an inability to follow instructions
2. Forgetfulness, repetition, and difficulties in decision making
3. Confusion, disorientation, and lack of awareness of time, place, and events
4. Radically diminished memory, depression, and overall weakness

Because Alzheimer's is a degenerative disease, the dying trajectory (see **Dying Trajectory**) for people diagnosed with the condition is most likely to be protracted, somewhat unpredictable, and involve long-term suffering and distress caused by the irreversible loss of mental as well as physical functioning. (People aged 65 and older can, on average, expect to live 4–8 years after diagnosis of Alzheimer's, though sometimes as long as 20 years). This places a tremendous burden upon those charged with caring for those with Alzheimer's, not only because of the behavioral disturbances wrought by the disease, but also because the gradual loss of the person with Alzheimer's produces a lingering and ambiguous dying that "cruelly smears death—and bereavement—across the years" (Sutcliffe, 2007). The grief experienced by those caring for someone with Alzheimer's—usually a spouse or close family member—is sometimes complicated and anticipatory, involving a "pulling away" from the person even before they have died. To this extent, Alzheimer's represents a kind of social death in which, as Jonathan Miller, former president of the British Alzheimer's Society put it, the person living with the disease comes to be viewed as "an uncollected corpse . . . which the undertaker has cruelly forgotten to collect" (Miller, 1990, in Howarth, 2007: 182). Similarly, the loss of the person living with Alzheimer's may be ambiguous for the person caring for them precisely because the beloved is physically present but psychologically absent.

As the population of the United States continues to age, Alzheimer's is set to affect an ever greater proportion of society. By 2050, it is estimated that the incidence of Alzheimer's among those aged 65 and older will triple, from 5.2 million people in 2012, to a projected 11–16 million people. Commensurately, and because many people with Alzheimer's require round-the-clock medical care and attention, it is estimated that associated health care costs will increase from 200 billion dollars in 2012 to 1.1 trillion dollars in 2050. Much of this care is provided in hospices and residential care facilities, such that by 2009, 6 percent of all people admitted to hospices in the United States had a primary diagnosis of Alzheimer's. For those who remain within the family home (some 60–70 percent of all Alzheimer's sufferers), the social, psychological, and financial burden on the 15 million Americans who provide unpaid care to them is especially high, often requiring caregivers to relinquish full-time paid employment in order to do so.

Alzheimer's does not affect all populations equally, affecting women more than men, chiefly because women live longer than men and the risk of Alzheimer's increases with age (two-thirds of Americans with Alzheimer's are women). The causes of Alzheimer's remain unknown and are likely the result of multiple factors rather than a single cause. While there is as yet no cure for Alzheimer's, notable cases such as those of President Ronald Regan and writers Iris Murdoch and Terry Pratchett have helped raise the profile of the disease. Since his diagnosis with Alzheimer's in 2007, Terry Pratchett has donated considerable time, energy, and money to ventures aimed at raising awareness and understanding of the disease—including a BBC documentary *Living with Alzheimer's;* while the 2001 movie *Iris,* starring Kate Winslet and Dame Judi Dench as Iris Murdoch, provided a tender and sensitive portrayal of a brilliant mind ravaged by Alzheimer's.

Michael Brennan

See also: Aging.

Further Reading

Alzheimer's Association. Alzheimer's Disease: Facts and Figures. *Alzheimer's and Dementia,* 8(2) (2012). http://www.alz.org/downloads/facts_figures_2012.pdf

Miller, Jonathan. "Interview." In *The Ruffian on the Stair,* edited by R. Dinnage. Harmondsworth: Penguin, 1990, cited in Howarth, Glennys, *Death and Dying: A Sociological Introduction.* Cambridge: Polity, 2007.

Sutcliffe, Thomas. "Malcolm and Barbara: Flawed but Virtuous." *Independent,* 9 August 2007.

AMERICAN INDIANS

Although there are more than 500 different indigenous American tribal groups in the United States, each with their own distinctive traditions, it is nevertheless possible to talk of commonalities representative of an "American worldview." Despite the fact that many centuries-old traditions have either changed or been forgotten altogether (due to the absence of a written history and European colonization), many beliefs and customs have persisted to the present day. These traditions permeate many aspects of life, including death, which, in native American culture, is regarded as very much part of life. In this vein, not only are life and death considered circular rather than linear, but the grief resulting from death is itself understood as present oriented. In contrast to dominant white culture, which focuses on the future without the deceased, native American culture focuses on life in the *present* without the deceased; whereby one is encouraged to live every day as though it is the last day of one's life, but to enjoy today more than yesterday and tomorrow more than today.

Spirituality and Death

Tribes show tremendous reverence and respect for life; and for the American Indian, death is not to be feared because it is viewed as not all that different from life.

Every part of all things—dirt, rocks, and trees—is considered sacred. Accordingly, the remains of the dead rest in sacred ground. Rather than disconnecting from the dead, American Indians continue to have an ongoing relationship with the dead, who are themselves believed to continue to love, care for, and protect the living (see also **Continuing Bonds**).

Most American Indians face death without fear or concern for their past actions. Death is viewed not as the termination of life but as merely a changing of worlds; an idea which is encapsulated in the notion that: "We live and then we live again." In this view, everyone is part of a larger whole and has a purpose and place in the world. Where one's purpose ends, so does one's life; death therefore fulfills one's destiny. Death in this sense is not considered a "defeat"; for we must all face death, and none are exempt. Neither is death viewed as the result of an offense against God or some other deity, but rather as the common fate of all. And while death affects those left behind, and is a painful separation for the living, survivors of the deceased can take comfort in the belief that they too will one day join the deceased.

Burial Practices

There is considerable variation in bereavement and burial practices among, and even within, the hundreds of native American tribes. The mortuary and burial practices of a tribe are affected by a number of factors, including: the cause of death, where the death occurred, as well as the age, sex, and social status of the deceased. It is also likely that climate, availability of materials to dispose of the body, and religious beliefs have, historically, been major determinants of how bodies of the dead were disposed of. Almost universally, however, tribes provide provisions for a spirit journey, whether for a single or group burial. What is also clear historically, is that tribal groups, even nomadic ones such as the Apache, did not abandon their dead but provided them with ceremonies and dignified disposal. In this tradition, Apache deceased are dressed in their finest clothes, wrapped in a blanket, where they are carried to the hills and buried in a crevice or shallow grave.

American Indian methods of disposing of the deceased reflect their attitudes toward the dead; so that, for example, cremation may be used and viewed as a way of sending the soul of the deceased skyward to an afterlife. Cremation may also be used to destroy the corpse in order to prevent the spirit of the deceased from coming back to inflict injury or harm upon the living. Mummification can be used to preserve the body from decay out of love and respect for the deceased, and is perceived as allowing the deceased to live on in an afterworld. It may also aid the grieving process to know that the body of the deceased has been cared for and preserved.

Tree burial, in which the body of the deceased is supported on, or attached to, the limb of a tree, provides another means of disposal and may have originated from living among trees and be seen as a way of returning to one's "roots." It may also be simply a way of returning the deceased to nature as quickly as possible by allowing animals, birds, and insects to consume the body. Tree burial and the use of burial scaffolds, in the which the body of the deceased is supported, may also provide a practical alternative to earth burial when in the winter months, because the ground may be frozen solid, it may be very difficult, if not impossible, to dig a grave.

Mound builders heaped rocks, soil, and the remains of burned buildings over the grave of the deceased so that, over time, the place in which the dead were interred became a raised piece of ground. Mounds may have been built to provide the deceased with the necessary provisions needed to make their journey to the afterworld, whether in the sky or the center of the earth. Mound building may also have been a method to keep the deceased (or the ghost of the deceased) from coming back to disturb (or haunt) the living. The rocks used in mound building may also have been intended to keep scavengers from ravaging the body of the deceased, and it is also conjectured that rocks were used to mark graves. The Sioux, for example, used grave posts to mark graves, which were inserted into the ground or supported with stones—the stones outlasting the markers. Some tribes, such as the Apache, disposed of their dead by leaving the body in the wickiup (a dome-shaped dwelling), which is then pushed down upon the body. Other groups placed the body in a canoe, cave, urn, or other vessel for disposing of the body of the deceased. Some would place the body in a hole in the ground and cover it with rocks or by pulling a fallen tree over it. For others, such as the Navajos, the actions of survivors after the death of a loved one are believed to influence the deceased's journey to the next world. Mortuary rituals and bereavement practices, therefore, come to assume great significance.

Bereavement Practices

The practice of leaving food and property for the deceased is common, perhaps out of fear that the deceased might return to disturb the living if items are not left for them. This practice may also have been born of a desire to honor and show great love and respect for the deceased by burying them with treasured items. The items buried with the deceased would often reflect their position and social role in society. So, for example, in the case of a child, one might leave toys, a cradle, and food; while in a warrior's grave, one might leave favored weapons, beads, medicine bags, tobacco, or paint; and in a woman's grave, one might leave food or tools for tanning or making pottery and baskets.

Most tribal groups dispose of their dead very quickly following death. Following disposal, some would bring gifts of food and other items for the spouse or family of the deceased, while others would have the spouse and family of the deceased give away the possessions of the deceased to those who attend the funeral and grieving ceremonies. A wake or some sort of ritualistic telling of tales and stories of the deceased would often follow the burial. Warrior tribes would often regal in tales of the bravery or prowess of the deceased, while sedentary tribes would tell tales of the lore of the tribe and the exploits of the deceased. Most tribes have men telling the stories, but some have women; and those who listen are expected to try very hard to stay awake for the telling of stories that may last for many hours. Those who get too sleepy may quietly slip away for a time and return silently later. Food, drink, and smoking are common practices, while some tribes play games. If games are played, the surviving spouse will typically not take part and close relatives are expected to remain in a state of mourning until the games are completed. For some tribes, this process may take days, while for others it may only last a short time.

Grief for American Indians is decidedly individual. Who died, one's relationship with them, how much experience one has with death, the spirituality of the griever, how traditional or "white" the griever has become, and whether one is a reservation or urban dweller, are all factors that may influence grieving. Importantly, the social status of the deceased will determine the extent and intensity of public grieving; yet what constitutes a high social status also differs among tribes. A tribal chief, a great hunter, a spiritual leader, or even a child, may be considered of high social status for one tribe, whereas another tribe may value and honor a grandfather, a story teller, or a holy person more highly. Generosity and sharing are strong cultural values among native American tribes and the amassing of money and possessions is not a traditional practice; instead goods are to be shared and savings are to be used. The give-away (or potlatch) ceremonies are still practiced among many groups (such as the Tanacross Athabaskans of central Alaska), as a means of redistributing wealth and objectifying the grief of the hosts.

Attitudes toward Dying and Death

Individuals from most tribes express a willingness to surrender to death at any time with little or no fear. The Lakota Chief Crazy Horse was noted for his chant before going into battle that, "Today is a good day to die." Indeed, every day is a good day to die if one has lived one's life to the full, and every day is to be lived *as if* it were one's last day. One does not, however, seek death before its time; nor does one avoid death or try to delay its occurrence.

Despite the generally accepting view of death among most American Indian groups, there are some, such as the Navajos, for whom death presents a degree of anxiety and fear. It is for this reason that Navajos are reported to favor bringing the sick and elderly into the hospital to die so that the family home is not polluted by the experience of death. It would appear that sedentary tribes, such as the Navajos and Pueblo, appear to be more fearful of the dead than are nomadic tribes, such as the Sioux and Apache. It has been suggested that this fear might stem from an apprehension that the spirit of the dead person may linger and remain to torment the living.

Gerry R. Cox and Michael Brennan

Further Reading

Carr, B.A. and E.S. Lee. "Navajo Tribal Mortality: A Life Table Analysis of the Leading Causes of Death." *Social Biology,* 25 (1978): 279–87.

Cox, Gerry R. "The Native American Way of Death." In *Handbook of Death and Dying,* Volume II, edited by Clifton D. Bryant (pp. 631–39). Thousand Oaks, CA: Sage, 2003.

Cox, Gerry R. and Andrea Sullivan. "Grief and the American Indian." *Grief Matters,* 14(3) (2011): 70–72.

Wilkinson, Charles. *Blood Struggle: The Rise of Modern Indian Nations.* New York: W. W. Norton, 2005.

ANCESTOR WORSHIP

Ancestor worship is one way the living continue their bonds with the dead. The term, however, is somewhat misleading because the dead are not worshiped in the sense that Christians, Muslims, or Jews worship their God; it simply means that the dead continue to have an ongoing role within the family, clan, or society. Ancestor rituals form a central part of all religious traditions at some points in their history, although it is not uncommon for the rituals to be suppressed or even forbidden at times when political rulers find that the ancestor rituals detract from their authority, for example, in Maoist China; or when religious leaders think the veneration of the dead detracts from veneration that belongs to God alone, for example, in medieval Europe when ancestors were replaced by Christian saints.

Ancestor worship is common throughout societies of southeast Asia, including Japan, Korea, and China, where it is a cornerstone of Chinese social structure, cultural beliefs, and religious practice; but it is also a characteristic of Maori culture in New Zealand and of some African tribal groups. The continued presence of ancestors in these societies is underscored by the moral influence that the dead continue to exert over the living. In these societies, funeral rites provide a ritual means by which living elders are transformed into ancestors. It is beyond the scope of this entry to describe the rituals and values in all of these cultures; it is nevertheless possible to use one of them, traditional Japanese

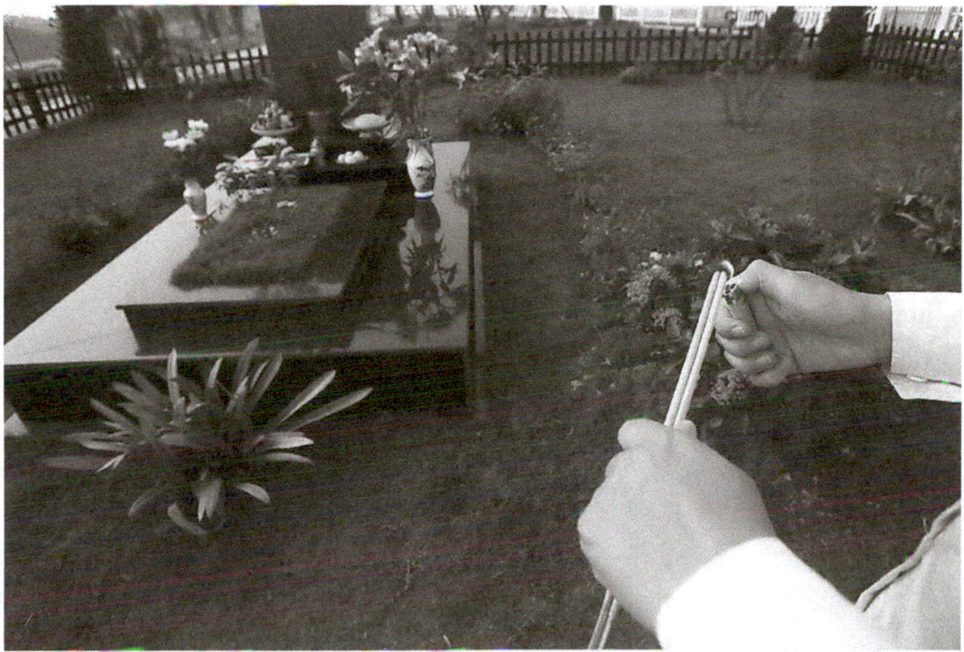

A Vietnamese employee who works in Lac Hong Vien cemetery burns incense for a customer's online order at the cemetery in Hoa Binh Province, Vietnam. The cemetery's online ancestor worship service is the first of its kind in Vietnam. Busy relatives can purchase graveside offerings for the dead by the mouse click. Cemetery staff bring the items to the tombs and send videos or photos of the display by e-mail. (AP Photo/Na Son Nguyen)

culture, to illuminate much about ancestor worship and the ongoing relationship between the living and the dead.

Where Are These, the Spirits of the Dead?

Deeply ingrained within Japanese culture, in ways that transcend formal religious institutions and traditions, the veneration of family connections central to Japanese ancestor worship predates the influence of Buddhism. In a modern and largely secular society, Japanese culture is characterized by a widespread belief in an afterlife in which the living will eventually be reunited with their ancestors. The familial connections between the living and the dead are emphasized by the notion of *kami*, in which the spirits of nature are dependent for their continued existence upon the actions of the living. By failing to nourish and sustain the spirits of nature, the dead may serve as a haunting presence with the power to cause problems for the living. The spirit world beyond this earthly existence cannot be described in anything but equivocal terms. In a spatial sense, it is simultaneously here and there; in temporal sense it is at once both then and now.

> The departed and ancestors always are close by; they can be contacted immediately at the household shelf, the graveyard, or elsewhere. Yet, when they return "there" after the midsummer reunion they are seen off as for a great journey. They are perpetually present. Yet, they come to and go from periodic household foregatherings. (Plath, 1964, 308)

A Ritual Place

One of the ritual places, is the *butsudan,* the buddha altar: a cabinet in traditional homes with incense burner, bell, candles, and the *ahai* (memorial tablets). Each morning, food and prayers are offered there. In their classic study of mourning rituals in Japan, Yamamoto and colleagues (1969) provide us with a detailed sense of what happens at the *butsudan* with the spirit of a beloved grandfather. They describe how the family altar serves as a "hotline" providing direct daily communication with one's ancestors. This altar offers the opportunity to ring the bell, light incense, and to talk over a current crisis with a person whom you have loved and cherished. Such a "hotline" was not only used in times of personal crisis, but functioned for the sharing of good news and positive feelings as well.

Thus, in a television drama, a young woman whose father had died waits for a letter telling her she has been hired for a job she really wants. When the acceptance letter arrives, she opens it, looks tearfully at her mother and rushes into the living room where she kneels before the *butsudan,* opens the doors, bows low, and holds up the letter to her father's photograph and tablet.

Ritual Time: *O Bon*

The rituals of *O Bon,* the major summer festival in Japan, welcome spirits of the dead for a three day visit. It provides for a periodic merging of two worlds (the living and the dead), solidifying the sense of ancestral continuity by reassuring the dead of the living's continued concern and care for their well-being.

After sunset on the first day, one lantern for each deceased member, and fires by the doorway, invite the spirits home. In early evening, family members gather to welcome the spirits back. The second day, people visit graves. Buddhist priests make rounds offering a brief prayer at each house. At the end of the third day, there is a large gathering in which the spirits are entertained before their departure. Formal farewells are said with expressions such as "Come back next year." In some areas, a candlelight procession moves toward the river where, one by one, representatives of each household place small boats, bearing the candles, into the current. As far as the eye can see, the flickering flotilla plies on. When the candle goes out, it is said, the spirit has been released to the other world.

Dennis Klass

See also: Continuing Bonds.

Further Reading

Geary, P.J. *Living with the Dead in the Middle Ages.* Ithaca, NY: Cornell University Press, 1994.

Gilday, E.T. "Dancing with the Spirit(s): Another View of the Other World in Japan." *History of Religions,* 32(3) (1993): 273–300.

Goss, R. and D. Klass. *Dead but Not Lost: Grief Narratives in Religious Traditions.* Walnut Creek, CA: AltaMira, 2005.

Goss, R. and D. Klass. "Spiritual Bonds to the Dead in Cross-Cultural and Historical Perspective: Comparative Religion and Modern Grief." *Death Studies,* 23(6): 547–67.

Plath, D.W. "Where the Family of God Is the Family: The Role of the Dead in Japanese Households." *American Anthropologist,* 66(2) (1964): 300–317.

Smith, R.J. *Ancestor Worship in Contemporary Japan.* Stanford, CA: Stanford University Press, 1974.

Yamamoto, J., K. Okonogi, T. Iwasaki, and S. Yoshimura. "Mourning in Japan." *American Journal of Psychiatry,* 125 (1969): 1661–65.

ANGELS

Many religions have a concept of spiritual beings that serve God and assist humanity. Belief in angels, derived from Zoroastrianism, influenced Israel during the exile and postexilic eras. The word itself is derived from the Greek word for messenger, as is the Hebrew (*mal'ak*) and the Arabic (*malak*). In the Hebrew Bible (Old Testament), angel or angels appears over 100 times. Angel(s) are mentioned in the New Testament over 150 times and in the Qur'an approximately 99 times. Angels have many functions: they praise God (Psalm 103:20), serve as God's messengers (Genesis 18: 1–10; Luke 1:11–2:14), guard the people (Psalm 91:11–12), and are instruments of God's judgment (Matthew 13:49–50). Many Christians, and all Muslims, believe that individual guardian angels are assigned to guard and guide individual human beings (Matthew 18:10).

With the exception of the orthodox, most Jews today consider angels symbolic. Although Rabbinic Judaism never adopted the idea of guardian angels, the fact that this Christian belief stems from the first century indicates that some Jews had adopted this understanding from Zoroastrianism. Today, Christians believe in the reality of angels; however, although Catholic Christianity presumes the reality of angels and promotes the understanding and devotion to guardian angels, the Catholic Church does not propose a position on angels that is binding on faith. Belief in angels is an essential tenet of Islam. Muslims believe that each person is assigned two angels: one to guard them during the day, and another to record the good and bad deeds of the day each night.

In the sixth century, an anonymous monk writing as Dionysius the Areopagite (today, called Pseudo Dionysius) listed nine kinds (choirs) of angels from the Bible. These fall into a hierarchy of Seraphim, Cherubim, and Thrones—who praise God and populate the heavenly abode; Dominions, Powers, and Authorities—who serve as God's agents throughout the heavenly and material universe; Principalities, Archangels, and Angels—who are God's soldiers or messengers to humanity.

Some angels are given names. The late postexilic Book of Daniel identifies the angels Gabriel and Michael. The angel Raphael is an important character in the deuterocanonical text of Tobit. Gabriel and Michael also appear in the New Testament: Gabriel announcing the conception of Jesus to Mary (Luke 1:19, 1:26), while Michael, who was identified in Daniel as a warrior angel, is said to be the leader of angelic forces who contend with the devil (Jude 1:9; Revelation. 12:7). In the Qur'an, Gabriel (Jibril) is the one who transmits the Qur'anic revelations to Mohammed over 23 years, and while Michael (Mika'il) is mentioned only once; in the Hadith (i.e., sayings, deeds, and stories of Muhammad) both are associated with Muhammad's night journey and ascension to heaven. Islam holds that these two angels will operate the scales of justice that weigh the good and evil deeds of humanity.

Recent research into contemporary mourning behavior suggests the continued influence of angels upon everyday thinking, indicating a widespread belief in angels—as providing care to both the dead and the living—even among those who claim to be nonreligious.

Regina A. Boisclair

Further Reading

Coudert, A. "Angels." In *The Encyclopedia of Religion,* 16 vols., edited by M. Eliade (pp. 282–86). New York: Macmillan, 1987

Walter, T. "Angels Not Souls: Popular Religion in the Online Mourning for British Celebrity Jade Goody." *Religion,* 41(1) (2011): 29–51.

ANIMISM

From the Latin *anima*, meaning soul or spirit, animism is the world's oldest form of religion, dating back 70,000 years and is still found today in about 7,000 cultures worldwide. It continues to be the only form of religion for most indigenous foraging and farming societies characterized by ecological sustainability. Such societies view nature as intrinsically spiritual: spirits are believed to be present in all objects encountered daily; natural and supernatural are not viewed as separate domains. Based on the belief that supernatural forces—known as souls or spirits—inhabit everything in nature, animate or inanimate, these spirits are believed to be capable of influencing human affairs. Humans, in turn, are believed to influence spirits through rituals and offerings. These rituals are usually led by a male shaman and female potter. English anthropologist E. B. Tylor was the first to document and analyze animism in his book *Primitive Culture* (1871). Tylor claimed animism explained the origin of all human religions. He believed that the first religious thought humans experienced was in dreams, which were no less real than was the waking world. People recognized a soul or spirit in all things, not distinguishing between animate and inanimate. Animism is viewed by many to be the basis for many major religions today, including Buddhism, Hinduism, Shintoism, and Neopaganism. Animism is a descriptor to a worldview of numerous and diverse religions focused on beliefs that objects in nature are inhabited by spirits and sacred forces, and all humans experience phenomena like dreams, visions, trances, and out-of-body experiences. These phenomena allow humans to be "here" and "there" simultaneously, connecting humans to the spirit world.

Andrea Malkin Brenner

See also: Religion; Totemism.

Further Reading

Clodd, Edward. *Animism, The Seed of Religion.* Frome and London: Butler and Tanner, 1905.

ANTHROPOLOGY

Anthropology is the study of human beings, with particular focus on the rituals, rites, and cultural practices that humans create in order to make their existence meaningful. Anthropology emerged in the late 19th century and was distinguished from its counterpart, sociology (whose focus was also the study of human society), by its focus on non-Western, preindustrial societies. Stimulated by innovative ideas of evolution, it flourished in the 20th century. It was influenced by numerous theoretical perspectives and has made two major contributions to an understanding of humanity: (1) the production of ethnographies—detailed accounts of how a people live, derived from months or years of fieldwork-based experience, and (2) a comparative method that sets these accounts alongside each other, providing "thick descriptions" of variation in life circumstances, geography, ecology, and climate.

Ethnographies inevitably depicted death. One group that developed theories to interpret these was largely French and sought to interpret "society," and death occurring within it, as a *total social process* rather than gather information about isolated exotic beliefs and practices. Emile Durkheim (1858–1917), a leading figure within this French tradition, made two significant death-related contributions, on suicide and mourning. *Suicide* (1897) described the bond between "individual" and "society," distinguishing between egoistic, altruistic, and anomic suicides. Suicide, Durkheim argued, was no random event. The "egoistic" reflected weak individual-society bonds, producing a sense that life was not worth living; the "altruistic" marked very strong bonds that, when beset by failure, status loss, or sense of honor, left suicide as a way out, while "anomic" suicide followed a sense of a breakdown of meaning and a purposelessness in life. Regarding mourning, Durkheim's famous study *The Elementary Forms of the Religious Life* (1912) emphasized the communal context and nature of mourning as a social performance rather than as an individually generated, self-focused, manifestation of feeling.

Robert Hertz (1882–1915), Durkheim's relative, developed the idea of double burial from southeast Asian ethnographies, distinguishing between the primary burial and decay of the corpse (the wet phase) and the secondary treatment of the resulting skeleton (the dry phase). This transformation marked the status change from life through death to becoming an ancestor; but it also allowed both for psychological changes associated with grief, as well as for changes of status among the living.

The issue of status change associated with death, and other aspects of life, was enhanced by Dutch anthropologist Arnold van Gennep's concept of *rites of passage*. This turns on the idea of the threshold (*limen* in Latin), with preliminal, liminal, and postliminal phases marking shifts in a person's status, with society leading a person from a pre-existing status, through an in-between (or liminal) stage, before granting a new social status. Traditional Catholic thought conceived of the dead as being in a liminal, in-between world of purgatory as a preparation for final incorporation into heaven, a view associated with prayers and other rites that link the dead and the living (see **Catholicism**). Protestants generally saw the dead as either asleep until their final resurrection or else as passing straight into heaven or hell (see **Protestantism**). In psychological terms, one contemporary trend speaks of continuing bonds existing between the living and the dead, emphasizing the role of a person's active memory and perceptions of the presence of the dead by the living. This contrasts with Sigmund Freud's view of grief as a process of separation and loss of prior attachments (see **Freud, Sigmund**). Victor Turner's later analysis of liminality (1969) spoke of *communitas* as a shared feeling of unity among ritual participants—in which traditional social distinctions of hierarchy and status were temporarily suspended—and is one way of analyzing mourning behavior.

Psychological factors, largely absent from van Gennep's theory of status change, did emerge later in Maurice Bloch's work on certain initiation rituals. His notions of "rebounding violence" or "rebounding conquest" identify the motif of "death" as a frequently occurring idea, a kind of natural symbol, describing how candidates undergo a "death" before being "reborn" into a new social status involving negative attitudes toward their former state. This death-rebirth motif is familiar in Christian notions of baptism and religious conversion, and in some Shamanic traditions. Similarly, life affirmation is also symbolized in postfuneral acts of ritual cleansing and funeral feasting. These echo Bronislaw Malinowski's earlier focus in *Magic, Science and Religion* (1948) on funerals as helping to manage emotions of hope and fear, and A. M. Hocart's (1883–1939) concern, in his essay "The Purpose of Ritual," with death rites as an opportunity to "seek life."

Subsequent anthropological studies have used many of these ideas in detailed ethnographies, for example, on contemporary American funerary behavior and on Hindu traditional and regional death rites and communication with the dead. Anthropological influences have also pervaded studies of ritual in theology, pastoral care, and death.

Douglas J. Davies

See also: Archaeology; Burial.

Further Reading

Bloch, M. *Prey into Hunter.* Cambridge: Cambridge University Press, 1992.

Bloch, M. and J. Parry. *Death and the Regeneration of Life.* Cambridge: Cambridge University Press, 1992.

Davies, D.J. *Death, Ritual and Belief,* 2nd edition. London: Cassell, 2002.

Durkheim, E. *The Elementary Forms of the Religious Life.* London: Allan Lane, 1976/1912.

Durkheim, E. *Suicide: A Study in Sociology.* London: Routledge and Kegan Paul, 1970/1897.

Hertz, R. "A Contribution to the Collective Representation of Death." In *Death and the Right Hand, 1905–1906,* edited by Rodney and Claudia Needham (pp. 27–86). New York: Free Press, 1960.

Hocart, A. M. "The Purpose of Ritual." In *The Life-Giving Myth and Other Essays* (pp. 46–52). London: Routledge, 2004/1952.

Malinowski, B. *Magic, Science and Religion.* London: Souvenir Press, 1974/1948.

Metcalfe, P. and Huntington R. *Celebrations of Death.* Cambridge: Cambridge University Press, 1991.

Parry, J. *Death in Banaras.* Cambridge: Cambridge University Press, 1994.

Turner, V. *The Ritual Process.* London: Routledge and Kegan Paul, 1969.

APOCALYPSE

The concept of apocalypse describes a cataclysmic end of the world, culminating in destruction, disaster, and death. As a prophetic narrative predicting impending doom and the ultimate destruction of humanity, the apocalypse has assumed widespread purchase and application in popular culture and imagination, where it can be found in movie and television storylines, media tropes, and religious as well as political discourses. Relating chiefly to *end times* and a battle of cosmic proportions between good and evil, the notion of apocalypse is an eschatological concept found in Christian theology, where it is contained chiefly in the book of Revelation of the New Testament of the Bible.

While questions of eschatology (combining the Greek words *eschatos* and *logos* and meaning the study of the *final days*) characterize all major religious traditions—especially the philosophical contemplation upon the ultimate destination and destiny of human beings following death, their salvation, and the afterlife—the notion of apocalypse has been uniquely interpreted in the Christian tradition as a revelation disclosing the return of Jesus Christ and the defeat of his enemies. References to the apocalypse can be found throughout the Bible: in Ezekiel (who issued harsh words of judgment to the Israelities), in Joel (who talked of a phoenix rising from the ashes), and in Daniel (who referred to the three who survived the fiery furnace), but the most foreboding apocalyptic warning is reserved for Book of Revelation of the New Testament and its description of Armageddon.

It is here, in Armageddon (combining the Hebrew for mountain, *har,* with Megiddo, a city in ancient Palestine), that the forces of good and evil converge for one last battle or judgment that will see the creation of a "new heaven and a new earth." Literal interpretations of this powerful and foreboding imagery have provided a central tenet of world-rejecting Doomsday cults and millenarian movements, whose shared belief in the impurity of earthly existence provides the pretext for a collision of forces that will pave the way for a new heavenly Kingdom of God. Such apocalyptic ideological thinking was a hallmark of the Peoples Temple in Jonestown, which culminated in the mass suicide of 900 followers of Jim Jones in November 1978; in the standoff between a Seventh-Day Adventist splinter group, the Branch Davidians, and U.S. authorities, resulting in the deaths of 74 of its members in Waco, Texas, in April 1993; and in the ritualized murder/suicides of members of the Order of the Solar Temple in Switzerland, Quebec, and France in March 1997.

For some individuals and groups, apocalyptic thinking provides the lens through which to view contemporary catastrophic events—from earthquakes and tsunamis, to 9/11 and Hurricane Katrina—as Biblical prophesies predicting impending doom and the end of the world. The location of Armageddon in what is today modern Israel has lent added political significance for fundamentalist and evangelical Christians to their view that perceives the Middle East to be the site of the final battle that will herald the Second Coming of Christ.

Such has been the power and influence of apocalyptic thinking upon American society that, according to Matthew Barrett Goss and Mel Gilles in their book *The Last Myth,* it has today thoroughly permeated mainstream secular culture. No longer the preserve of the evangelical Christian right, they argue that apocalyptic thinking routinely functions as a narrative that unites all Americans, and can be extended to issues of concern to the political liberal/left, such as global warming and climate change, in ways that govern and shape not only our understanding of worldly events but also our response to them.

Michael Brennan and Richard B. Gilbert

See also: Cults; Epidemics and Plagues.

Further Reading

Barrett Goss, Matthew and Mel Gilles. *The Last Myth: What the Rise of Apocalyptic Thinking Tells Us about America*. New York: Prometheus Press, 2012.

Walliss, John. *Apocalyptic Trajectories: Millenarianism and Violence in the Contemporary World.* Bern: Verlag Peter Lang, 2004.

ARCHAEOLOGY

Archaeology is the study of past human societies through an examination of the physical remains which have survived. As a subdiscipline of anthropology, archaeology is interested not only in the recovery of the physical remains of past cultures, but rather in how these remains can allow archaeologists to investigate and understand the various cultural practices of past peoples, and when possible, individuals within the culture being studied. With its focus on past cultures and peoples, archaeology would appear, by definition, to be a study of death, since the cultures and people under investigation are no longer living. In reality, however, archaeology is the study of the living, since the goal of the discipline is to reconstruct the living, vibrant culture from its "dead" remains.

At the core of the science of archaeology is the concept of *context*. While archaeologists can study individual artifacts (pots, arrowheads, beads, baskets, coffins, etc.), each artifact studied in isolation does not provide sufficient information to reconstruct past cultural practices. To obtain the most information from the items archaeologists excavate from the ground, it is necessary to fully examine the context in which the artifacts or other physical remains are found. By fully knowing, recording, and analyzing the context; the location where an item is found; the type of soil or sediment from which it is removed; as well as the associations an item has with other nearby artifacts, archaeologists are much better able to compile clues from the past so as to reconstruct a much fuller and accurate picture of the lives of past peoples.

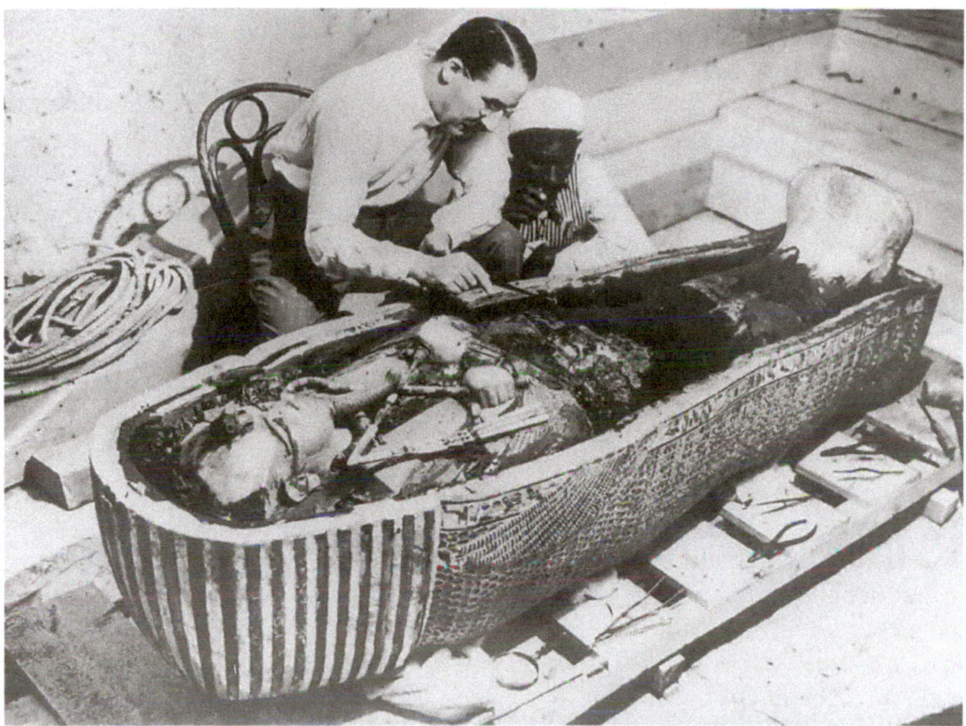

British archaeologist Howard Carter and an assistant, seated beside the coffin of King Tutankhamen, remove the consecration oils which covered the third or innermost coffin. During Carter's tenure as an investigator for the Egyptian Antiquities Service, he supervised many important excavations, including his famous discovery of the tomb of the "boy-king" Tutankhamen. (Library of Congress)

While archaeologists look at the full spectrum of past activities and behaviors, it is through the study of the dead and the cultural practices associated with death and dying, and disposal of the dead, that archaeologists can reconstruct aspects of a living society in the past. Through the excavation and study of human remains, archaeologists can gain information about the past at a variety of levels, namely, the individual, family, community, and larger society. From the study of an individual's mortal remains—whether in the form of frozen or mummified flesh or in a skeletal state—archaeologists can learn a great deal about an individual's life. For instance, using an analysis technique known as bone isotope analysis, archaeologists can determine where an individual grew up, as our bodies incorporate into the makeup of our bones and teeth various chemicals and concentrations of chemicals from the groundwater we drink. Therefore, it is possible to determine if a Roman soldier found buried in York, England, was born and grew up in the local area around York prior to joining the Roman military forces, or rather, was from one of the Roman Empire's provinces in North Africa. This same technique can allow archaeologists to reconstruct the diet of an ancient individual as certain plants and animals contribute higher quantities of certain chemical isotopes than others, and the more we eat of that species or set of species, the more of those compounds we subsequently incorporate into our physical makeup. Such an analysis can help to determine whether a population was agriculturally based or relied on wild resource for their diets.

Within our skeletons, we also preserve a record of illnesses we may have had as well as any injuries. It is possible to see if a past individual suffered from malnutrition, anemia, tuberculosis, arthritis, as well as variety of other ailments. Perhaps even more interesting is the ability to determine the possible occupations past individuals were engaged in. Repetitive activities performed over long periods of time can leave tell-tale signs in our skeletons. Individuals who repeatedly carry heavy loads show signs of this in deformations of their vertebrae, while cowboys and mounted cavalry soldiers will show signs of long-term horseback riding by the presence of enlarged muscle attachment points in their upper leg bones.

It is also possible to determine in some cases the actual cause of death in an individual through studying the long-preserved physical remains of their skeletons, and in good preservation conditions, hair and other body parts. Death as a result of violence, either intentional or unintentional, will leave traces in the skeletons in the form of bone breaks, cut marks on bones, or marks from specific types of weapons like clubs and bullets.

Archeologists are not only interested in reconstructing aspects of single individuals. By studying the ways in which societies dispose of their dead, they can reconstruct how the society was organized. Was it, for example, egalitarian or a highly structured hierarchical society with a supreme ruler? When an individual dies, it is their family and/or community who buries them. The way the body is treated, where it is buried, next to whom it is buried, the position of the body, whether items are placed in the grave with body or not, can all be related to that particular individual's standing in the community/society, as well as the religious beliefs of their culture. The type and size of grave are a reflection of the amount of time, labor, and resources expended on its creation and can be directly related to the individual's wealth and/or status within his or her society. If archaeologists excavate a cemetery and find that only the oldest individuals have elaborate graves or many objects placed in their graves, then it might be assumed that status within this past society was based on one's lifetime deeds and achievements. If, on the other hand, both old and very young have elaborate graves with many rich offerings, then it is most likely that within this society, status is based not on one's achievements and abilities, but rather on one's bloodline or lineage.

The orientation of a grave and the placement of the body within the grave can tell us some things about the religious beliefs of the culture. Early Christian burials were typically aligned east-west, with the head to the west so that when they arose on Judgment Day they would be facing God. Early ancient Egyptians were buried with their heads to the south, with face turned toward the west welcoming the coming afterlife and their joining the gods in that realm. When archaeologists encounter limited numbers of graves that are different from the others in a cemetery or those in a particular society—a few oriented with their heads to the west when all others are to the east, or with some buried spatially segregated from the rest—it may signify that these individuals were viewed as somehow different from other members of society. Perhaps they were buried with their heads to the west because they were shamen or priests who were seen as belonging to both the living world as well as to the other realm. Being buried segregated from everyone else might signify the commission of a social or religious crime, as was the case with individuals who completed suicide being denied burial in consecrated cemeteries in Christian societies.

David A. Anderson

See also: Anthropology.

Further Reading

Bahn, Paul. *Written in Bones: How Human Remains Unlock the Secrets of the Dead.* Richmond Hill, ON: Firefly Books, 2003.

Pearson, Mike Parker. *The Archaeology of Death and Burial.* College Station: Texas A&M University Press, 2000.

ARIÈS, PHILIPPE

French social historian Philippe Ariès (1914–1984) made a very significant contribution to the study of death and dying by exploring changes in the attitudes and practices surrounding human mortality over a thousand year period. Ariès's first significant contribution to scholarship, however, came not in the field of death and dying but in the historical study of childhood, where he was able to demonstrate that the concept of childhood, as we know it, is a relatively recent invention. Not until the 17th century, Ariès reveals, did a period of "childhood"—in which children were spared the hardships and responsibilities of adult life—come to be seen as separate from, and as a precursor to, adulthood. Instead, children were exposed to the same experiences as adults—including work, violence, and death—and were regarded as "little adults," in which they were not only dressed as miniature adults, but were expected to behave like adults.

This interest in childhood, a concept that in Western societies appears both sacrosanct and unchanging, led Ariès to explore death and dying as another area of human life that appeared immutable and, in modern Western societies, had become a topic that was deeply taboo. As in *Centuries of Childhood,* where Ariès successfully laid bare many of the taken-for-granted assumptions about childhood by demonstrating that how children were viewed in the past had undergone a fundamental transformation, so in his historical study of human mortality Ariès was able to show how attitudes toward death had undergone a "brutal revolution" by which death and dying had been "furtively pushed out of the world of familiar things" (Ariès, 1974, 85, 105).

Aside from more than a dozen academic papers on death and dying, Ariès's most lasting and significant contribution to understanding the evolution in attitudes toward human mortality can be found in two books: *Western Attitudes Toward Death,* published in 1974, and *The Hour of Our Death,* which appeared first in French as *L'homme devant la mort,* and then published in English in 1981. Together, these two books provide unprecedented insight into how, over the course of several centuries, death had gone from something that was both "familiar and near," arousing no great terror or fear, to something that by modern times was so frightfully abhorrent that we dare not any longer call it by its name, but rely instead upon a range of euphemisms and metaphors by which we attempt to deny, conceal, and hold death at arm's length.

In all, Ariès claimed to have identified five prevailing patterns of attitudes and practices surrounding death, each loosely corresponding to a particular time period. These five patterns are described by Ariès as (1) tame death, (2) death of self, (3) remote and imminent death, (4) death of other, and (5) death forbidden and denied. In the first pattern, "tame death," Ariès outlines an attitude in which death was openly accepted with a sense of resignation and inevitability, in which people were not only fully prepared for death when it came, surrounded by neighbors, friends, and family (including children), but, in some instances, embraced it as part of a journey from this earthly existence to the afterlife. For those who died in battle, death was perceived as an honorable and noble event, while for others death was a "beautiful" and transcendental event that transformed the often decaying and disease-ridden body into one of sublime beauty. Underscored by a framework of Christian religious thinking that helped make sense of human mortality and suffering, death in medieval Europe was viewed as a "release" from earthly existence; the reward for having lived a pious life. Images of the dead during this period routinely portray the dead as if they are sleeping, positioned in a restful and recumbent position as if awaiting spiritual awakening.

In the second pattern, "death of self," Ariès describes the steady growth in anxiety about death, where passage to the afterlife becomes less assured and more firmly premised on notions of Judgment Day that rely on moral assessments about the life one has lived. It is during this period that we see the emergence of *ars moriendi*, a new genre of literature providing instruction on "the art of dying," including the necessity of repentance as a means of securing passage to the afterlife.

In "remote and imminent death," Ariès outlines an ambivalent attitude toward death in which death becomes both a topic of intrigue but also of repulsion. As the dominance of religious frameworks for making sense of death begin to fade, and as the growth of science accelerates during the 18th century, curiosity about the human body (including processes leading up to and following death) intensifies; as does a fear of dying, which, in the Age of Enlightenment, is no longer reassured by the religious beliefs of earlier centuries.

By the 19th century, a concern with the fate of one's own soul following death has given way to anxiety about how we will cope following the death of our loved ones and what Ariès calls "death of other." It is here in the Victorian era, accompanied by the rise of the Romantic movement in literature and art, that the modern concept of bereavement truly emerges and is marked by intense feelings of loss and grief. Romantic expressions of grief can be found in poetry and paintings in which heaven is depicted as human centered (anthropocentric), a place where romantic unions and family relations cut short by death can be resumed, where the dead are not "lost" but "gone before."

Finally, by the 20th century, death had become "forbidden and denied," removed fully from public view where it was screened off behind closed doors in hospitals and nursing homes. Surrounded by a cultural taboo that placed strict limits on the expression of death and grief, death in this era became invisible, viewed not as beautiful but as disgusting and nauseating. Here, the "beautiful death" has given way to the "ugly and hidden death, hidden because it is ugly and dirty" (Ariès, 1981: 569). Death in Ariès's historical analysis has thus gone full circle: from a position in the past when it was "tame" and evoked no great fear or consternation, to a situation in modern times where, under certain medical conditions and in the absence of religious frameworks for making sense of it, it has become "wild."

Ariès's work can today be considered part of a classical canon of literature within death studies, which emerged in the second half of the 20th century as a critique of the impoverishment of death and dying in the modern era. His historical analysis, however, is not without criticism. Two criticisms stand out as worthy of attention. The first challenges Ariès's claims about attitudes toward death in the wider West, on the basis of what are essentially French data, as over generalized. The second suggests that Ariès mistakes literary and artistic *representations* of death and dying in ancient times for actual experiences and attitudes. Here, critics contend that these depictions are themselves idealized wish fulfillments that help betray the brutal reality of death in medieval society.

Nevertheless, Ariès's impressive and groundbreaking body of work stands as an important reminder that attitudes toward death, like many other social phenomena, are never static but are continually evolving.

Michael Brennan

See also: Ars Moriendi; Death Denial; Taboo.

Further Reading

Ariès, Philippe. *The Hour of Our Death.* New York: Oxford University Press, 1981.

Ariès, Philippe. *Western Attitudes toward Death: From the Middle Ages to the Present.* Translated by Patricia M. Ranum. Baltimore: Johns Hopkins University Press, 1974.

ARS MORIENDI

Derived from Latin and meaning literally "the art of dying," *ars moriendi* refers to a genre of devotional Christian literature that emerged in the late Middle Ages and was intended to provide practical guidance for the sick and dying on what they should do in order to die well. This body of literature was most widespread in European societies of the 14th and 15th centuries amid a period when public anxiety about death and dying was at its greatest, stimulated no doubt by the prevalence of death due to famine, warfare, and plague—which helped to ensure that death was a ubiquitous feature of the medieval landscape.

The popularity of such instructional literature during this time can also be explained by a shift in beliefs, from a widespread conviction that salvation was a collective event, to a belief that each individual would have to face judgment for his deeds during life. One of the first of these texts, which was published anonymously in the Netherlands around 1430, spawned other practical guides that were used not just by the sick and dying but by those caring for them, as well as by preachers when putting together sermons on how to attain the "good death." These texts included Thomas Lupset's *The Waye of Dyinge Well* (1534); Thomas Beacon's *The Sicke Mannes Salve* (1563); and Jeremy Taylor's *The Rule and Exercises of Holy Dying* (1651).

As arguably the most notable text within this genre, Taylor's book, like others of its kind, emphasized the idea that death, when it was near, should be embraced willingly and gladly. Taylor strongly recommended *memento mori* ("remember death"), insisting that others assist the dying while in their death throes, thereby providing not only support to the dying, but at the same time learning in advance how to prepare themselves for death when it eventually came. In this context, dying well routinely entailed repenting for sins committed during life, affirming one's religious faith, and begging forgiveness in order to help secure salvation and ensure safe passage to the afterlife.

Michael Brennan

See also: Deathbed Scene; Memento Mori.

Further Reading

Vogt, Christopher P. "The Art of Dying (*Ars Moriendi*)." In *Encyclopedia of Death and the Human Experience*, edited by Clifton D. Bryant and Dennis L. Peck (pp. 70–72). Thousand Oaks, CA: Sage, 2009.

ART AND LITERATURE

Since the beginning of time, artists and writers in every era and culture have been occupied with the subject of death and dying, portraying deathbed scenes, suicides, massacres, plagues, natural disasters, burials, grievers, and the afterlife in literal and figurative ways. The genres of relevant arts include, but are not limited to, poetry, narratives, memoirs, essays, and novels (broadly defined as "literature"), architecture, dance, sculpture, music, painting, theater, film, photography and comics. What Franz Kafka said of a book—"to be the axe to thaw the frozen sea within us," could be applied to any one of these genres.

Engaging in any of the arts, whether as initiator or observer, is in itself a creative act, and is often catalyst enough to assist in the search for meaning, to enable grief, facilitate renewal, and initiate change. The engagement (be it reading or writing, viewing or drawing, listening or enacting), to varying degrees, involves attention, analysis, identification, catharsis, and insight. The beauty of the process is its openness to interpretations, to the way any of us takes it in and uses it for oneself, in both personal and professional contexts.

In the Old Testament, Job laments that death is a one-way street from which there is no return. In prose, poetry, etching, and watercolor, the entire Book of Job's undeserved suffering is illuminated and illustrated. In the New Testament, we are told at least three times that Jesus literally shed tears of grief, and in the shortest sentence in the Bible, it is exquisitely stated that "Jesus wept." Bible stories and the Crucifixion have inspired old masters, visual artists, filmmakers, and musicians to this day.

"Out, Out Brief Candle"

The metaphor of the candle, representing the fragility and brevity of life, has often been used in the arts. In Shakespeare's play *Macbeth,* the protagonist's despair at the untimely death of his wife concludes in his soliloquy that after all our "strutting and fretting" on the stage "life is meaningless." Yet in sonnet *LXXIII,* acknowledging the fact that though expiration will be the final fate, Shakespeare focuses on the flame's final spurt of color and energy: on the glowing of a fire that, "consumed by that which it was nourished by," propels us heed, to *carpe diem* (seize the day), and "to love that well which thou must leave ere long," in other words, to love that which, ultimately, we must give up because it's existence is finite.

In contemporary music, one of the best-selling songs of all time, *Candle in the Wind,* has also paid homage to life's brevity and fragility in three different

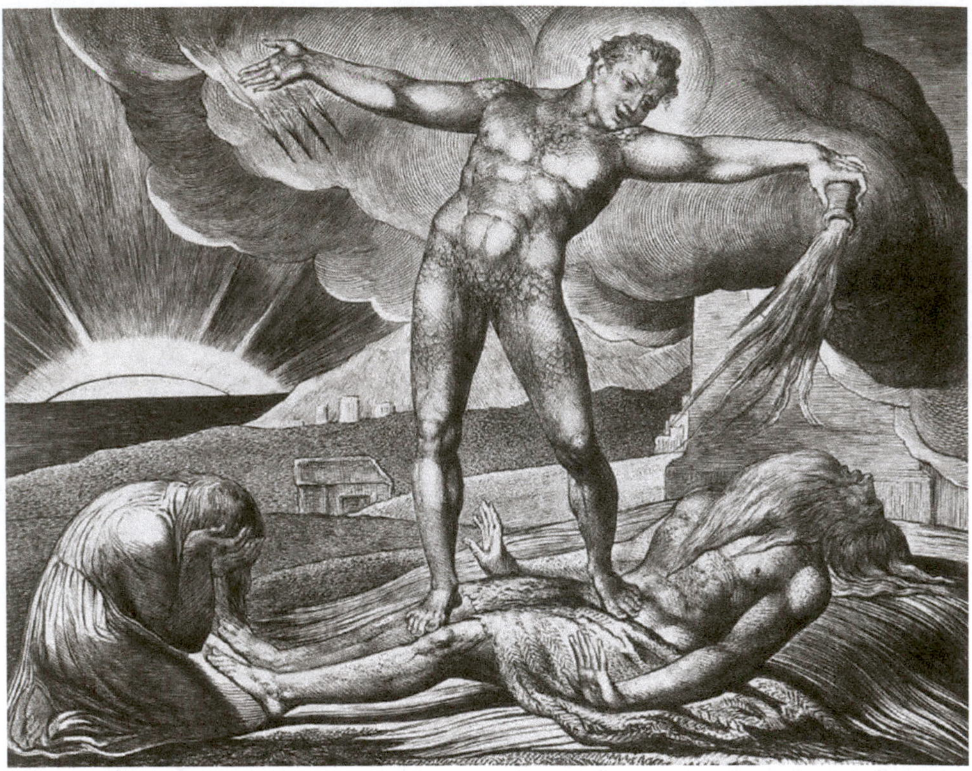

William Blake, *Satan Smiting Job with Sore Boils*, circa 1826. Ink and tempera on mahogany. (Courtesy of The Tate Collection)

momentous occasions. The opening lyrics of the original song, written in 1973, by Elton John and Bernie Taupin, were clearly about film star Marilyn Monroe: "Goodbye Norma Jean/Though I never knew you at all." In 1990, Elton John dedicated the song to Ryan White, the youngster who contracted AIDS through a tainted hemophilia treatment and was subsequently expelled from school because of the disease. After the death of this young AIDS activist, Congress enacted the Ryan White CARE Act, which is funded to this day. Later, rewritten to honor the death of Princess Diana in 1997, Elton John performed a reedited version at her funeral in Westminster Abbey.

This haunting tribute—"Your candle burned out long before your legend ever did"—to three young, misunderstood, and mistreated human beings, applies (and draws upon the metaphor of the candle as a signifier of life's finite existence) to another artist as well: the painter Vincent Van Gogh. Don McLean's song, *Vincent*, with its open line of "Starry Starry Night" is a reference to Van Gogh's painting, *The Starry Night.* The candle appears in several of Van Gogh's paintings: in *Open Bible, Extinguished Candle and Novel* (1885), painted in memory of his father, possibly acknowledging their contrary religious beliefs, yet reminiscent of the 17th-century vanitas theme (see **Images of Death**); and in *Gauguin's Chair* (1888), in which are two naturalistic novels and a burning candle.

Another metaphor widely used in the arts personifies death as it also challenges death. John Donne's holy sonnet X (1633) opens with the lines "Death be not proud, though some have called thee/Mighty and dreadful, for, thou art not so." *Death Be Not Proud* is the title of John Günter's memoir chronicling his adolescent's son's struggles to overcome a brain tumor and his ultimate death. Widely read in high school classes, the book, published in 1949, was made into a film which debuted in theaters in 1975. Perhaps the most current and well-known allusion to this metaphor is Margaret Edson's (1999) Pulitzer Prize–winning play *Wit,* most often styled as "W;t." In this drama, the main character, Vivian Bearing, PhD, is a single 50-year-old professor of metaphysical poetry, diagnosed with stage IV metastatic ovarian cancer. In 2001, the play was adapted into an Emmy Award–winning cable television film, directed by Mike Nichols with Emma Thompson cast in the role of this exacting, strict professor. In the play and the film, the entire action takes place in the protagonist's hospital room. Currently, local professional theater companies at medical centers throughout the United States and Canada invite medical students, house staff, and other health care providers to attend readings of the play followed by structured discussions of the play's themes. More than conventional educational methods, this experiential activity appears to be resulting in increased skill in caring for dying patients.

Personifications of death appear often in Emily Dickinson's poetry. "Because I could not stop for death/he kindly stopped for me." In one of her most famous poems, Dickinson has death dialogue directly with the spirit, which ultimately is triumphant. As death "argues from the ground," "the spirit turns away/Just laying off for evidence/an overcoat of clay."

Thus, the arts, in a manner different from—but no less penetrating than—clinical analysis, both reduce and at the same time heighten reality by giving it another dimension. Back to Shakespeare's *Macbeth:* "Give sorrow words. The grief that does not speak/whispers the o'er fraught heart and bid it break."

Sandra L. Bertman

Further Reading

Artsology: http://www.artsology.com/death-portrayed-in-art.php

Bertman, S. L. *Dying, Bereavement and the Healing Arts.* London: Jessica Kingsley, 1997.

Bertman, S. L. *Facing Death: Images, Insights and Interventions.* New York: Taylor & Francis, 1991.

Bertman, S. L. *Grief and the Healing Arts.* Amityville, NY: Baywood, 1999.

ASSASSINATION

Assassination is a type of causing death. The term, however, is ambiguous. On some occasions its use is on a par with usage of "murder," while on others it is on a par with ordinary uses of "killing" (which may be either noncommittal with respect to the moral evaluation of the act under consideration, or convey that the act is morally justifiable).

Compare the meaning of "killing" with the meaning of "murdering." Each of these terms denotes an act that causes the death of a person. There is, however, a major difference between "killing" and "murdering": whereas the latter denotes an unjustifiable act of causing death, the former may be understood as denoting a justifiable act of causing death or denoting an act of causing death without conveying any evaluation of the extent to which the act is justifiable.

When U.S. president Barack Obama announced the death of Osama bin Laden, he said he can report "that the U.S. has conducted an operation that killed Osama bin Laden" and added that "justice has been done." In contrast, Ismail Haniyeh, the head of Hamas in the Palestinian Gaza Strip, said, according to a May 2, 2011 Reuters report, that he "condemn[s] the assassination and the killing of an Arab holy warrior." Noam Chomsky's reaction, on May 6, 2011, was that: "It's increasingly clear that the operation was a planned assassination, violating elementary norms of international law. . . . In societies that profess some respect for law, suspects are apprehended and brought to fair trial. I stress 'suspects.'" In the last two reactions to the operation that caused the death of Osama bin Laden, "assassination" is a pejorative notion. Both convey the view that assassination is on a par with murder. Arthur Kaplan, ethicist at the University of Pennsylvania, was asked whether the killing of Osama bin Laden constituted assassination, and if so, was it morally right? Did it "serve justice?" In response, he argued that American values, in some instances, permit retribution without due process. In this reaction to that operation, "assassination" is not a pejorative notion, since in some instances it is considered justifiable.

We are concerned here with defining "assassination" without making a moral evaluation of any particular act. What, then, is an *assassination* (when the term is used in the noncommittal sense)? Definitions of some notion of assassination abound, but most of the suggested definitions are not especially helpful, because they capture the meaning of "assassination" in the pejorative rather than the noncommittal sense. According to the *Merriam-Webster Online Dictionary,* "to assassinate" means "to injure or destroy unexpectedly and treacherously." Whatever we take "treacherously" to mean, it is clearly a pejorative term, the use of which renders the suggested definition of "to assassinate" inappropriate for our noncommittal purposes.

A survey of descriptions of acts as "assassinations" in the noncommittal sense, and of suggested definitions of the term, leads to a family of features of assassination, which include the following:

- A Target: killing a person; killing a political leader; killing a noncombatant; killing selectively
- A Plan: killing intentionally; killing in a premeditated manner
- A Purpose: killing for political, ideological, or religious purposes
- A Manner: killing unexpectedly; killing by a person not in uniform; killing secretly (i.e., without admitted national responsibility); killing by clandestine means

Trying to use this list of features in order to formulate a definition, we have to disregard features that are common in assassinations, but are not necessarily conditions that *have* to exist for an act to constitute an assassination. For example, an assassination of a person can be publicly announced by a state as intended (rather than remaining a state-kept secret). One can imagine the Allies during World War II making such an announcement concerning Adolf Hitler. An operation of assassination can be carried out by a military force performing a targeted killing mission. The assassination (in the noncommittal sense of the term) of Osama bin Laden was done by a Seals team, a unit in the U.S. Navy. A March 2003 air strike on Saddam Hussein's Presidential Palace in Baghdad was also presumably a nonclandestine attempt to assassinate (in the same noncommittal sense) Saddam Hussein.

Two of the features within the above-named category of "target" are also problematic. Identifying the target as a "political leader," though often an existing characteristic of assassination, is not necessarily the case on other occasions. First, the term "political" usually excludes military leadership, but this is not always the case. A person in the position of political leadership may at the same time serve in a military capacity as well. The president of the United States, for example, is both formally and practically the U.S. commander in chief, whom it would be inaccurate to describe as a "noncombatant" during a war or armed conflict in which U.S. military forces are involved. Moreover, on some occasions the person under consideration is an operative leader but not a political leader. In a November 3, 2002 operation in Yemen, a U.S. citizen was killed by a missile fired (presumably) from a CIA drone. He was described by the U.S. administration as playing a leading role in Al Qaeda's 2000 attack on the USS *Cole*. In a September 30, 2011 operation, also in Yemen, another Al Qaeda–affiliated U.S. citizen was killed, described by President Obama as one who "took the lead in planning and directing efforts to murder innocent Americans." In both cases, the persons were operative leaders, but not political ones. Hence, the feature referring to killing of a "political" figure cannot be used in a strict definition. However, it can be replaced by another feature, which seems to capture its essential element, namely, the killing of a prominent person.

A working definition of "assassination," in the noncommittal sense of the term, could, therefore, be *an act of killing a prominent person selectively, intentionally, and for political, ideological, or religious purposes.*

Distinctions

Operations of targeted killing are ostensibly similar to assassinations: they are acts of killing a person, selectively and intentionally. However, the person killed in such an operation is not necessarily a prominent person. In the context of fighting terrorism, the target is often a person who plays a crucial role in creating jeopardy, such as a person who produces explosive belts intended to be used in suicide-bombing operations, but who is not, nevertheless, considered prominent. More importantly, in the same context, targeted killing is meant to be performed for self-defense, unlike assassination, which is carried out for other purposes.

On some occasions, acts of killing a person, whether as assassination or as targeted killing, are described as "extrajudicial executions." This term is used to convey a criticism of the act under consideration, on grounds of it being carried out without due legal process. However, unlike extrajudicial executions, assassination and targeted killing operations do have firm legal grounds; for, strictly speaking, they are seldom extralegal and there is no impropriety in their being extrajudicial.

Justification

Assassination has been commonly taken to be unjustifiable. A 1973 UN Convention bans murder and other crimes against "internationally protected persons," including heads of states, prime ministers, as well as ministers of foreign affairs and diplomatic agents. In the United States, there have been several executive orders that banned assassination. The first, the 1976 EO 11905, signed by President Ford, ordered that "no person employed by or acting on behalf of the U.S. Government shall engage in, or conspire to engage in, political assassination." The 1978 EO 12036, signed by President Carter, and the 1981 EO 12333, signed by President Reagan, ban assassinations in general.

On the other hand, under some circumstances, assassination, as it is defined here, may be justifiable—morally, ethically, and legally. If the political purpose of assassination is to bring about a change in the system of powers in the arena of international relationships or within a state, then it is unjustifiable. However, if the political purpose is, for example, gaining victory in a war against an aggressor and assassination is the last resort, then assassination may be carried out and be justified.

Asa Kasher

Further Reading

Chomsky, N. "My Reaction to Osama bin Laden's Death." Guernica: A Magazine of Art and Politics. http://www.guernicamag.com/daily/noam_chomsky_my_reaction_to_os/

Herman, S. *The Classic Guide to Famous Assassinations.* Newhaven, UK: Golden Guides Press, 2012.

Kasher, A. and A. Yadlin. "Assassination and Preventative Killing." *SAIS Review,* 25(1) (2005): 41–57.

Pape, M. S. "Can We Put the Leaders of the 'Axis of Evil' in the Crosshairs?" *Parameters* (2002, Autumn): 62–71. http://www.carlisle.army.mil/USAWC/parameters/Articles/02autumn/pape.pdf

"U.S. Drone Strikes: Memo Reveals Case for Killing Americans." *BBC News,* February, 5, 2013. http://www.bbc.co.uk/news/world-21333570

AUTOEROTIC ASPHYXIA

Autoerotic asphyxia involves the practice of starving the brain of oxygen (cerebral hypoxia) in order to stimulate a heightened sense of sexual gratification. This self-directed sexual practice typically involves methods that include the use of ligatures to induce strangulation; the placing of airtight materials (such as plastic bags) over the head; as well as the use of solvents, anesthetic gases, and chemicals (such as amyl nitrite) that work to produce a psychoactive effect by helping to remove oxygen from the brain and induce a brief euphoric and semihallucinogenic state. Although the practice was first formally identified by researchers in 1902, it has a much longer provenance and can be found in anthropological literature and the work of the 18th-century French aristocrat, Marquis de Sade (1740–1814), who became renowned for his sadistic and sexually explicit writing.

While the main aim of autoerotic asphyxia is the satisfaction of sexual desire, one unintended risk for those practicing it, is death resulting from a lack of oxygen supply to the brain. However, because it is a highly secretive activity practiced only in seclusion, authorities charged with investigating the causes of death, such as police, coroners, and forensic pathologists, often wrongly misinterpret the evidence as suicide. This is often not helped by the fact that friends and relatives of individuals who die as a result of autoerotic asphyxia may attempt to hide or conceal the various accoutrements that accompany it for the fear of embarrassment and shame surrounding it.

Tell-tale clues that can help forensic investigators distinguish autoerotic asphyxia from suicide include the presence of pornographic material; the use of bondage and other sexual paraphernalia; evidence of masturbation and incomplete hanging; doors to a property which are barred from the inside; the use of rope or ligature which has a release mechanism so that the individual can regulate the amount of asphyxia; evidence of wear on the strangulation device suggestive of repetitive use for sexual purposes; and the use of padding on the ligature in order to conceal evidence of marks around the neck.

Because of the secrecy surrounding autoerotic asphyxia, it is difficult to ascertain with any degree of certainty or precision the numbers or types of people regularly involved in it. There is, however, some evidence to suggest a much higher prevalence among men than women (with a male-to-female rate of practice believed to be greater than 50:1), and higher prevalence among white men under the age of 30. In North America, it is estimated that approximately 1,000 deaths per year can be attributed to accidental deaths resulting from autoerotic asphyxia and that this figure has increased in the last 25 years, perhaps due to a curiosity to try the practice inspired by greater media reporting. In recent decades, two high profile cases of fatalities resulting from autoerotic asphyxia have included the death of Michael Hutchence, lead singer of the Australian rock band INXS, in 1997, and the death of the British Conservative politician and journalist Stephen Milligan in 1994. In the case of Hutchence, although the coroner ruled his death as the result of suicide, friends and family have claimed it was more likely the outcome of autoerotic asphyxia.

One intriguing and unresolved dimension of autoerotic asphyxia is the apparent intimate relationship between sex and death. This has led some to speculate that the evidence of images of death and dying found at the scene of fatalities involving autoerotic asphyxia is itself used by practitioners as a source of sexual gratification. Another possibility is that the very idea of the potential risk of death associated with the activity may, for some practitioners, be sufficient to produce and enhance sexual orgasm.

Michael Brennan

See also: Sex and Death.

Further Reading

Byard, Roger W. "Autoerotic Death: A Rare but Recurrent Entity." *Forensic Science, Medicine, and Pathology,* 8(4) (2012): 349–50.
Sheleg, Sergey and Edwin Ehrlich. *Autoerotic Asphyxiation: Forensic, Medical and Social Aspects.* Tucson, AZ: Wheatmark Inc., 2006.

AUTOPSY

An autopsy or postmortem is a medical examination of the body of a deceased person. It differs from an anatomical dissection of a dead body—which is designed to help us understand more about the human condition—in that the purpose of an autopsy is to determine the cause of death. The dissection of dead bodies has been carried out for centuries, beginning with the ancient Greeks who dissected the bodies of dead animals to gain knowledge of the workings of their internal organs. During the 17th and 18th centuries in Europe, anatomical dissections where undertaken on human bodies and detailed drawings made of the human skeleton, muscle groups, blood systems, and organs. One well-known book of such anatomical sketches is *Gray's Anatomy,* which was an important source of education for the developing medical and surgical professions. It was during the 19th century that Thomas Hodgkin, an English physician who gave his name to Hodgkin's disease, developed the systematic study of "morbid anatomy." The aim was to use the detailed examination of the body of the deceased as a means of understanding more about the person's disease condition prior to death and, in this way, to attempt to determine the cause of death.

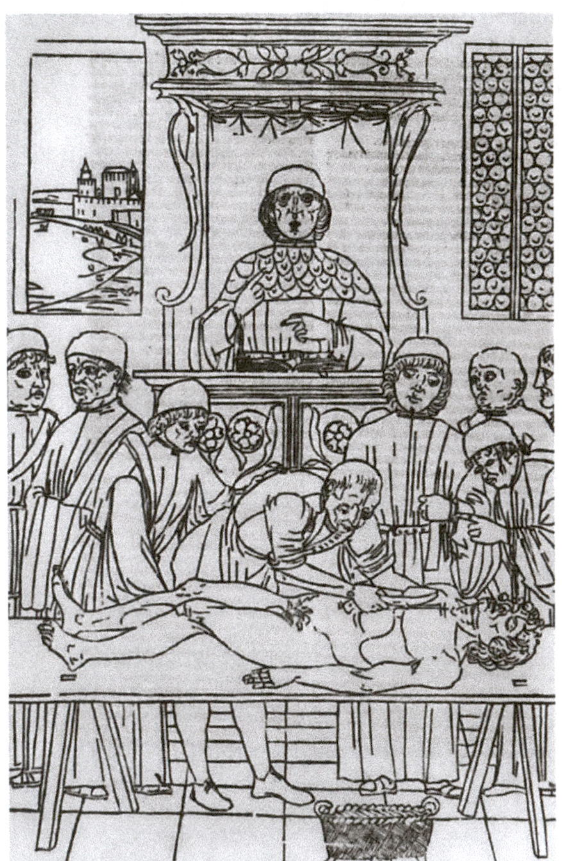

Man performing autopsy on cadaver lying on table as eight other men look on, 1495. Wood engraving. (Library of Congress)

Nowadays, autopsies are usually only performed on people who have died suddenly or in violent circumstances, or those where the cause of death is unknown or controversial in some way—for example, if there is a suggestion of foul play or of medical negligence. Given the extent of contemporary medical knowledge of the nature of disease, the autopsy provides important information for the family of the deceased and also for society at large. In some cases, it may alert us to new diseases or to potential pandemics; for example, if a person has died suddenly as a result of traveling overseas and been exposed to a fatal illness that might spread to traveling companions or unprotected people in their home country.

The autopsy is central to the medical examiner or coroner's (see **Coroner/Medical Examiner**) investigation of the cause of death, and the report of the pathologist (the medic who carries out the autopsy) will be made available to all the interested parties (including the family) and may be read out in court. This can cause distress to the family and friends of the deceased person, especially if the death occurred in violent circumstances. It can, however, also be an invaluable source of information for them, particularly if the autopsy reveals some underlying risk factor that points to a genetic disposition to a potentially fatal disease. Nevertheless, families can be extremely upset at the thought of their relative undergoing a postmortem examination and there are individuals and groups that object to autopsy on cultural or religious grounds. Christian Scientists and Jehovah's Witnesses, for example, are usually opposed to autopsy. Some religions, such as Islam and Judaism, believe that it is important to keep the body complete after death and that an autopsy is, therefore, a violation of the body. Hindus have fewer objections to autopsy provided that all the organs are returned to the body afterward. For others, it is deemed to be crucial that the funeral is held as quickly as possible and autopsy inevitably causes delay.

Over recent years, the idea of autopsy has been popularized by television shows such as *CSI, Law and Order, Silent Witness,* and *Cold Case,* whose storylines tell of complicated crimes being solved through knowledge and technological advances in forensic science (see **Forensic Science**). While these shows are highly entertaining and raise popular expectations about the ability of forensic pathologists to detect hidden factors that lead to the identification and conviction of murderers, they far outweigh reality and have been described as bearing "as much resemblance to reality as a badger does to a stealth bomber." Nevertheless, they engage audiences in the value of science and have led many young people to consider a career in forensic science. More realistic versions of autopsy have been offered in HBO's *America Undercover* documentary series, *Autopsy* and, in the United Kingdom, in the Channel 4 (2002) documentary, *Anatomy for Beginners*, in which anatomist Gunther von Hagens and pathologist John Lee performed the first public autopsy in the UK in over 150 years.

Glennys Howarth

See also: Body Worlds Exhibition; Cadavers.

AWARENESS CONTEXTS

The term "awareness contexts" was developed by American sociologists Barney Glaser (1930–) and Anselm Strauss (1916–1996) in their study of patients with terminal conditions who were dying in hospital settings. Their study was based on the qualitative research method known as ethnography, in which researchers gather information about a small group through direct observation and by immersing themselves in the social interactions that are the object of investigation. On the basis of their research into hospital patients in the San Francisco Bay area, Glaser and Strauss identified four different awareness contexts that helped shape patients' experiences of dying: *closed awareness, open awareness, suspected awareness,* and *mutual-pretence awareness.*

In *closed awareness* contexts, patients were kept in ignorance of their impending death by medical staff who skillfully avoided answering questions or engaging patients in conversations that might reveal the terminal nature of their condition. In these contexts, patients did not—and, indeed, could not—conform to the social norms expected of dying patients because they did not know they were dying. Medical staff preferred *closed awareness* contexts for three main reasons: (1) because a prognosis of how long a patient had left to live could not be predicted with any degree of certainty; (2) for fear that disclosing such information to patients who were dying would lead to psychological distress and depression; and (3) because medical staff were themselves spared the emotional distress of breaking such bad news to patients. However, *closed awareness* contexts were difficult to maintain and often gave way to one of the other three awareness contexts.

In contrast, *open awareness* contexts, in which all parties knew and acknowledged that the patient was dying, were easier for patients and medical staff to navigate and were also thought to avoid some of the negative consequences of *closed awareness* contexts for patients, such as social isolation, loneliness, and a feeling of betrayal by medical staff at not having been told the truth about their condition (see **Social Death**).

Glaser and Strauss's work in this area is significant for two main reasons. First, as a contribution to sociological thinking (see **Sociology**), their research illustrated that a patient's behavior during terminal illness is a learned (or "socially constructed") response that emerges from the context of particular types of social interaction. Second, as a contribution to the study of death and dying, Glaser and Strauss's research demonstrated the benefits of effective and honest communication with dying patients about their condition so that they may be better prepared and accepting of their impending death. Glaser and Strauss's work has provided the basis for subsequent studies of dying within medical settings and has contributed to the development of the hospice and death education movements in the United States (see **Death Education; Hospice Movement**).

Michael Brennan

Further Reading

Glaser, Barney G., and Anselm L. Strauss. *Awareness of Dying.* Chicago: Aldine, 1965.
Glaser, Barney G., and Anselm L. Strauss. *Time for Dying.* Chicago: Aldine, 1968.

B

BANSHEES

Banshees are female harbingers of death, derivative of Irish and Scottish folklore. In both traditions, when a banshee is seen or, more often, heard, it is an omen of death either for the person who witnessed the banshee or for someone in their family. The Irish variety of banshee is called the bean sidhe and the Scottish variety is known as the bean nighe.

Bean Sidhe

In the Irish tradition, the bean sidhe is often portrayed both as a disembodied female soul and as a kind of fairy. She is also known as The Female Fairy, The Lady of Death, The Angel of Death, The Woman of Peace, The White Lady of Sorrow, and The Nymph of the Air. Banshees take a particular, and by some accounts, exclusive, interest in the old aristocratic families of Ireland. The banshee remains connected to the family for as long as that family survives and heralds the death of each of its members. This type of banshee is not concerned at all with newer aristocratic families, so as old family lines die out, banshees disappear with them. The bean sidhe's connection to powerful families of Ireland is such that the only time one might hear the sound of multiple banshees is when someone of great importance is about to die.

The bean sidhe takes different forms, depending on her motives. She is always someone who is strongly connected to a particular family, either through great affection or great anger. Her sound and appearance vary depending on her motivations. If she is affectionate toward the family, she might sing on the occasion of an impending death. Her song will be soothing and reassuring, a welcome into the next world. Many traditional Irish songs claim to have the song of the banshee as their basis. This type of singing is known as "keening."

If the banshee is angry, it may be because of some great injustice done to her while she was alive. In this case, she will not sing or keen, but will instead let loose the scream of a fiend—a demonic howl meant to terrify the person who is about to die and their family. She will remain connected to the family forever; her desire for vengeance is such that she wants to bring misery to all the descendants of those who wronged her.

Though reports of the sighting of the bean sidhe are rare, tradition holds that if she is peaceful she will appear as a beautiful maiden, and if she is angry she will appear as a haggard crone.

Bean Nighe

The bean nighe is a Scottish banshee; a washerwoman that is found at deserted streams, washing the bloody clothes of those who are about to die. Bean nighes are commonly held to be the spirits of women who died during childbirth when the veil between this world and the next is particularly thin. Bean nighes often appear as crones. Legend has it that if a person is able to sneak by the bean nighe undetected, she must grant that person three wishes.

Rachel Robison-Greene

Further Reading

Eason, C. *A Complete Guide to Faeries and Magical Beings: Explore the Mystical Realm of the Little People.* York Beach, ME: Red Wheel/Weiser, 2002.

McAnally, David Rice. *Irish Wonders: The Ghosts, Giants, Pookas, Demons, Leprechawns, Banshees, Fairies, Witches, Widows, Old Maids, and Other Marvels of the Emerald Isle/Popular Tales as Told by the People.* New York: Weathervane Books, 1977.

BEREAVEMENT

Bereavement is the term that denotes having irretrievably lost someone or something of value. While the word is commonly reserved to refer to the death of someone, what has been lost can also include material possessions or intangible realities, such as one's reputation, thereby generating a grief-like response. The term grief is used less exclusively to denote the emotional and behavioral reaction to loss, including (but not limited to) bereavement, whereas the term mourning typically describes the outward manifestation of grief in a variety of social and cultural practices and contexts. Bereavement, grief, and mourning are thus intricately interwoven, and discussions of bereavement lead naturally to discussions of grief and mourning (see also **Grief; Mourning**).

Two powerful explanations of bereavement and its outcomes have influenced scholars and clinicians, one by the founder of psychoanalysis, Sigmund Freud (see **Freud, Sigmund**), and the other by the British psychiatrist, John Bowlby. Freud described grief as the normal, yet deeply painful response to being bereaved. Freud explicitly asserted that grief's anguish would mislead some observers to label the reactions pathological, but that in reality the torment of grief involves not only the *normal response* to the loss of someone loved but also the *process of recovering* from the condition of being bereaved. Freud indicated that the process of recovering from bereavement is drawn out and filled with distress. He identified three tasks that the griever must endure: (1) they must allow themselves—consciously and fully—to experience the agony that their loss causes; (2) they must detach themselves emotionally from the person who has died; and (3) they must create a mental representation of the person who has died, a representation that permits remembering the person without experiencing the anguish that their death has elicited. Freud suggested that grievers needed time to carry out the painful tasks of grieving, and he warned that grievers do not—and indeed, should not—be referred for professional help (Freud, 1957/1917).

American psychiatrist Erich Lindemann (1900–1974) had a considerable influence in promoting Freud's understanding of bereavement. In the early 1940s, Lindemann and his team of clinicians were working with people traumatized and bereaved by the deaths of nearly 500 people in a Boston nightclub fire. Looking for a framework to help guide interventions with these people, Lindemann turned to Freud's account of bereavement and, in effect, institutionalized the process that Freud had described. Lindemann called it "grief work," and this approach has remained the leading explanation for what recovery from bereavement entails. Among the tasks that a griever must accomplish in completing grief work, Lindemann noted such actions as accepting the distress that bereavement causes, expressing feelings of guilt, talking openly about one's feelings, and appraising one's relationship with the person who has died. Lindemann reshaped Freud's explanation in two key ways: (1) by asserting the need to talk about one's grief as a core requirement and (2) by suggesting that bereavement was a condition treatable by therapeutic intervention.

Attachment Theory

Bowlby derived his theory of bereavement from his work to understand the reactions of British children separated from their families during World War II. The British government had evacuated children from major cities into rural areas of England in order to prevent them from being killed or maimed in the German bombing of metropolitan areas. The children were cared for by strangers and Bowlby turned to attachment theory to explain children's responses to, at first, being separated from their parents and, eventually, at then being reunited with them. He recognized through his clinical observations that he had discovered a powerful mechanism for explaining the human response to bereavement. In short, Bowlby argued that bereavement caused by the death of a person occurs because attachment bonds had been irreparably sundered. Correspondingly, in the absence of attachment to someone, a person would not become bereaved when that person died.

Bowlby's use of attachment theory is complex and involves appeals to both ethology (the study of animal behavior in natural settings) and evolutionary theory; for instance, Bowlby maintained that attachment bonds were a result of human evolution that enabled infants to survive into adulthood because mutual attractions developed between infants and caregivers. Individuals construct their own expectations about human relationships due to the quality of attachments formed with caregivers, and these attachment expectations (which Bowlby termed "schemas") influence a person's ongoing relationships over a life span. There is a similarity between Bowlby's emphasis on these early attachment experiences and Erik Erikson's notion of the first psychosocial crisis in identity formation; namely, whether or not, and the extent to which, personal experiences help foster a sense of trust between an infant and the external world.

Bowlby described the process of recovering from bereavement as occurring in four distinct phases: (1) *numbing,* during which the bereaved person seems unable to comprehend the loss; (2) *yearning* and *searching,* during which the person becomes preoccupied with thinking about the deceased individual and desiring their return; (3) *disorganization* and *despair,* during which the person gradually succumbs to a realization that the loss is permanent; and (4) *reorganization,* during which the person begins reclaiming relations with the world, with other people, and with oneself. What occurs during these phases is completely compatible with Freud's and Lindemann's understanding that recovery from bereavement requires considerable "grief work" and will not simply happen by itself.

Stage Theories of Bereavement

Building directly on Lindemann's legacy, Worden has developed a four-task framework for dealing with bereavement. Initially, these four tasks were (1) accept the reality of the loss; (2) work through the pain of one's grief; (3) adjust to an environment in which the deceased is missing; and (4) withdraw one's emotional energy from the deceased and (re)invest it in other relationships. Worden, however, has since rephrased task 2 to read "*process* the pain of grief." He has rephrased task 4 a further two times. The first rephrasing was "to emotionally relocate the deceased and move on with life," and has subsequently become "to find an enduring connection with the deceased in the midst of embarking on a new life." In addition, Kenneth J. Doka has further suggested that people engage in a fifth task; namely, in rebuilding their spiritual worldviews and assumptions which are sometimes shattered by the sense of shock, pain, and incredulity caused by some types of bereavement.

Continuing Bonds

Worden changed the wording of task 4 due to his growing awareness that ongoing attachments with the deceased are far more common than had first been recognized. One publication in particular forcibly challenged the assertion that normal bereavement entails withdrawing all emotional and psychic attachments to the deceased. This book, *Continuing Bonds: New Understandings of Grief,* published in 1996 by Dennis Klass, Phyllis Silverman, and Steven Nickman, presented research data which asserted that, at the very least, a corrective was needed to the assumptions that normal responses to bereavement require relinquishing emotional bonds with the person who has died. The concept of "continuing bonds" was rapidly accepted within scholarly and clinical circles until, eventually, almost a wholesale reversal in clinical thinking had occurred, whereby ongoing attachments to the deceased, which were once considered unhealthy or "pathological," were now considered healthy and normal. Research data have now tempered the sweeping prescription that maintaining bonds is expected of all grievers; rather, and as demonstrated by Stroebe et al. (2010), it is now understood that secure attachments forged during life lend themselves to remaining attached following death, but that insecure attachments require letting go of one's ongoing bonds.

Dual Process Model of Bereavement

The dual process model of coping with loss, as developed by Margaret Stroebe and colleagues in the Netherlands, has also recently entered mainstream thinking about bereavement. This model accepts the grief work theory up to a point; however, a modification has been introduced. Clinical observation of bereaved people reveals that they engage in, and oscillate between, two distinct behavioral processes: at times they engage in direct, purposeful confrontations with the distress that bereavement causes, but at others deliberately avoid such confrontations and instead engage in being alive in the world. The first process is called *loss orientation,* and it confirms assumptions underpinning grief work theory, while the second is referred to as *restoration orientation.* The dual process model insists that people recover from bereavement by engaging in both processes and that they do so naturally and intuitively. Insisting that recovery from bereavement requires solely confronting one's loss is, according to the dual process model, counterproductive and at odds with how people actually behave when bereaved.

Analysis of longitudinal data with many older adults whose spouses had died has further led George Bonanno (2009) to postulate recently that human responses to bereavement take the form of one of three distinct trajectories: a person's bereavement responses follow either: (1) a "resiliency trajectory," (2) a "recovery trajectory," or (3) an "enduring grief trajectory." The *resiliency trajectory* describes people who very quickly return to normal functioning following the death of a loved one. Bonanno noted that a plurality of persons, perhaps even the majority, exhibit this response to bereavement. It is not that these people are unmoved by bereavement, but that what has happened has not challenged what they fundamentally understand and believe about the world, and thus they do not struggle to come to terms with the death.

The *recovery trajectory* describes people who struggle with the death of a loved one, who experience acute grief that subsides within six to eight weeks, but who grapple for up to two years following the death with distress over the loss. Around 40–45 percent of people demonstrate this response to bereavement, and it is plausible that such persons are the ones who come to the attention of professional counselors and therapists. These people engage in grief work, especially the *loss orientation* and *restoration orientation* identified in the dual process model of coping.

The *enduring grief trajectory* describes a small proportion of bereaved individuals, somewhere between 10 and 14 percent, for whom acute grief never lessens. We have come to think of these people as experiencing complicated bereavement (i.e., grief reactions which deviate from normal patterns of grieving through their intensity and duration, and which threaten to overwhelm and debilitate the griever, leading to maladaptive behaviors that inhabit the successful resolution of grief). People whose bereavement constitutes an *enduring grief trajectory* do not recover unless they are provided with professional help and support. Fortunately, evidence-based practices have been developed that effectively work with people mired in an *enduring grief trajectory.*

Two overall approaches to grieving have been identified. One involves the open, conscious, desired sharing with others of what a person is experiencing. Here, the focus is on talking about feelings, and the primary strategy, described as an "intuitive" approach to grieving, is to experience fully the distress that bereavement causes and is thus consistent with theories of grief work. The second approach, referred to as an "instrumental" approach to grieving, focuses cognitively on bereavement. The primary strategy here is to identify and solve problems and to master the situation in which one finds oneself; people employing the instrumental approach to grieving are generally reluctant to discuss their feelings. While these two approaches to grieving have been linked respectively to how females and males deal with bereavement (see **Gender**), evidence also shows that not all females are intuitive grievers and not all males are instrumental grievers (Doka and Martin, 2010).

Other contemporary approaches to explaining bereavement include the growing emphasis on psychological constructivism, which asserts that the central issue at stake in bereavement is meaning-making (Neimeyer, 2001). There has also been the application of existential phenomenology to explain that grieving requires people to "relearn" their relationships with others, with the world, and with oneself (Attig, 2010).

David E. Balk

See also: Freud, Sigmund; Grief; Mourning.

Further Reading

Attig, T. *How We Grieve: Relearning the World,* 2nd edition. New York: Oxford University Press, 2010.

Bonanno, G. A. *The Other Side of Sadness: What the New Science of Bereavement Tells Us about Life after Loss.* New York: Basic Books, 2009.

Doka, K. J. and T. L. Martin. *Grieving beyond Gender: Understanding the Ways Men and Women Mourn.* New York: Routledge, 2010.

Freud, S. "Mourning and Melancholia." In *The Standard Edition of the Complete Psychological Works of Sigmund Freud,* Vol. 14, edited and translated by James Strachey (pp. 243–58). London: Hogarth Press, 1957/1917.

Klass, D., P. R. Silverman, and S. L. Nickman (eds.). *Continuing Bonds: New Understandings of Grief.* Philadelphia: Taylor & Francis, 1996.

Neimeyer, R. A. (ed.). *Meaning Reconstruction and the Experience of Loss.* Washington, DC: American Psychological Association, 2001.

Stroebe, M. and H. Schut. "The Dual Process Model of Coping with Bereavement: Rationale and Description." *Death Studies,* 23(3) (1999): 197–224.

Stroebe, M., H. Schut, and K. Boerner. "Continuing Bonds in Adaptation to Bereavement: Toward Theoretical Integration." *Clinical Psychology Review,* 30 (2010): 259–68.

Worden, J. W. *Grief Counseling and Grief Therapy: A Handbook for the Mental Health Practitioner,* 4th edition. New York: Springer Publishing Company, 2009.

BIOETHICS

Bioethics deals with questions of the "rightness" and "wrongness" of conduct in medicine and the life sciences, and is especially pertinent to a range of end-of-life issues, including adjudications over the "right to die." It can be viewed in a technical sense primarily as an academic subdiscipline that arises from ethics, a major branch of philosophy, and is predominantly practiced by those who have basic philosophical training and are seen as engaging in a type of applied philosophy. Widespread bioethical education means that most modern health care providers are imbued with the principles of bioethics. Most societies are becoming more diverse and multicultural, and no single religious tradition can be relied upon for the regulation of conduct. Appeal is thus made instead to consensus guidelines (public statements formulated by medical experts on particular aspects of medical knowledge), law, and a new secular bioethics.

There is a potentially confusing interplay between the concepts of ethics and morality that philosopher Ronald Dworkin helps clarify: ethical judgments are about what individuals do to live well in their own lives, and moral judgments concern how we should treat other people. Medicine has for centuries generated codes of conduct based on the Hippocratic tradition, thus constructing its own moral milieu.

Bioethics as a Conversation Space

Ethics and bioethics can also be seen as a space for conversation and exchange between the professions and academic traditions engaged in the life sciences, together with the broader community. Everyone has a stake not only in what medicine and science do, but also in why and which conduct is permitted. In this sense, it is a multidisciplinary space, where all scholarly perspectives have a contribution to make, especially law, theology, and philosophy, and now more prominently, sociology.

Public engagement is also necessary, as external scrutiny of the otherwise closed world of science is one of the main ways through which conduct is regulated. In this respect, bioethics is akin to politics, and in a democracy derives its authority from public scrutiny.

Bioethics can therefore be seen as both a discipline, perhaps more of an interdisciplinary endeavor, and a public forum. It deals with the "interstitial" space between academic domains and the public or "laity" who are uninitiated in the technical or academic sense, but offer the perspective of the "man on the Clapham omnibus" of the English common law tradition, or jury member; where common sense and nonexpert input are both valued and potentially decisive, and give authority to bioethical scrutiny. This is necessary because one cannot leave these matters up to the experts involved, as they are interested parties, and cannot stand back and offer unbiased deliberation and decision making. In other words, medicine and science cannot be left to self-regulate, their morality cannot solely arise intrinsically from practice, or be dependent on the good character and personal integrity of the practitioners involved.

Historical Considerations

The origins of the modern bioethics movement can be traced to the calamitous events and consequences of World War II, together with the subsequent spurt in medical progress from the 1940s onward. The Doctors' Trial at the Nuremberg Tribunal in August 1947 revealed the direct and enthusiastic involvement of doctors in grotesque medical experimentation, involuntary euthanasia, and other crimes against humanity committed by Nazi Germany. These gave rise to an international concern to ensure that such events could never be repeated. The Nuremberg Code laid down 10 points to govern future medical research, and thus began a large and sustained growth in research ethics. To this day, Human Research Ethics Committees (HRECs) and their resourcing have been a major part of bioethics growth. HRECs are also a source of authority and legitimization of research conduct. Bioethics is now composed of a broad front to scrutinize medicine from the outside and make it "accountable." Meanwhile, medical practitioners and their chief representative and regulatory bodies continue to defend the notion (and the best elements of its tradition) of the medical profession as a "liberal" independent self-governing profession, especially in countries that have British institutional histories. Incidentally, the social philosopher and political scientist Ralf Dahrendorf (1929–2009), held that it was the absence of this professional independence that left the German medical world vulnerable to subversion.

Bioethics and Death

Medical and biological progress means that bioethics is predominantly concerned with matters pertaining to the beginning and end of life. All countries are struggling to respond to the health and social needs of an aging population, particularly with regard to chronic disease journeys and death preparation. Decision making with patients and families as death approaches often becomes constructed as an ethical issue or dilemma, with autonomy as the most valued attribute of good decision making. In fact, death is not automatically a priori (intrinsically or self-evidently) an ethical issue, and often the choices are limited. Bioethics makes a significant contribution to analysis and arbitration in end-of-life issues, but is not equipped to help people deal with the realities of finitude and the trials of dying. The issue of whether individuals can have assistance to die (voluntary euthanasia, physician-assisted suicide, and assisted suicide) preoccupies contemporary debate on death-related issues in most countries, and hence is a common subject for bioethical scrutiny. Bioethics grapples frequently with these issues, and provides a space within which heated debate can find structure and fair process. Narrative ethics and sociology also give valuable channels for the expression of patient and family voices.

Michael Ashby

See also: Definitions of Death; Euthanasia; Physician-Assisted Suicide.

Further Reading

Ashby, M.A. "The Futility of Futility: Death Causation Is the 'Elephant in the Room' in Discussions about Limitation of Medical Treatment." *Journal of Bioethical Inquiry,* 8(2) (2011): 151–54.

Beauchamp, T. L. and J. F. Childress. *Principles of Biomedical Ethics.*, 5th edition. New York: Oxford University Press, 2001.
Dworkin, R. *Justice for Hedgehogs.* Cambridge, MA: Belknap, Harvard University Press, 2011.
Jonsen, A. R. *A Short History of Medical Ethics.* New York: Oxford University Press, 2000.
Singer, P. (ed.). *A Companion to Ethics.* Oxford: Blackwell, 1991.
Steinbock, B. (ed.). *The Oxford Handbook of Bioethics.* Oxford and New York: Oxford University Press.

BODY DISPOSAL

The need to properly dispose of a dead body has been a feature of human society for millennia. The most common forms of disposal are burial and cremation (see **Burial; Cremation**). While burial usually involves interring the remains in soil, that is, in a grave in a cemetery or churchyard, the term can also refer to any method used to remove the dead body from sight. In earlier times, this may have involved placing the body in a cave or underground burial barrow designed for the purpose. In ancient societies, bodies, especially those of important members of society, might be buried in flamboyant tombs—the most famous of which are the pyramids of ancient Egypt. Other notable forms of burial are bodies interred in catacombs found particularly in Italy but also in other countries in Europe and South America. Catacombs are narrow underground tunnels with built-in niches or shelves where the bodies are placed (see also **Charnel Houses**). The most famous catacombs are located in Rome, where they were introduced around the second century and are thought to have been a response to the shortage of land and, possibly, as a place where persecuted Christians could bury their dead in secret. In Europe in the Middle Ages, and up until the mid-19th century, bodies might also be buried under the floorboards of Christian churches and in crypts designed for the purpose. It was believed at the time that the closer to the altar a person was buried, the closer they were to God, and thus to a place in heaven. Needless to say, this form of burial was usually reserved for the wealthy and influential.

Contrary to popular belief, cremation is an ancient form of bodily disposal that has been used across the world for the last 20,000 years. Cremation uses heat to dispose of the corpses of the dead. In some cultures and religious traditions, this is achieved by placing the body on a pyre (a flammable heap of wood and other materials) and setting fire to it. In contemporary Western societies, cremation uses technology to burn the body in a furnace powered by gas or electricity and takes place in a building designed for the purpose—a crematorium. As a form of disposal, cremation was outlawed for centuries in Christian societies, as it was believed to be important to keep the body whole if a person was to achieve resurrection in the next life. It was not until the beginning of the 20th century that the practice of cremation became legal. Rates of cremation differ dramatically between countries and this is largely dependent on religious beliefs and cultural traditions. For example, around 71 percent of disposals in the United Kingdom use cremation, compared to 24 percent in the United States.

More recently, other novel and innovative forms of bodily disposal are being introduced. For example, natural or woodland burial grounds have been created, which emphasize environmental factors, and usually involve the corpse being placed in a cardboard (or similar material) coffin with a tree planted in place of a headstone (see also **Green Burials**). It is also possible to donate your body to science or to von Hagens's Body Worlds for "plastination" (see **Body Worlds Exhibition**) to have it freeze dried or liquefied or, for a price, to have cremated ashes fired into space (see also **Cremains**).

Glennys Howarth

BODY WORLDS EXHIBITION

Body Worlds is a rather controversial traveling exhibition of human bodies that have been preserved using the technique of "plastination." The exhibition was created and is owned by the German anatomist Gunther von Hagens. He was also the developer of plastination, which is a process whereby the water and fats in the dead body are removed and replaced by plastics. The result is a body or a body part that does not smell, will not decay, and will also retain most of its original properties. The purpose of the exhibition is stated as the desire to educate people about the workings of the human body and so to help them gain better awareness of healthy life choices. While the makeup of the exhibitions vary, they usually entail the display of around 25 full-body plastinates and hundreds of organs or organ systems displayed in glass cases. The full-body exhibits are commonly shown in positions that demonstrate the workings of particular organs or systems within the body; for example, a pregnant woman whose womb is exposed to reveal her unborn child. Other exhibits feature diseased organs alongside healthy organs to show the impact of unhealthy practices; for example, a liver with cirrhosis or the lungs of a smoker.

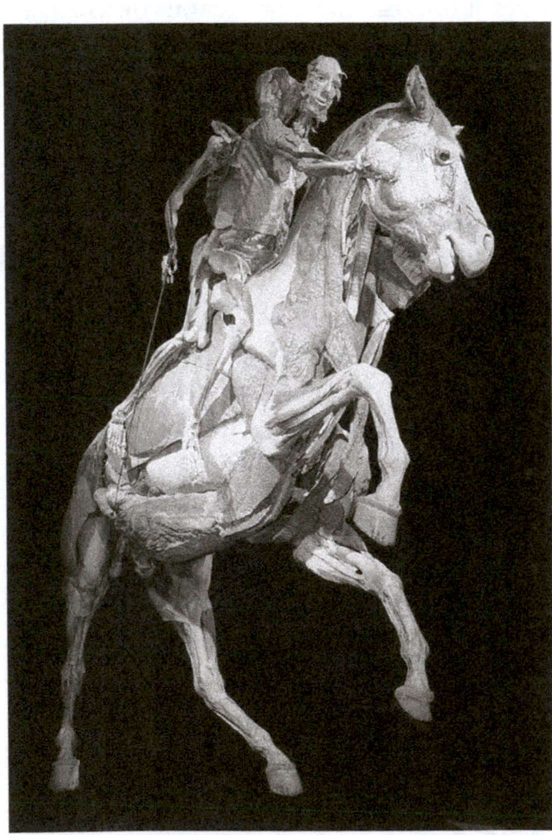

Horse and rider, preserved through plastination, on display during Gunther von Hagens's exhibition, Body Worlds & The Mirror of Time. (Rune Hellestad/Corbis)

Body Worlds has been visited by over 30 million people around the world and was first presented in Tokyo in 1995. It subsequently traveled to numerous venues in North America, Europe, and Asia. Body Worlds has always been at pains to state that the bodies used for plastination are acquired via a body donation program whereby individuals believe that their bodies may be useful after death. The success of Body Worlds has led to a number of other organizations producing their own exhibitions of plastinated bodies using cadavers donated to medical science, or more controversially, unclaimed bodies from countries such as China.

The source of bodies for plastination is a major concern and legislation has been proposed and enacted in numerous countries to guard against the importation of bodies for exhibition that were acquired without due regard for the ethical practices surrounding informed consent (see **Informed Consent**). The difficulty in relying on such legislation is the almost impossible task of proving that bodies were donated in full knowledge of how they might be used in the exhibition. One factor that exacerbates this problem is that in order to retain the privacy and anonymity of donors, von Hagens refuses to link the plastinated bodies with the donor's documentation. While this could be argued to be laudable, it merely adds fuel to those who challenge the legal source of the bodies.

The ethical issues associated with whether the donor gave fully informed consent are unlikely to be resolved in the near future. These exhibitions, however, are also subject to other criticisms. Religious groups have argued that the display of human remains is objectionable and runs counter to the reverence that should be shown for the human body. Some have gone as far as to claim that the display of human bodies for commercial gain can be compared to displays of pornography. Indeed, von Hagens's 2009 exhibit of a plastinated couple having sex was received in many quarters with horror and disgust. In the United Kingdom, the Bishop of Manchester launched a campaign against the opening of Body Worlds in the city, arguing that the exhibitors were essentially "body snatchers" (see **Grave Robbing**) and were depriving medical science of bodies and organs that could be used in transplant surgery to save lives. The Bishop was also responsible for a petition to the U.K. government demanding a review of the law that allowed traveling exhibitions of human corpses. Concerns have also been raised about the educational benefit of the exhibition and the potential for distress that might be caused to children who view the exhibits. So, while some schools are keen to take their students to the exhibition, others, particularly in the United States and the United Kingdom, have decided against such field trips.

A further challenge to the exhibition was raised by Megan Stern who argued that the displays perpetuated gender stereotypes. She pointed to the fact that male plastinates tended to be shown in active roles, while females where displayed in passive roles emphasizing beauty, grace, or reproductive systems.

Glennys Howarth

Further Reading

Stern, Megan. "Shiny, Happy People: 'Body Worlds' and the Commodification of Health." *Radical Philosophy,* 118 (March/April) (2003): 2–6.

Walter, Tony. "Body Worlds: Clinical Detachment and Anatomical Awe." *Sociology of Health and Illness,* 26(4) (2004): 464–88.

BUDDHISM

The human encounter with death plays a fundamental role in the beginning of Buddhism. Awareness of death is one of the four sights—an old man, a sick man, a corpse, and a wandering ascetic—that convinced Siddhartha Gautama to renounce his life of comfort and pleasure and set forth in search of liberation from *samsara,* the endless cycle of birth and death. As recorded in the Pali canon (the scriptures of the Theravada school), Prince Siddhartha declares that it was his acceptance of the inevitability of his own death that proved determinative in his decision to renounce his wealth and position as heir to the throne. That Siddhartha's quest for awakening is essentially a quest for a solution to the cycle of endless death (and rebirth) is seen also in the fact that one of the definitions of *nirvana,* the soteriological goal of early Indian Buddhism, is "the deathless state." Death, therefore, takes center stage in the origins of Buddhism, and as it grew into a world religion, the tradition developed a number of teachings and practices on death, offered various death rituals and services within its specific host cultures, and formulated ethical perspectives on issues such as suicide and euthanasia.

Contemplative practices on death and dying play an important role in all three of the main Buddhist traditions: Theravada, Mahayana, and Vajrayana. The general purpose of these various practices is to remind practitioners, both monastics and lay, of the "three marks of existence"—suffering, impermanence, and no-self—and of the urgency of striving for liberation. A focus on two specific traditions—Theravada Buddhism and Tibetan Buddhism—proves illustrative. The foundation of Theravadin practices comes from the *Satipatthana Sutta* or *The Foundations of Mindfulness,* one of the most well-known suttas (discourses of the Buddha) in the Pali canon, in which the Buddha instructs a group of *bhikkhus* to compare their own body with that of a decaying corpse found in a charnel ground. Building on this, *The Visuddhimagga* or *Path of Purification,* the authoritative commentary on meditation in Theravada Buddhism written by the fifth-century monk, Buddhaghosa, contains two forms of death contemplations. One is the *asubha-bhavana* or "meditation on the foulness of the body," which includes a detailed visualization of a corpse undergoing various stages of decay, and the reflection that the same process will inevitably inflict one's own body. The other is the *marana-sati* or "(eightfold) mindful contemplation on death," which evokes a realization on the inevitability of one's own death. Influential Theravadin monks such as the 20th-century Thai forest reformer Ajahn Mun and his student Ajahn Chah have continued this emphasis on death meditations by encouraging practitioners to visit charnel grounds and cemeteries, and one often finds human skeletons in the meditation halls of Thai forest monasteries.

Tibetan Buddhism is also a rich resource for Buddhist teachings and practices on death. In addition to death contemplations designed to motivate practitioners to fully utilize the auspiciousness of one's "precious human rebirth" toward liberation, the tradition offers a number of practices designed to work directly with the actual death process, which is considered an extremely potent opportunity for spiritual awakening. The most well-known of the former category comes from the Lam-Rim (gradual stages of the path) tradition and is called "the nine-round meditation on death." It consists of three main contemplations: (1) death is certain, (2) the time of death is uncertain, and (3) the only thing that will help us at the time of death is our state of mind.

Examples of the second category are found within the bardo literature, which contains a number of practices that familiarize the practitioner with the death process so that one will be able to gain control and harness its spiritual potency. The most prominent of the bardo texts is *The Liberation through Hearing in the Intermediate State,* known in the West as *The Tibetan Book of the Dead.* The highest aim of the bardo practices is to recognize the "Clear Light Mind" that manifests in the bardo state, and thereby gain liberation; they are also commonly used to guide the deceased through the intermediate bardo state and secure a good rebirth. Mention should also be made of *phowa,* an advanced practice that aims at the transference of consciousness, either to a Buddha realm or a better rebirth at death.

As Buddhism traveled across Asia, it also developed a number of distinct funeral ceremonies and death rituals in dialogue with the indigenous death practices and beliefs of its various different host cultures (Stone and Walter, 2008; Gouin, 2010). In Japan, for example, by the seventh century, Buddhist rituals had become established as the preeminent methods for consoling what were believed to be the lingering spirits of the dead. A popular contemporary Japanese Buddhist death ritual is *mizuko kuyo,* a memorial rite dedicated to a fetus lost through miscarriage, stillbirth, and abortion, which centers on the Mahayana bodhisattva *Jizo,* who is believed to protect children. Jeff Wilson (2009) has traced the American adaptation of the "water-baby ceremony," showing how a ritual that functions primarily in Japan as a shame based-practice that aims to placate the potentially wrathful fetal spirit, has been reconstituted in American Zen communities as an affirmation of female agency focused on the spiritual healing of the grieving mother.

Within the field of Buddhist ethics, there has been significant reflection on death-related issues, such as suicide and euthanasia (Harvey, 2000). With rare exception, suicide is seen as an essentially negative, futile act that would generate bad karma and lead to more future suffering in one's next rebirth. However, in line with Buddhist understandings of karma, the intentionality behind the action is also important. For example, the self-immolation of Vietnamese monks in protest against the oppression of Buddhists by the United States-backed regime of Catholic dictator Ngo Dinh Diem, and more recently of Tibetan monks and nuns protesting the Chinese occupation of Tibet, have been interpreted, drawing on Mahayana literature, as great acts of compassion and self-sacrifice for the benefit of other sentient beings.

The ongoing dialogue between Buddhism and death and dying can also be seen in the increasing role the tradition is playing in hospice care in the West. In 1987, the Hartford Street Zen, whose founding member Soto Zen priest Issan Dorsey died from AIDS in 1990, opened the Maitri Hospice Center to care for those dying from the disease. It was the first Buddhist hospice in the United States. A number of Buddhist organizations such as the Zen Hospice Project in San Francisco, California, have since developed Buddhist end-of-life care programs and chaplaincy training. Buddhism has also significantly influenced the nonsectarian death awareness or conscious dying movement (Levine and Levine, 1989).

Ann Gleig

See also: Death Awareness Movement; Reincarnation.

Further Reading

Buddhist Hospice Dictionary: http://www.buddhanet.net/hospices.htm

Garces-Foley, K. "Buddhism, Hospice, and the American Way of Dying." *Review of Religious Research,* (44)4 (2003): 341–53.

Gouin, Margaret. *Tibetan Rituals of Death: Buddhist Funerary Practices.* London: Routledge, 2010.

Halifax, J. *Being with Dying.* Boston: Shambhala, 2009.

Harvey, P. *An Introduction to Buddhist Ethics: Foundations, Values and Issues.* Cambridge: Cambridge University Press, 2000.

Levine, S. and O. Levine. *Who Dies? An Investigation of Conscious Living and Conscious Dying.* New York City: Anchor, 1989.

Perreira, T. R. "'Die Before You Die': Death Meditation as Spiritual Technology of the Self in Islam and Buddhism." *The Muslim World,* (100)2–3 (2010): 247–67.

Sogyal, Rinpoche. *The Tibetan Book of Living and Dying.* San Francisco: Harper San Francisco, 1984.

Stone, J. and M. N. Walter (eds.). *Death and the Afterlife in Japanese Buddhism.* Honolulu: University of Hawaii Press, 2008.

Wilson, Jeff. "The Great Matter of Life and Death: Death and Dying Practices in American Buddhism." In *Religion, Death and Dying,* Vol. 3, edited by Lucy Bregman (pp. 149–70). Westport, CT: Praeger, 2009.

Wilson, Jeff. *Mourning the Unborn Dead: A Buddhist Ritual Comes to America.* Oxford: Oxford University Press, 2009.

BURIAL

The rites and rituals concerning final disposition of the body help maintain a positive relationship with ancestral spirits, reaffirm social solidarity, and restore group structures that are severed by death. In some cultures and religions, an individual is considered to be composed of several elements (body and soul), and each element may have a different fate after death. The actual disposal of the body, be it burial, cremation, or decomposition, is believed to divide these elements. For example, in India, when a son breaks the skull of his father on the funeral pyre (a combustible pile for burning a corpse), he is demonstrating that the body no longer has any value—because it is worn out—but the soul lives on (see **Hinduism**).

Earth burial as a method of final bodily disposition is by far the most widely used in the United States. It is used in approximately 65.3 percent of the 2.43 million American deaths annually. Almost without exception, earth burial takes place within established cemeteries. In some instances, earth burial can take place outside of a cemetery if the landowner where the interment is to be made, and the health officer of jurisdiction, grant their permission. In 1997, comedian and actor Bill Cosby acquired permission from local authorities to bury his son Ennis on the grounds of his estate. By law, cemeteries have the right to establish reasonable rules and regulations to be observed by those arranging for burial in them. A person does not purchase property within a cemetery, but rather purchases the "right to interment" in a specific location within that cemetery. Most cemeteries require that the casket or coffin be placed into some kind of outer receptacle or burial vault. The cemetery will also control how the grave can be marked with monuments or grave markers.

The length of time for final decomposition of the body will vary depending upon the condition of the soil or ground (mummies buried in the sands of Egypt never decompose), while an adult body that has not been embalmed but is buried six-feet deep in ordinary soil, without a coffin, would usually take between 10 and 12 years to decompose to a skeleton.

Cross-Cultural Comparisons

Some societies keep corpses in or near the home of the deceased. The Yoruba of Nigeria, for example, dig the grave in the room of the deceased. In Uganda, a Lugbara male is buried in the center of the floor of his first wife's hut. The Swazi of Africa bury a woman on the outskirts of her husband's home.

To assure that the spirit will be reborn, some societies go to great lengths. For example, the Dunsun of northern Borneo kill animals to accompany the deceased on the trip to the land of the dead. The Ulithi in Micronesia place a loincloth and a ginger-like plant in the right arm of the deceased so that gifts can be presented to the custodian at the entrance of the other world. For the Zinacantecos of Mexico, a chicken head is put into a bowl of broth beside the head of the corpse. The chicken purportedly leads the "inner soul" of the deceased. A black dog then carries the "soul" across the river.

The Russian Orthodox community in Oregon shares this concern for the rebirth of the spirit and constructs the grave site to accommodate that rebirth. All the graves are lined up facing east, with an Orthodox cross at the foot of each grave. At the Second Coming, the dead will rise from the grave and stand next to the cross, facing east, toward Christ.

As with the Zinacantecos of Mexico, a chicken is used in the burial rites of the Yoruba in southwestern Nigeria. A man with a live chicken precedes the carrier of the corpse, plucking out feathers and leaving them along the trail for the soul of the deceased to follow back to town. Upon reaching the town gate, the chicken is killed by striking its head against the ground. The blood and feathers are then placed into the grave so that others will not die. A second chicken is killed, and its blood is put into the grave so that the soul of the deceased will not bother the surviving relatives.

In the old days of the Wild West in the United States, one was buried "6 feet under with his boots on." It is true that graves were 6 feet deep in earlier periods of U.S. history, but efficiency (and perhaps agnosticism regarding the belief in ghosts) dictates that today graves are less than 6 feet deep—typically around 4½ feet with 18 inches of soil above the top of the casket/vault. With the sealed, heavier caskets of today—often placed within a steel or concrete vault—it is not necessary to place the body so deep in the ground, as was the case with the unsealed pine box of an earlier period.

The Kalingas of the Philippines bury adults in graves 6 feet deep and 3 feet wide. The Mardudjara aboriginal inhabitants of Australia dig a rectangular hole about 3 feet deep, line the bottom with leafy bushes and small logs, and then place the body inside it. Similarly, the Semai of Malaya dig the grave 2–3 feet deep.

Alternatives to the Typical Earth Burial

A less common form of burial is burial at sea or water burial. This form of burial can involve the submerging of the entire body, weighted down so as to prevent the body from resurfacing. However, more commonly, burial at sea involves the scattering of cremated remains over fresh or salt water.

Although earth burial is the dominant practice in the United States, for Protestants, Roman Catholics, Jews, and Muslims, the number of cremations has increased dramatically in the last two decades. During the past two decades, the number of cremations has more than doubled from approximately 20 percent to 40 percent currently. In the Western states of Nevada, Oregon, Washington, Hawaii, and Arizona, more than 60 percent of all deaths involve cremation (see also **Cremation**).

Many people choose to memorialize the site of disposition because they find comfort in knowing that there is a particular place to visit when they wish to remember and feel close to the person they have lost, regardless of whether the remains are in fact located at that particular place.

Earth burial is always more expensive than cremation and would be the most expensive form of bodily disposition; the typical cost of a simple "no-frills" cremation is approximately 40 percent of the cost of the traditional funeral service with burial. The range of burial plots (which could be used for traditional earth burial or cremated remains) range in price from $50 in a country church grave yard to $5,000 in an urban cemetery. More expensive alternatives include mausolea and outdoor above-ground crypts (buildings or wall for above-ground accommodation of a casket). A private family mausoleum can cost in excess of $1 million in an elite urban cemetery (such as the Mars Mausoleum in Lakewood Cemetery in Minneapolis for the founder of the Mars Candy Company).

Some have suggested that there is a need for alternatives to traditional earth burial because of a lack of space in urban areas. In some city cemeteries, grave plots are rented for a definite period of time (a practice found in Chicago, New Orleans, New York, and other large urban areas where burial space is at a premium). When the lease expires on these plots, if the family does not renew the lease, bodies are often "dug down" and new burials are put on top of the old ones or they are destroyed and/or reburied in another unmarked location in a land fill.

San Francisco between 1920 and 1940 moved its major cemetery to Colma, California. It did so because the city passed an ordinance in 1900, which outlawed the construction of any further cemeteries within the city (chiefly due to increased property values which made the cost of using city land for cemeteries prohibitive). The city then passed another ordinance in 1912 evicting all existing cemeteries from city limits. Colma is a small in town in San Mateo Country, California, at the northern end of the San Francisco Peninsula in the San Francisco Bay Area. The town was founded as a necropolis in 1924. With most of the town dedicated to cemeteries, the population of the dead outnumbers the living by more than a thousand to one. At the 2010 census, the population was 1,792. This has led to it being called "the city of the silent." It also has provided the basis to the town's humorous motto: "It's great to be alive in Colma."

However, there is a current trend for some people to opt for a less expensive earth burial known as Green Graveyards as a natural and ecologically friendly form of bodily disposal (see **Green Burials**). Ramsey Creek Cemetery of Westminster, South Carolina, is the nation's first contemporary green graveyard. The dead are buried in biodegradable caskets and placed in graves that are mounds of earth dotted with wildflowers and marked with flat stones engraved with the names of the dead. The costs associated with green graveyards are considerably lower than that of traditional lawn cemeteries because they avoid the need to purchase a vault or grave liner and maintenance of the graveyard does not involve the costs of mowing and fertilizing lawns.

Michael R. Leming

See also: Body Disposal.

Further Reading

Elvig, P. "Burial Laws." In *Encyclopedia of Death and the Human Experience,* edited by Clifton D. Bryant and Dennis L. Peck (pp. 127–30). Thousand Oaks, CA: Sage, 2009.

Iserson, K.V. *Death to Dust: What Happens to Dead Bodies?* Tucson, AZ: Galen Press, 2001.

Metcalf, P. and R. Huntington. *Celebrations of Death: The Anthropology of Mortuary Ritual.* Cambridge: Cambridge University Press, 1991.

Parker Pearson, M. *The Archaeology of Death and Burial.* London: Stroud, 1999.

Stewart, D.J. "Burial at Sea: Separating and Placing the Dead during the Age of Sail." *Mortality,* 10(4) (2005): 276–85.

Stewart, D.J. "Burial at Sea." In *Encyclopedia of Death and the Human Experience,* edited by Clifton D. Bryant and Dennis L. Peck (pp. 123–25). Thousand Oaks, CA: Sage, 2009.

C

CADAVERS

Cadavers, also known as corpses, remains, or "stiffs," are dead human bodies most often intended for medical dissection and anatomical study. Prior to the Renaissance, the preeminent anatomist Claudius Galen (ca. AD 130–210) based his observations about the human body on animal dissections. To this day, gems of anatomical study are the accurate human body illustrations of Andrea Vessalius and Leonardo da Vinci.

In the 19th century, the growth of medical science led to a greater demand for cadavers. Fresh bodies were sought for dissection and this was often met by body snatchers, grave robbers who sold bodies at handsome fees (see also **Grave Robbing**). Because of the lucrative but illicit trafficking in stealing fresh corpses from graves and mortuaries (and the public outcry following the trial of William Burke and William Hare for murdering people in order to sell their corpses), the Anatomy Act of 1832 was passed in Great Britain, permitting the legal acquisition by medical schools of unclaimed bodies from prisons, hospitals and workhouses.

Organ donation, an organ or biological tissue gifted to a living recipient in need of a transplantation, may be obtained from a living or newly dead person (see **Organ Donation/Transplantation**). Embalming, the process of preserving a human body to ensure a better presentation during funerals or wakes, delays the decomposition (see **Embalming**). Currently, cadavers for medical education and research are embalmed body donations, anatomical gifts arranged prior to death. Many medical schools end the dissection experience with a memorial service celebrating the lives of the body donors.

Though used to introduce the history of medicine, Rembrandt's "Anatomy Lesson of Dr. Nicolaes Tulp" (1632), introduces the luxury of aesthetic distance and invites analysis of the concepts of detached concern and medical gaze as it captures a variety of coping concerns among medical students. This painting is not only appropriate for stimulating reflective practice, it is also is an example of a criminal, Aris Kindt, newly executed for the event of a public dissection.

Not only anatomists but also artists had a need to understand the inner workings of the human body. In *The Agony and the Ecstasy,* biographer-novelist Irving Stone chronicles Michelangelo's experience. The young artist's questions and concerns parallel almost exactly those of the medical student. While medical students often wonder about the personal lives of their cadavers and how they came to be body donors, Michelangelo wonders, "What had this unfortunate creature done that he should now, without his knowledge and consent, be mutilated." Stone adds, "His first feeling was one of pity for the dead man." While

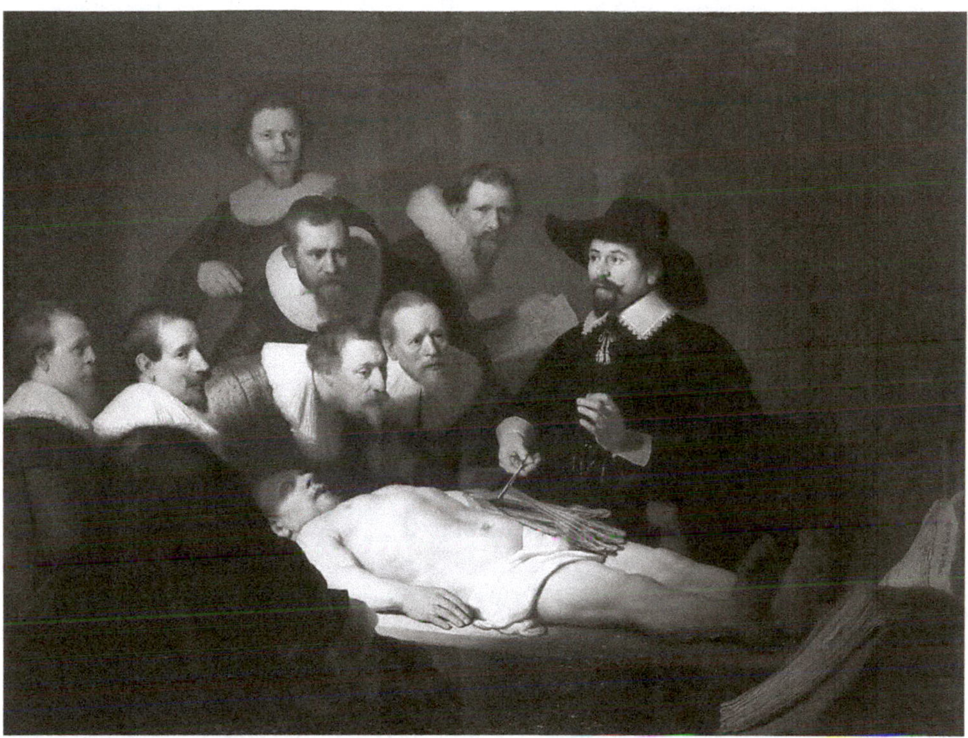

Rembrandt's *The Anatomy Lesson of Dr. Nicolaes Tulp*, 1632. (National Library of Medicine)

physicians are concerned that their license permits them to maim, desecrate, and violate another human being's body in the name of medicine, so Michangelo, too, questions whether he is "obsessed" and has the right to do such things in the name of sculpture. At one point, the effect of dissecting the human face is so ghastly that he must abandon the task. Eventually returning to it, he is "overcome with a sense of guilt" when he cracks open the skull. And when the medical students' self-doubt, discomfort, and horror evolve into fascination, excitement, and joy in the discovery of the intricate beauty of the human frame, so too does Michelangelo feel the thrill of his first look at the human brain and at holding a human heart in his hands: "As quickly as it had come, the fear departed. In its place came a sense of triumph. . . . He felt the happiness that arises out of knowledge, for now he knew about the most vital organ of the body, what it looked like, how it felt."

Simulated learning environments are becoming substitutes for cadaver dissection, but there is much debate as to whether viewing prosections (dissected parts of a cadaver) or interacting with computer-based modules is as effective in capturing the dimensions of the anatomy experience.

Sandra L. Bertman

See also: Autopsy; Body Worlds Exhibition.

Further Reading

Bertman, S. L. "From the Very First Patient to the Very Last: Soul Pain, Aesthetic Distance, and the Training of Physicians." In *Death and the Quest for Meaning,* edited by S. Strack (pp. 163–92). Northvale, NJ: Jason Aronson, 1977.

Bertman, S. L. *One Breath Apart: Facing Dissection.* Amityville, NY: Baywood, 2009.

Mahadevan, Vishi. "Dissection." In *The Oxford Companion to the Body,* edited by Colin Blakemore and Sheila Jennett (pp. 219–21). Oxford: Oxford University Press, 2001.

Stone, I. *The Agony and the Ecstasy.* Garden City, NY: Doubleday, 1961.

CANCER

Cancer is an umbrella term that refers to a group of diseases that are characterized by the proliferation of abnormal cells that invade and disrupt normal cell structures. Cancers are generally named after the body part in which the cancer is identified, so that, for example, a cancer in the breast is known as breast cancer. Cancer is the second leading cause of death in the United States, accounting for the estimated 580,350 people who are projected to die from it in 2013. Rates, as well as types, of cancer vary according to social and demographic characteristics. All age groups and sexes are affected by cancer, although most cases of cancer (about 77 percent) are diagnosed in adults aged 55 and upward. Cancer, nevertheless, is also the second leading cause of death in young people, accounting for approximately 12,500 children and adolescents who are diagnosed with it annually. Young people and adolescents are more likely to be diagnosed with leukemia (a cancer of the white blood cells) than other types of cancer. Among women, the most common form of cancer is breast cancer, while among men prostate cancer is the most commonly diagnosed malignancy. For both men and women, lung cancer has the highest rate of mortality.

Cancer is caused by a range of factors, both external (i.e., environmental) and internal (i.e., heredity). Environmental factors are estimated to account for between 75 and 80 percent of cancers, while hereditary factors are estimated to account for between 5 and 10 percent. The largest preventable cause of cancer is tobacco, which is estimated to account for more than 30 percent of all cancer deaths and for between 80 and 90 percent of deaths from lung cancer. Screening and early detection are essential in improving the chances of surviving cancer, which, with effective treatment, are greater now than they have ever been. Indeed, while cancer has often functioned as a metaphor for death, health care professionals and advocates of greater patient knowledge and empowerment have worked tirelessly to convey the message that cancer is not necessarily the death sentence it once was.

There are five major categories of cancer, including the following:

- Carcinoma: cancer that begins on the skin or the tissues that line the internal organs
- Sarcoma: cancer that begins in bone, cartilage, fat muscle, blood vessels, or some connective or supportive tissue
- Leukemia: cancer that starts in blood-forming tissue such as the bone marrow and causes large numbers of abnormal blood cells to be produced and enter the blood

- Lymphoma and myeloma: cancers that begin in the cells of the immune system
- Central nervous system cancers: cancers that begin in the tissues of the brain and spinal cord

What is clear from these distinctions is that the categories form a typology of the sorts of body tissues that give rise to the abnormality. The question as to how cancer develops may be elucidated by the following analogy. What should occur in the body is much like the replacements of goods on a grocery store shelf. When groceries are purchased by customers, the shelves are restocked with replacements. For the most part, this is an orderly process. So, too, when cells in the body progress through a cycle of development and senescence (growing older and dying), the process is orderly. It is when the cell is altered and produces changed (and abnormal) cells that cancer is said to occur. Often, one of the first questions from the person so affected is "has it spread?" And while the health care practitioner is also concerned about this, another question that may affect the response to the query about spread is also of consequence and that is the tumor grade. This question is of significance in that a low-grade tumor in which cells are well differentiated is deemed to be less aggressive, meaning it will grow more slowly, than one where the cells are poorly differentiated (a high-grade tumor) and growth will occur more rapidly. Cancer staging, on the other hand, takes into account the extent of the tumor, and whether there is lymph node involvement. The latter indicates the potential for spread through the lymphatic system from the initial site to other parts of the body and is known as metastasis. A sentinel lymph biopsy examines the lymph node to which cells from a tumor in a given site are most likely to spread.

Spread may be categorized as follows: in situ or restricted to the layer of cells containing the initial abnormality; localized or contained within a specific organ where the abnormality originated; regional, which indicates spread to nearby lymph nodes; and distant, which indicates spread to distant organs or lymph nodes or to the bone. Staging considers tumor grade as well as a number of other factors gleaned from physical examination, laboratory tests, imaging studies, and surgical and pathology reports. The latter include observations made during surgery at the operative site and, subsequently, of tissue specimens removed (biopsy) for pathological examination. Biopsies to obtain specimens for examination also occur using a needle to aspirate or withdraw tissue or fluid as well with other instruments to access different parts of the body.

Laboratory tests include the identification of abnormal or normal (in excess) substances found in body fluids. The normal substances may be present in higher quantity in response to the tumor. More than 20 tumor markers are now being used to detect tumors as well as to measure the progress of treatment. For example, prostate-specific antigen (PSA) is used to diagnose and to evaluate the success of treatment in prostate cancer.

There are a wide array of approaches to cancer treatment beyond radiation therapy and chemotherapy including angiogenesis inhibitors, biological therapies, bone marrow transplantation, cryosurgery, the use of lasers, photodynamic therapy, hormonal therapies, and targeted cancer therapies. The type of therapy used is dependent on the type of tumor, its location, and staging. Combinations of types of therapy may be used concurrently or sequentially. Again, the decision as to the best approach is dependent not only on the characteristics of the tumor but also of the host. That is, does the person with cancer have other debilitating diseases? Is the individual pregnant or someone who wants to maintain her fertility? What is the age of the individual? What does the individual want for herself? The decision as to the best therapy for a given individual needs to be made in consideration of the individual as well as the cancer.

The future of cancer therapies is likely to include an emphasis on more targeted therapies that destroy only the malignant cells and not those that are healthy. Both health care providers and patients need to consider the quality of life of the individual, both when receiving therapy and thereafter. An investigational drug promising an additional six months of life, of which five months necessitate hospital care for the therapy and its side effects, may not be deemed of value to all patients. For other individuals, the chance of remission, let alone cure, may be worth the duress of treatment no matter how onerous. Information as to what may be expected during, and from, treatment is essential to decision making. Some individuals may elect for complementary and alternative (CAM) therapies in concert with medical therapies or in lieu of those. The importance of rigorous investigation of any such therapies cannot be overstated if patients are to have access to data for informed decision making (see also **Informed Consent**).

Cancer is of concern worldwide. It is not a disease of resource-adequate nations alone but is observed in resource-limited nations as well. The causes of cancer include smoking, exposure to chemicals, radiation, and other carcinogens. The challenge is to reduce the exposure to known carcinogens and to share the research findings of cancer treatments, whatever their origin, so that incidence of cancer is reduced worldwide.

Inge B. Corless

Further Reading

Almeida, Craig, A. and Sheila A. Barry. *Cancer: Basic Science and Clinical Aspects.* Hoboken, NJ: Wiley-Blackwell, 2010.

Armstrong-Coster, Angela. *Living and Dying with Cancer.* Cambridge, UK: Cambridge University Press, 2004.

http://www.cancer.gov/cancertopics/cancerlibrary/what-is-cancer

Sontag, Susan. *Illness as Metaphor.* New York: Vintage Books, 1979.

CANNIBALISM

Cannibalism, also known as *anthropophagy,* is the act of eating parts of the human body, including, but not limited to, flesh, blood, and muscles. Reports of cannibalism exist throughout the world and are usually focused on groups of people whom the Western perspective considers "barbarians." Societies that practice cannibalism and cannibalism-related incidents are often viewed by social scientists in one of three ways: (1) as a way of satisfying mythical and overarching psychosexual fantasies and desires, (2) as an adaptation to hunger or other material deficiency, or (3) as part of the overall universal order and normative function in a society. Events and societies where cannibalism has been practiced have a number of similar traits: they are politically homogeneous and the local government is supreme; they have a history and culture of maternal dependency; there is a cultural history of oral aggression; there is a taboo against sexual intercourse; and there is a significant level of food stress, in particular, protein. There are a number of notable incidents in the last two centuries which indicate the existence of emergency cannibalism, such as the Donner Party of American pioneers in 1846 in Sierra Nevada and the crash of an F-227 airplane in the Andes Mountains of Argentina in 1972 carrying members of the Uruguayan Rugby Team. The majority of early accounts of alleged cannibals were based on an ethnocentric colonial viewpoint. This has made it difficult to definitively establish the cannibal ritual of the literal eating of the flesh and blood of a fellow human being. However, new research and accounts have established that ritual cannibalism probably occurred, and still occasionally occurs, in areas such as Papua New Guinea and Polynesia. Cannibalism also exists in cultures in the form of mythology such as witches, werewolves, and vampires consuming blood or human flesh for power and other nefarious purposes.

Andrea Malkin Brenner

Further Reading

Askenasy, Hans. *Cannibalism: From Sacrifice to Survival.* Amherst, NY: Prometheus Books, 1994.

CAPITAL PUNISHMENT

Capital punishment (often referred to interchangeably as the death penalty) has been practiced by all known societies at some point or other during the course of history. It has been used, and in some parts of the world (including the United States) continues to be used, for a variety of offenses. Taking a variety of forms (including hanging, gassing, burning, drowning, stoning, shooting, and beheading), capital punishment has been used for crimes including murder, rape, treason, and in medieval times was used against those accused of heresy and witchcraft. Even today, in some countries that practice it, the death penalty has been used for adultery, "apostasy," and as recently as June 2012, was used in Iran to execute four people accused of "enmity against God and corruption on earth."

While in the past the use of capital punishment was more widespread, today the overall global trend in terms of the number of executions and states that retain the death penalty on the statue books is generally a downward one. Figures from the human rights organization Amnesty International show that in 2012, 682 people were executed (in 21 countries) and 1,722 people were sentenced to death (in 58 countries). This compares with the 1,813 people who were executed (in 31 countries) and the 3,857 people who were sentenced to death (in 64 countries) just over a decade earlier in 1999. This decline is further indicated by figures

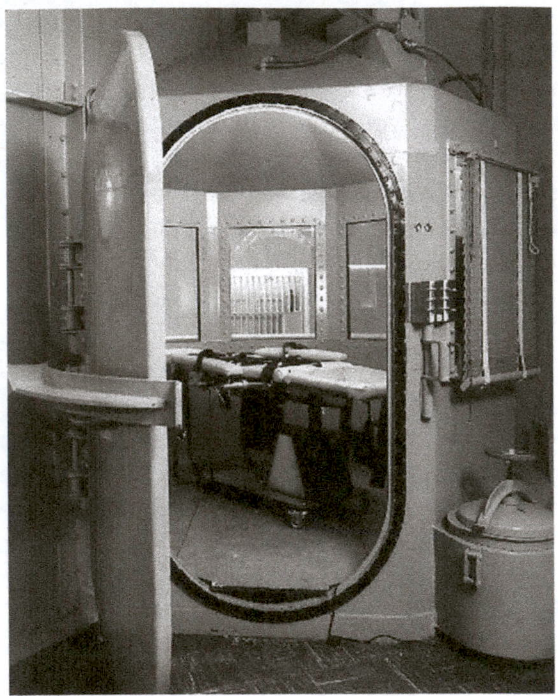

Lethal injection chamber used for executions at San Quentin State Prison in California. (California Department of Corrections)

which show that more than two-thirds of countries in the world have now abolished capital punishment, the most recent of which was Latvia in January 2012. As of December 31, 2012, 97 countries had formally abolished capital punishment for all offenses. This marks a significant increase on the 80 countries that had abolished capital punishment for all offenses some 10 years earlier in 2003 and the just 16 countries that had abolished it for all offenses in 1977.

Globally, the majority of executions in the world are concentrated in just five countries: China, Iran, Iraq, Saudi Arabia, and the United States. In China, information on the number of executions is not freely available and is considered a state secret. Since 2009, Amnesty International has stopped publishing estimates on the annual number of executions in China because of the lack of reliable data, though available information continues to indicate that China executes more people than the rest of the world combined. In the Middle East and North Africa, 99 percent of all executions are performed by just four states: Iran, Saudi Arabia, Iraq, and Yemen. In the Americas, the United States is the only country to continue to use capital punishment; it was abolished by Venezuela as early as 1863 and by Argentina as recently as 2008. In Western Europe, the move away from capital punishment in most countries had become well established during the second half of the 20th century. Since the fall of communism and the breakup of the Soviet Union, many Eastern European states have also become abolitionist, such as Poland, where capital punishment was abolished in 1997, and Estonia and Lithuania, where it was abolished in 1998.

In the Unites States, 43 people (in nine states) were executed in 2012 and the number of death sentences handed down (77) was the second lowest since 1976, when the U.S. Supreme Court reaffirmed the constitutionality of the death penalty. In April 2012, Connecticut became the 17th state to abolish capital punishment and in November of the same year California narrowly failed in a ballot initiative to abolish the death penalty. Among the nine states that performed capital punishment in 2012, Texas executed the most prisoners (15), followed by Arizona, Mississippi, and Oklahoma, each of whom executed six prisoners. The number of prisoners "on death row" (i.e., under sentence of death) in 2009 was 767,434. There have long been concerns expressed about the disproportionate number of African Americans and those from the poorest and most socially disadvantaged communities who continue to make up the ranks of those awaiting execution.

In the longer term, the gradual shift away from capital punishment in most Western societies can be seen as part of a wider process of social transformation occurring within Western European societies from the late 18th century onward. The emergence of political philosophies which championed individual human rights, challenges to the despotic authority and dominance of clerical rule (often underscored by the Old Testament injunction of "an eye for an eye"), and shifting sensibilities toward death and dying are all factors that have contributed to the demise of judicial killing as a form of punishment. Part of this shift is also attributable to changing views about crime and punishment itself, away from retributive forms of punishment designed to inflict maximum pain and suffering upon the perpetrator of crime (as both vengeance and as a deterrent to others), toward the "carceral society," replete with prisons and "correctional" facilities designed to not only deny criminals their liberty but remedy them of their criminal ways by subjecting them to new disciplinary regimens of power and surveillance. Where the death penalty was retained in these societies, the means of execution itself became more "humane," was increasingly performed behind "closed doors," and less as gruesome public spectacle. In France, for example, the introduction of the guillotine was considered a swifter, more merciful killing; while states in the United States that continue to use capital punishment do so through the use of electrocution and lethal injection, with only the victims, their families, and the prison staff in attendance.

Capital punishment is still a sharply divisive and controversial issue in the United States. Opinion poll data indicate that support for the death penalty has fallen since the mid-1990s (when it peaked at 80 percent), and has stabilized in the second decade of the 21st century around the low to mid-60s. In 2012, 63 percent of the population said they were in favor of capital punishment. Supporters claim that it serves as the ultimate deterrence against capital crimes, while those opposed to it claim it is ethically wrong, financially costly, and provides no safeguards against evidence that may subsequently come to light proving the innocence of those sentenced to death.

Michael Brennan

See also: Homicide.

Further Reading

Amnesty International. *Death Sentences and Executions 2012*. London: Amnesty International Publications, 2013. http://www.amnesty.org.uk/uploads/documents/doc_23136.pdf

Garland, David, Randell McGowen, and Michael Meranze (eds.). *America's Death Penalty: Between Past and Present*. New York: New York University Press, 2011.

Hood, Roger and Carolyn Hoyle. *The Death Penalty: A Worldwide Perspective*, 4th edition. Oxford and New York: Oxford University Press, 2008.

Prisoners under Sentence of Death. U.S Census Bureau, Statistical Abstract of the United States: 2012. http://www.census.gov/compendia/statab/2012/tables/12s0351.pdf
Sarat, Austin and Jürgen Martschukat (eds.). *Is the Death Penalty Dying? European and American Perspectives.* Cambridge: Cambridge University Press, 2011.

CARDIOVASCULAR DISEASE

Cardiovascular disease refers to a class of diseases that involve the heart or blood vessels (arteries and veins), often involving narrowed or blocked blood vessels that can lead to chest pain (angina), heart attack (myocardial infarction), or stroke. Other conditions affecting the heart muscle, valves, and beating rhythm are also considered forms of cardiovascular disease. The term "cardiovascular disease" is commonly used interchangeably with "heart disease." Although the term technically refers to any disease affecting the cardiovascular system, it is also used specifically to refer to heart problems resulting from atherosclerosis (hardening of the arteries).

Atherosclerosis is a condition that develops when plaque builds up on the walls of the arteries, making them more rigid, narrow, and harder for blood to flow through. If a blood clot forms near a narrowed artery, it can block or dramatically restrict the flow of blood, leading to a heart attack or stroke. Cardiovascular disease is treated medically by cardiologists, vascular surgeons, neurologists, thoracic surgeons, and interventional radiologists.

Cardiovascular diseases include the following:

- Aneurysm
- Angina
- Arrhythmia
- Atherosclerosis
- Cerebrovascular accident (stroke)
- Cerebrovascular disease
- Congestive heart failure
- Coronary artery disease
- Heart valve problems (stenosis, regurgitation, and prolapse)
- Myocardial infarction (heart attack)
- Peripheral vascular disease

Risk Factors

The primary risk factors for cardiovascular disease can be divided into two main groups:

1. **Uncontrollable risk factors**
    - Family history of heart disease
    - Male sex
    - Older age
    - Post-menopausal
    - Race/ethnicity: African Americans, American Indians, and Mexican Americans have higher risks

2. **Controllable risk factors**
    - Unregulated diabetes
    - A diet high in fat, low in fiber, and whole grains, and fewer than five portions of fruits and vegetables daily
    - Elevated levels of stress, anger, and anxiety
    - LDL or "bad" cholesterol levels exceeding 160 mg/dL
    - Hypertension (high blood pressure) exceeding 139/89 mmHg
    - Low HDL or "good" cholesterol levels less than 40 mg/dL for men or 50 mg/dL for women
    - Obesity: body mass index (BMI) exceeding 30.0
    - Physical Inactivity: less than 30 minutes of vigorous activity most days of the week
    - Smoking

Morbidity and Mortality

Cardiovascular disease is the leading cause of death in the United States. Over 80,000,000 adults in the United States have some form of cardiovascular disease. One in every three deaths is from heart disease and stroke, which equals approximately 2,200 deaths per day. Problems relating to cardiovascular disease are also the leading cause of disability, preventing people from working and enjoying family and recreational activities. According to the American Heart Association, some progress is being made on reducing death rates from cardiovascular disease: the death rate from heart diseases declined 27.8 percent from 1997 to 2007, while the death rate from stroke rate fell 44.8 percent. However, in the same time period, the total number of inpatient cardiovascular operations and procedures increased 27 percent. These procedures have helped extend the average age of death from cardiovascular disease to 75 years, but this is still well below the 2010 average life expectancy of 78.3 years in the United States. In 2010, heart disease and stroke hospitalizations cost the United States more than $444 billion in health care expenses and lost productivity, far exceeding any other condition (including cancer), according to the Centers for Disease Control and Prevention. These problems are not unique to the United States; cardiovascular disease is the leading cause of death and disability in the world. Although a large proportion of cardiovascular disease is preventable, it continues to increase because preventative measures are inadequate.

Treatment Options

By the time heart problems and the symptoms of cardiovascular disease are identified, the underlying cause (atherosclerosis) is often quite advanced, having progressed undetected for considerable time. Thus, there is an increased emphasis on preventing atherosclerosis by modifying controllable risk factors, such as diet, physical activity level, and avoidance of smoking. Cardiovascular disease, unlike many other chronic medical conditions, is treatable and sometimes reversible, even after a prolonged period of disease. Treatment for cardiovascular disease involves an emphasis on diet, exercise, and reducing stress. The key focus in recent years has been largely on prevention, promotion of health education, and raising of awareness so that people can make better lifestyle choices.

Tim Thornton

See also: Alcohol; Cancer; Disease; Epidemiology; Health Promotion; Tobacco.

Further Reading

http://www.cdc.gov/heartdisease/
http://www.heart.org/HEARTORG/
http://www.mayoclinic.com/health/heart-disease/DS01120
http://www.who.int/cardiovascular_diseases/en/

CATHOLICISM

Catholic, a word meaning *universal,* is one of the four "marks" or essential characteristics of the church listed in the Nicene Creed. By the end of the first century, the term "Catholic Church" began to name institutional Christianity in recognition of its mission to all peoples.

Catholics believe that Jesus appointed St. Peter as the church's foundation and that his leadership continues with the Bishops of Rome. In the seventh century, the Bishop of Rome came to be called Pope (from the Latin *papas,* Greek πάππας—a child's term for father). Today, the Pope serves as worldwide leader of the Catholic Church. Catholics ground their beliefs in Biblical Scriptures, as listed by the Council of Trent, as well as Sacred Tradition, defined and interpreted by the magisterium (teaching office) and a charism (an extraordinary power or gift) given to the church by Christ to teach with binding authority.

After severance from the Eastern (Orthodox) Churches in 1054, the term "Catholic Church" identified Christianity in the West. In the 17th century, the term "Roman Catholic Church" emerged to distinguish it from churches of the Reformation, emphasizing the Roman church's claim to a historic link to St. Peter, martyred in Rome, and underscoring the church's central administrative officer and offices in Rome. Today, the terms *Catholic Church* and *Roman Catholic Church* are used synonymously. It is the largest branch of Christianity and the world's second largest religion.

Early Christians appropriated the idea that human mortality was God's punishment for the disobedience of Adam and Eve from late post-exilic Israel. The experience of, or faith in, Christ's resurrection connected with an emerging belief in a future resurrection and an afterlife of reward or punishment. Early Christians held to a belief in immortality of the soul, a concept developed among Hellenized Jews. While early Christians were convinced that Christ's second coming, followed by a general resurrection of the dead, was imminent, Catholics today have marginal concern for Christ's second coming. Like the early Christians, Catholics today affirm that their faith in Jesus's life, death, and resurrection effects forgiveness of sins, acquittal, salvation, and eternal life.

The early Christians' solidarity with deceased Christians, especially martyrs, developed into the belief in the communion of saints, linking the Church

Triumphant—those in heaven—with the Church Militant—the Christians on earth. By the fifth century, Purgatory, a place or condition of temporary purification of souls unworthy to enter heaven immediately after death, became in the West a standard option to afterlife. However, Purgatory was never accepted in the East and was later rejected by Reformers. While Catholics believe that souls in Purgatory can do nothing for themselves, souls do benefit from prayers of the living and can intercede to God to assist the living who pray for those in Purgatory.

Christians have always accepted the reality of hell, although early Christians were not obsessed with damnation. They sensed Christian life as a right relationship with God, empowered by the Spirit in anticipation of being raised to the experience of God "face to face." By the Middle Ages, emphasis on human sinfulness and "the four last things" (death, judgment, hell, and heaven) reflected a society burdened by terrified consciences magnified by lethal plagues that persisted into the 18th century.

Until very recently, Catholics assumed that all who were not baptized were damned. The only exceptions were unbaptized children, deemed consigned for eternity to limbo, a place of natural peace. The existence of limbo was never an official Catholic teaching, and Catholics today tend to presume that a good God would not deny right-living non-Christians, let alone children, the possibility of heaven. Although they affirm the reality of Purgatory and hell, today's Catholics tend to emphasize the hope of eternal life with God.

Catholics believe that life is a gift from God; the faith is committed to protection and enhancement of life from conception to natural death, even as the faithful profess that afterlife in union with God is life's ultimate goal. Death today is no longer considered life's most terrifying reality. Factors contributing to this include widespread infant survival and unprecedented longevity. More significant, however, is the prospect of dementia among the elderly and advanced medical technology that is capable of extending biological life beyond cognitive faculties, which are often considered fates worse than death.

Catholics are obligated to care for their physical well-being, but dying Catholics are not obligated to make use of extraordinary forms of medical intervention. Recent teachings indicate that, once initiated, tubal nutrition and hydration constitute ordinary care that may only be discontinued under limited circumstances. As medicine advances and issues related to aging become more nuanced, it is likely that more attention will be devoted to defining and refining ordinary from extraordinary care.

Pastoral practices for the dying and the bereaved, developed at various times throughout history, continue to influence the church today. Early Christian reverence for mortal remains of martyrs evolved into a cult of relics of the saints. While this reverence was prominent in the Middle Ages, which saw considerable abuses, Catholic churches continue to revere relics, placing relics of saints in or under altars.

The earliest ministry to the dying provided for reception of the Eucharist, called *Viaticum* (food for the journey), at the last possible moment before death. By the eighth century, however, the practice of anointing the sick came to be perceived as effecting forgiveness of sins to be administered *only* by a priest. It was then called Extreme Unction and offered as the Last Rite to the dying after the absolution of confessed sins and the reception of *Viaticum.* Catholics today identify all three sacraments as Last Rites that may be administered separately and even on several occasions.

Regina A. Boisclair

See also: Heaven; Hell; Purgatory.

Further Reading

Boisclair, Regina. A. "The Rituals for Dying, Death, and Bereavement among Roman Catholics and Eastern Orthodox Christians." In *Religion, Death and Dying*, Vol. 3, edited by Lucy Bregman (pp. 41–62). Westport, CT: Praeger, 2009.

CAUSE OF DEATH

Cause of death is a means of communicating how an individual's life came to an end. Determination of the cause of death is the fundamental duty of the attending physician in cases where the subject has been regularly followed by a doctor and where no foul play is involved. If either condition is not met, the case falls under the statutory jurisdiction of the jurisdiction's medicolegal death investigator (MDI), which may be a medical examiner, coroner, or rarely, a justice of the peace. An official cause of death is required for completion of the death certificate, allowing survivors to settle the estate.

Less commonly, but more significantly, in cases where foul play is involved, having a specific determination of the means by which someone was dispatched (i.e., put to death) facilitates the criminal prosecution. If no specific cause is readily apparent after a thorough investigation and examination, the cause may be certified as due to "unspecified violence," as often happens in cases of severely decomposed remains where the occurrence, if not the specific type, of foul play is readily apparent. Related, and often confused, concepts include *manner of death* and *mechanism of death.* Manner relates to the circumstances under which a cause of death came to be. Mechanism of death refers to the mechanics of how a cause acted to end life.

Generally, simplicity of understanding, logical flow from available data, and especially objectivity are essentials in effective death certification. In all cases, cause, manner, and mechanism are all opinions based on the certifier's education, training, and experience in interpreting available information. Should additional information become available, these opinions may be reevaluated in light of existing and amended opinions, and revised death certificates and autopsy reports may be issued.

Manner of death is primarily investigative shorthand. The purpose is to provide a brief general description of how a death came to be. Classically, there are five categories—natural, accident, suicide, homicide, and undetermined—although some jurisdictions allow a sixth—therapeutic misadventure. Death by natural causes is self-explanatory, in that no foul play is suspected and includes all the specific myriad diseases that might prove fatal. The most common single cause of natural death consistently remains cardiac disease, although infections and cancers are also prevalent. Unnatural manners of death include the remainder (and although precise definitions vary by local custom and practitioner, it is advantageous for the practitioner to develop internal consistency in order to assure reproducibility). *Homicide* means literally death at the hand of another. *Accident* may be defined as an unforeseen, and reasonably unforeseeable, specific outcome of action(s) ending in death. For example, individuals travel by automobile on a daily basis and would have no reason to believe that, on a specific day and at a specific point in time, their life would be ended by a car crash. *Suicide* refers generically to death by one's own hand, for example, by a self-inflicted gunshot wound. The *undetermined* category is reserved for those cases which, based upon available information and to a reasonable degree of certainty, do not neatly fit into any of the former categories. This is often due to a lack of investigative data or other vital information.

In some jurisdictions, the MDI assigns this manner to certain *types* of deaths, commonly drug overdoses, arguing that there is no certainty as to how to account for the excessive drug level, be it inadvertent or willful (i.e., suicide or homicide). In some areas, the inadvertent and undesired outcome of a medical procedure may be classified as "therapeutic misadventure." This might occur when a rare but known complication of a medical procedure results in death. In those areas where such an option is not available, because the complication is expected and due directly to the surgery necessitated by the original condition, the proper manner certification follows the original underlying cause. That is, but for the original disease, treatment would not have been needed.

Another related issue is the requisite reasonable degree of certainty and exactly what that means. Most MDI certifiers use "a reasonable degree of medical certainty" as a standard in issuing opinions. In undetermined cases, the data is equivocal and/or *no* component is more likely than not. Reasonable probability means simply that one event is more likely than not—that is, a greater than fifty-fifty chance. *Beyond a reasonable doubt* is another vague and unquantified concept, but is generally felt by the MDI to be close to certainty (the legal bar is far lower).

In all cases, the *cause* is the initial event that set in motion the unbroken chain of events which eventuated in the victim's death. Time is not a component of the process; a death may follow immediately or days or even decades after the initiating insult. As long as the temporal chain of causation and relation is unbroken and logical, the initial insult and outcome are linked. Thus, a quadriplegic shot 20 years earlier may die from pneumonia related to the paralysis and the death certified as due to the complication of the original gunshot wound. The *mechanism of death* would relate to the systemic infection and resultant inadequacy of air exchange or "respiratory failure." The *manner* would be properly designated homicide. In most instances, the relative contribution of an unnatural component supercedes the natural; thus, if an injury is involved in the death, even as an "other significant condition," then the manner of death would revert to the investigative reason for the initiating trauma.

A fascinating internal inconsistency is the insistence by some practitioners on using the concept of "intent" only in determining suicide but specifically excluding the same in classifying homicide. This also ties into the concern with levels of certainty. As intent could be considered a relative commodity defying metrics, it becomes hard to determine the precise degree to which an individual intended the specific outcome of an act. For example, in homicide cases, the legal system specifically determines an assailant's intent in assessing the degree of criminal culpability (i.e., "degree" of murder, manslaughter, or justifiable homicide). Likewise, in cases of questioned sexual violation, the courts determine whether or not a "rape" occurred—the physician is unable to speak specifically to a subject's or victim's intent, despite the degree and nature of injuries present or absent. Only in cases of self-killing does the certifier commonly express the decedent's intent by means of notes recovered, threats, etc. Where notes are absent (as occurs in many, if not most, suicides), the certifier often speaks of "intent being inferred in the act." Intent is at issue in a minority of cases, where the victim is not actually intending to complete suicide but is rather using threats and attempts as a cry for help. For example, taking a bottle full of pills and calling for help with the intent of being rescued. Should help not come, then the outcome, although specifically unintended, is the same. Thus a different, or perhaps more fundamental (but more complex), definition of suicide is in order—commission of a volitional act, over which the victim has control, wherein the imminent threat of serious self-harm up to, and including death, is or should be known to the perpetrator.

James Claude Upshaw Downs

See also: Coroner/Medical Examiner; Death Certificate; Homicide.

Further Reading

DiMaio, V. J. and D. DiMaio. *Forensic Pathology: Practical Aspects of Criminal and Forensic Investigations,* 2nd edition. Boca Raton, FL: CRC Press, 2001.

Hanzlick, R., J. C. Hunsaker, and G. J. Davis. *A Guide for Manner of Death Classification.* National Association of Medical Examiners, 2002. http://www.charlydmiller.com/LIB03/2002NAMEmannerofdeath.pdf

Hoyert, D. L. and J. Xu. Deaths: Preliminary Data for 2011. National Vital Statistics Reports, 61(6) (2012). U.S Department of Health and Human Services, Centers for Disease Control and Prevention, National Center for Health Statistics, National Vital Statistics System. http://www.cdc.gov/nchs/data/nvsr/nvsr61/nvsr61_06.pdf

National Center for Health Statistics. Physicians' Handbook on Medical Certification of Death, 2003 Revision, Department of Health and Human Services. National Center for Health Statistics, Centers for Disease Control and Prevention National Center for Health Statistics, Hyattsville, MD. http://www.cdc.gov/nchs/data/misc/hb_cod.pdf

Spitz, W. U. and D. J. Spitz. *Spitz and Fisher's Medicolegal Investigation of Death: Guidelines for the Application of Pathology to Crime Investigation,* 4th edition. Springfield, IL: Charles C. Thomas, 2006.

CEMETERIES

Cemeteries are formal burial locations where a number of interments have taken place. The term is normally reserved for those burial areas not associated with Christian churches, which are termed graveyards or churchyards. Another generic phrase is burial ground. Cemeteries are the site of inhumations (the ritual placing of a corpse in a grave), with or without coffins, or burial of cremated remains, often in some form of container.

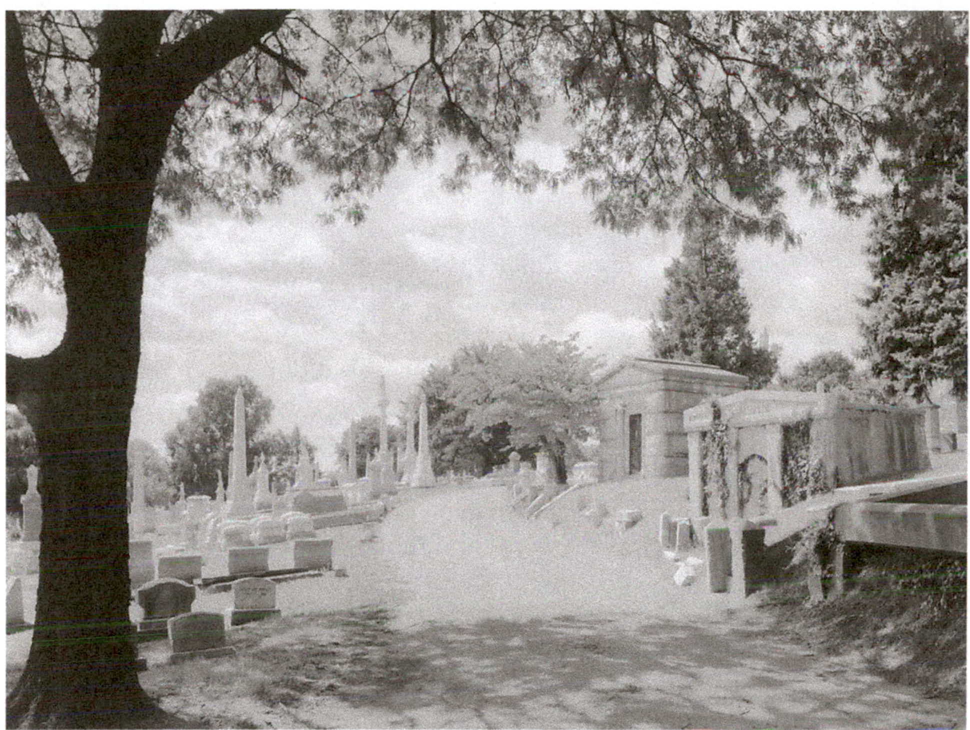

Laurel Cemetery in Philadelphia, 1979, from the Historic American Buildings Survey. (Library of Congress)

Ancient Cemeteries

Ancient cemeteries are often investigated by archaeologists who can learn much about past cultures from the layout of graves and any grave markers, the formal arrangements of the burials, and the treatment of the bodies. In addition, the skeletal remains can provide information on life expectancy, diet, illnesses through life, and sometimes cause of death. In many cultures, burials were accompanied by grave goods—objects deposited in the grave. These are often ceramic vessels, jewelry, weapons, and tools, and can also include food offerings.

The Origin of Modern Cemeteries

In the Middle Ages, all Christian burials in and around churches and monasteries were controlled by the Church, apart from the burials of those excluded from society, such as criminals or suicides, who were deposited elsewhere as part of their punishment. All burials were inhumations, and rarely had any grave goods; only the wealthiest had coffins. Jews always had their own cemeteries, but due to persecution these were not always allowed in every town that had a Jewish population.

Modern cemeteries are normally owned and managed by local government agencies or private companies. This arrangement originated in the later 18th century in Europe when overcrowding of urban graveyards, caused by the massive increase in populations during the Industrial Revolution, put the existing arrangements under extreme stress. Previously, burial had been at sufficient intervals across the churchyard that when an interment took place, the earlier burials would have decayed by that time, leaving only bones. These could either be pushed to one side in the grave, or removed and placed in pits or buildings termed ossuaries. As the numbers dying increased, reuse of particular grave spaces became more frequent, and there was insufficient time for the previous interment to decay. Indeed, as burial in mass graves with little backfill between them began to be used for the poorer classes, there was insufficient soil with the necessary bacteria to perform the expected degradation, leading to bodies remaining largely intact in the ground.

The 18th-century Enlightenment brought increased scientific understanding, new philosophical attitudes to the body, and more varied beliefs about death and the afterlife. This encouraged many to challenge the domination of the churches in the control of burial, but the ecclesiastical authorities resisted relaxation of the existing controls as the fees associated with burial were an important source of income. The introduction of cemeteries took place across Europe at different times, depending on population densities and the power of the local established church, whether Protestant or Catholic.

One of the first countries to develop secular cemeteries was France where the anticlericalism that formed part of the ideology of the French Revolution took control of burial away from the church. For this reason, and to remove the health risks associated with overcrowded cemeteries, existing burial grounds were closed and new cemeteries opened outside the towns and cities. In Paris, the existing graveyards were cleared, and many of the bones were used to line tunnels and chambers cut under the city to quarry rock for many of the buildings. These macabre subterranean spaces were used for parties and have subsequently become a tourist attraction and are still partially open to the public.

Several clear regional styles of cemetery developed across Europe and North America and in European colonies, while parallel developments, appropriate to cultural priorities, developed in the Middle and Far Eastern states. In France, cemeteries in the countryside around Paris were constructed for burial, the most famous being Père Lachaise (opened in 1804) and Montmartre (1825). The former in particular was considered a landscaped idyllic setting, which provided an internationally influential style of garden cemetery that was emulated, first in Britain, and then across North America, where by the 1860s there were over 60 such cemeteries in American cities. Although appearing to be rustic and rural, such cemeteries were in practice carefully plotted out with many grave spaces available for sale or lease. Many European cemeteries offered relatively short leases, often 25 years, after which remains were removed and placed in ossuaries, allowing the frequent reuse of space. In Britain, longer leases of 99 years were the norm, and perpetual use was typical in North America. In these cases, the grave spaces were not available for reuse, so more land was required as the original cemeteries became full; these could be adjacent extensions, or the cemeteries could be closed and new ones opened elsewhere. Moreover, as the garden cemeteries filled up, their rural appearance was lost as the green open spaces were covered with monuments. Exceptions are those few cemeteries that invested their income such that they could maintain open areas and landscaping, as is the case with Mount Auburn, Boston. Here impressive monuments are set within plantings of specimen trees, which support a wide range of wildlife, all within a beautifully managed historic cemetery.

In Mediterranean Europe, burial below ground in earth graves was one option, but for those with more resources the alternatives were burial within a family mausoleum or partially sunken tomb, or placement in an above-ground chamber for one or two coffins. These *loculi*, as they are often called, were built against the walls of the cemetery, with tombs and earth graves in the center; some cemeteries have many such walled areas and in the 20th century detached blocks of *loculi* were built. The niches housed coffins end on, and could be sealed with a commemorative panel. The structures for *loculi* could be five or six inches high, requiring special lifts to hoist the coffins up to be placed in the niches, and ladders for relatives to place flowers on the front of the panel. These burial arrangements are still in use in many Mediterranean countries today. In North America, the same use of *loculi* was established in New Orleans, where several of the old cemeteries in the city (including St. Louis Cemetery No. 1, 1789 and No. 2, 1823) have such arrangements. While this is explained locally as being a solution to the high water table, making the placement of bodies in earth graves difficult, it is more likely that this reflects the cultural traditions of the Mediterranean being transferred to North America.

There are also several regional forms of cemetery found across North America. One of the most widespread is of the Upland South Folk Cemetery tradition, found from Texas to Virginia. While elements (including some of the tomb forms) reflect European origins, this was a local development where the management of the landscape with scraped bare earth was a key feature, though this has declined in recent years. Cemeteries can also be distinctive according to ethnicity, such as Spanish-Mexican, Chinese, and African American cemeteries. Each has distinctive monument forms, layout, and traditions of grave decoration and maintenance. Many groups have special grave cleaning and social events on All Saints' Day (November 1), the most famous being the Mexican Day of the Dead (see **Day of the Dead**).

A very influential cemetery form that was developed in North America, but has subsequently been copied in some other parts of the world with varying degrees of success, is the lawn-park cemetery. These landscaped spaces are not dissimilar to garden cemeteries, except that monuments were much more closely controlled and an open aspect maintained. This became most developed with the further development of the memorial park at Forest Lawn, Glendale, California, in 1913, where only small tablets flush with the ground are allowed for most graves, keeping a very open, uncluttered appearance, and allowing easy mechanical grass cutting to keep maintenance costs low.

At every stage of cemetery development, there have been criticisms regarding the exploitation of the bereaved, the controlling power of burial authorities, and the ways in which cemeteries reflect the values and practices found throughout society. This should not be surprising. Variation in ethnic or religious identities and practices, as well as changing attitudes to death, the body, and the role of graves and grave visiting, all play their part in the design, management, and ongoing use of cemeteries.

Problems with Historic Cemeteries

Cemeteries in Britain and North America, once full, generated no income, so management costs could not be recouped. This led many cemetery companies to file for bankruptcy or not maintain those areas which were full, letting them become overgrown. These often became locations for antisocial and criminal behavior, but also havens for wildlife, as the land around the cemeteries became engulfed in urban sprawl. Many old cemeteries are locked and inaccessible, although some have been taken over by local government authorities or charitable trusts to maintain the cultural and ecological value of the sites and make them a valuable resource in an urban environment.

Many cemeteries have become abandoned over time, and their locations and extent are either uncertain or forgotten completely. When development takes place and such cemeteries are located, the burials require clearance and descendant communities may be involved in this and the subsequent reburial. For some cultural and religious groups, disturbance and reburial are not a concern, but for others it is a critical matter. In North America, the disturbance of native American remains has often been a matter of controversy, and this has been addressed by legislation in the Native American Graves Protection and Repatriation Act (NAGPRA). Many of the lost burial grounds belonged to poor communities, and are frequently those of African Americans. The discovery of some of these has also had political and wider cultural consequences. The disturbance and partial removal of the African burial ground in New York was one such cemetery that generated a great deal of protest and criticism, although it is now a national monument.

Modern Cemeteries

Many contemporary cemeteries are old ones that continue to be used, often with extensions to provide more space for burial. Where land is cheap and easily available, extensive landscaping is still incorporated, but in most cases modern urban cemeteries are designed to have a grid of tightly packed burial plots, reducing the amount of vegetation to soften the visual impact. Grounds maintenance costs are managed by controlling planting on the plots and through the provision of packages paid for by the bereaved, either annually or as perpetual care with an up-front sum invested to provide for long-term management. Many modern cemeteries also have a crematorium that provides a steady income. In North America, the remains of the corpse after cremation are often called cremains (see also **Cremation**;

Cremains); in other parts of the world they may be called ashes. The cremated remains can be taken away by the bereaved to be kept or scattered wherever they feel fit, leaving no permanent public memorial, or can be placed in suitable small cemetery plots or within structures termed *columbaria,* where niches similar to the *loculi,* but much smaller, are provided. These can be against external walls, as freestanding structures, or within buildings that may even have crypts for additional remains.

In some cities, there is once again a burial crisis as existing cemeteries become full and all surrounding land has been developed. Cemeteries often have to be placed ever further from where the bereaved live, creating tensions in grieving and grave-visiting patterns. In some countries, cremation has eased the pressure on cemetery spaces, especially where the remains are scattered, but in multicultural communities and other contexts where religious and cultural requirements make interment of the body in the ground essential, new burial crises are developing in the 21st century.

Conclusion

Cemeteries are an effective solution to the issues of body disposal and allow for varied forms of commemoration and grave visiting. There is considerable variation in form and management over time and space, reflecting the societies and cultures they served. As such, they are informative of past and present attitudes to death, and reveal priorities in the expression of identities, including those of kinship, ethnicity, and religion. Some old cemeteries are now important in heritage tourism even if their role in burial has ended (see also **Dark Tourism**).

Harold Mytum

See also: Body Disposal; Burial; Charnel Houses; Green Burials.

Further Reading

Curl, J. S. *The Victorian Celebration of Death.* Newton Abbot, UK: David & Charles, 1972.
Linden-Ward, B. *Silent City on a Hill. Landscapes of Memory and Boston's Mount Auburn Cemetery.* Columbus, OH: Ohio State University Press, 1989.
Meyer, R. E. (ed.). *Cemeteries and Gravemarkers: Voices of American Culture.* Ann Arbor, MI: UMI Research Press, 1989.
Meyer, R. E. (ed.). *Ethnicity and the American Cemetery.* Bowling Green, OH: Bowling Green State University Popular Press, 1993.
Mytum, H. *Mortuary Monuments and Burial Grounds of the Historic Period.* New York: Kluwer/Plenum, 2004.
Sloane, D. S. *The Last Great Necessity. Cemeteries in American History.* Baltimore: Johns Hopkins University Press, 1991.

CHARNEL HOUSES

A charnel house (or ossuary) is a building for the storage of human bones and skeletal remains. Although predominantly a feature of medieval European societies, charnel houses have existed throughout history in a variety of cultures. They can be found, for example, among the prehistoric peoples of what is today Maryland, the Hopewell societies of Southern Ohio, and the Iroquoian and Southeastern Algonquian native American tribes. While many of these mortuary structures were periodically dismantled or burned to the ground, one such structure was discovered by archaeologists at Spiro, Oklahoma, dating back to AD 1200–1350. Elsewhere, charnel houses are a characteristic of locations where arid or rocky terrain have made earth burial difficult, such as in Greek islands that constitute the Aegean archipelago, or at the foot of Mount Sinai, the site of Saint Catherine's Monastery, which still has a working charnel house.

In medieval Europe, where charnel houses were born chiefly of a shortage of burial space, once cemeteries became full and corpses had decomposed, the bones were exhumed and placed in charnel houses. Revealing much about the shift in attitudes and cultural sensibilities toward death in Western societies, charnel houses were once a central part of public life, where they functioned as places for people to meet, conduct business, dance, gamble, and engage in merriment. In contrast to Western attitudes toward death in the 20th century, with its sharp separation of the living from the dead (who were viewed as repugnant), charnel houses provided an opportunity for the living to not only commune with the dead but also with death more generally, where the aesthetic, and sometimes convivial, display of human corpses served a *memento mori* function by reminding the living of their own mortality.

Michael Brennan

See also: Body Disposal; Dance of Death; Memento Mori.

Further Reading

Koudounaris, Paul. *The Empire of Death: A Cultural History of Ossuaries and Charnel Houses.* London: Thames & Hudson, 2011.

CHILDREN

Today, researchers believe that children of all developmental levels understand death to some degree. It is important to realize that each child is unique and each death is unique, so a variety of factors and levels of maturity can influence a child's understanding of death. These factors may include children's experiences with death and dying, the openness of their family members in discussing death with them, their cognitive functioning, personality, and cultural and religious upbringing. However, there are some general characteristics that can help us understand how children respond to death.

Infants—Toddlers

While infants and toddlers do not have the verbal ability to express their questions or concerns, they do respond to the absence of a significant person in their lives. They also intuit, and respond to, the feelings of those around them. They do not understand the finality of death or its implications for their lives, but they do respond to the loss. Responses tend to be in terms of a regression in behavior (bedwetting, for instance) or refusing to eat or feed oneself.

An infant or toddler who suffers the death of a primary caregiver is unable to express the loss of the attachment; however, he or she may exhibit separation anxiety and cry for the return of the caregiver. Families tend to believe that these children are too young to understand and so may minimize or ignore their expressions of grief. Developmentally, these children are building trust and the loss of an important person can interfere with the growth of trust in adults and the environment.

Children of this age group need reassurance that they will be cared for. They respond well to consistency and familiar faces. They need both physical and emotional comfort.

Preschoolers

Young children may be able to recognize what "dead" means, but cannot understand that death is permanent and universal. They are, by nature, egotistical and often feel that they have "caused" a death by what they were thinking or doing. Researchers call this "magical thinking."

Children in this age group tend to believe that death is temporary and reversible. They may have difficulty expressing their feelings and their questions regarding death. They may experience anxiety about their own bodies and regression in terms of bedwetting and sleep disturbances.

These children need exact language and age-appropriate answers. They may need explanations over and over again. They can require help learning language to express their feelings. Like their younger counterparts, they benefit from a consistent schedule.

School-Age Children (Kindergarten through Fourth Grade)

Developmentally, children in this age range can differ dramatically, though most understand that death is final. They often believe that death can happen to others, but not to themselves or to people in their own family. Children who experienced a death as infants, toddlers, or preschoolers may regrieve this death as they begin to understand that the person who died will never be with them again physically.

Children in the school-age category tend to be able to use vocabulary that indicates that they understand death more accurately than those in earlier stages. However, it must always be remembered that every child is different. Children at this age are not always able to think abstractly and so may be confused by abstract ideas and words.

This is often the age where children see death as the "boogey man" or as some kind of monster. Because children in this group are often concerned with fairness and equity, they often see death as retribution for some evil doing. They are beginning to understand the difference between living and nonliving things. At this time of life, children frequently believe that death is contagious and so would avoid a child who had experienced a death so that "it won't happen to me." School-age children may withdraw or be anxious when a death occurs. Nightmares and night terrors can occur in some children. These children benefit from detailed answers to questions and consistent explanations of the death. They also profit from the chance to see adults mourning, and benefit from being given permission to grieve in their own ways.

Children with Developmental Disabilities

Children with cognitive disabilities may have difficulty understanding death and the grieving process. K. A. Oltjenbruns (2001) says that children must understand three concepts regardless of their age:

1. Dead people are nonfunctional
2. Death is not reversible
3. Death is universal and inevitable

Not understanding any of these concepts can certainly complicate the way that a child accepts a death and grieves the loss of a loved one. It is important to realize that even if a developmentally disabled child does not fully understand death, the child does experience separation and pain from that loss. Grief in the developmentally delayed or disabled should not be ignored or minimized.

Death Rates among Children in the United States

While the infant mortality rate of the United States has dropped in recent years, the most up-to-date figures from the Center for Disease Control (CDC) for 2010 note that the infant mortality rate was 6.06 infant deaths per 1,000 live births, lower than in previous years. The Central Intelligence Agency's *World Fact Book* lists the United States as 175th of 222 countries for infant mortality (see also **Infant Mortality**).

The leading cause of death in children between the ages 1–14 years is unintentional injury. Among this age group in the United States, the leading unintentional injury is motor vehicle accidents. Cancer was the second leading cause of death in this age group. In 2007, about 1,300 children aged 1–14 years died from cancer, representing 12 percent of deaths in this age group. In 2007, the cancer death rate was 2.3 deaths per 100,000 children, 15 percent lower than 10 years earlier, in 1997. Congenital malformations, deformations, and chromosomal abnormalities were the third leading cause of death in this age group, representing 9 percent of deaths. About three-fifths (59 percent) of deaths in this age group from congenital malformations were among children 1–4 years of age. Death rates from congenital malformations decreased 16 percent between 1997 and 2007.

Homicide was the fourth leading cause of death, accounting for 7 percent of deaths in this age group. Children 1–4 years of age accounted for 53 percent of homicide deaths in this age group. Homicide rates among children aged 1–14 years decreased 13 percent between 1997 and 2007. Heart disease was the fifth leading cause of death for children in this age group in 2007, accounting for 414 deaths, representing 4 percent of all deaths in children 1–14 years of age.

Unintentional Injuries

While in the United States, motor vehicle accidents are the leading cause of unintentional injuries in children 1–14 years of age, other causes of unintentional injury and death include drownings, burns, falls, and poisoning. In 2008, the United Nations Children's Fund (UNICEF) proposed interventions to prevent or minimize all of these possible causes of death. They include safety standards, engineering measures, environmental measures, legislation and standards, education, and ways to treat children in these circumstances. Two additional interventions include active adult supervision and providing education to children and caregivers at "teachable moments"—timely opportunities, for example, when an injury has occurred or could have occurred.

Homicides

While the deaths of children from disease and unintentional injury are decreasing in number, the deaths of children from homicide are increasing in the United States (see **Homicide**). Young children are the victims of family members, most frequently being beaten, shaken, or suffocated. However, children aged 6–11 die as a result of maltreatment, the use of firearms, sexual abuse, and multi-family homicides.

Children with Life-Limiting Illnesses

Before the 1970s, it was generally believed that children under the age of 10 neither understood nor experienced anxiety at the prospect of their own death. Research with gravely ill children during that decade, however, showed that children much younger than 10 were aware that they were dying, even when families and caregivers tried to protect them from this information. These children experienced loneliness, anxiety, and fear in this situation.

Frequently, dying children's awareness of their prognosis was at odds with their parents' beliefs about their child's awareness. Even when families and medical personnel provided minimal or no information to these children about their condition, the children acquired information about their disease on their own. Many of the children kept their knowledge secret to protect their loved ones.

Practitioners who work with gravely ill children encourage communication between patients, families, and health care workers. Both art therapy and music therapy are ways to promote effective communication. What to tell the child and how much to tell the child depend greatly on the child's age, cognitive and emotional functioning, family structure, and previous experiences of loss.

Healthy siblings must also be considered when a child is dying. They too depend on parents for support and nurture, while possibly being worried that they too may become ill and die. In addition, siblings may resent the amount of attention and care that are provided to the dying child.

Dying children, like adults, are concerned that they will be comfortable and safe during the dying process. Those who participate in the dying child's world need to reassure the child and provide support, comfort, and presence in the child's life.

Jane Moore

See also: Adolescents; Death Education.

Further Reading

Corr, C.A. and D.E. Balk (eds.). *Children's Encounters with Death, Bereavement, and Coping.* New York: Springer, 2010.

Health, United States 2010. http://www.cdc.gov/nchs/data/hus/hus10.pdf

National Association of School Psychologists. Helping Children Cope with Loss, Death, and Grief: Tips for Teachers and Parents. http://www.nasponline.org/resources/crisis_safety/griefwar.pdf

Oltjenbruns, K.A. "Developmental Context of Childhood. Grief and Regrief Phenomena." In *Handbook of Bereavement Research: Consequences, Coping, and Care,* edited by M.S. Stroebe, R.O. Hansson, W. Stroebe, and H. Schut (pp. 169–97). Washington, DC: American Psychological Association, 2001.

Walter, C.A. and J.L.M. McCoyd. *Grief and Loss across the Lifespan: A Biopsychosocial Perspective.* New York: Springer, 2009.

World Factbook: https://www.cia.gov/library/publications/the-world-factbook/rankorder/2091rank.html

Xu, J., K.D. Kochanek, S.L. Murphy, and B. Tejada-Vera. Deaths: Final Data for 2007. *National Vital Statistics Reports,* Vol 58 no 19. Hyattsville, MD: NCHS; 2010. Available from: http://www.cdc.gov/nchs/data/nvsr/nvsr58/nvsr58_19.pdf.

CHRISTIANITY

Christianity is the largest religion today, counting approximately one-third of the world's population among its members. This entry focuses on beliefs that all Christians hold regarding the person and mission of Jesus Christ, his death and resurrection, and the impact of these for Christians' own expectations for death and afterlife. The central Christian assertion is that "God was reconciling the world to Himself in Christ" (2 Cor. 5:19). Through the death and resurrection of Jesus of Nazareth, God's Son, humanity has been freed from sin and death, and receives salvation and eternal life. While Christians have many interpretations of these basic beliefs, these are the foundation of the religion.

Christians inherit the Hebrew Bible, now known as the Old Testament, in which the story of God's creating the world, choosing a people for himself, and guiding that people so they could become "a light to the nations" is told. Christians read Hebrew Scriptures this way, so that the continuing story of salvation history culminates in the figure of Jesus. Christians accept the New Testament, the writings of the early Christian communities about Jesus and his importance. Jesus, a prophetic preacher-teacher and healer, is proclaimed by Christians as the promised Messiah, the holy king, and deliverer (the title "Christ" signifies this role). While others expected a national liberator, Jesus as Messiah was persecuted, tried, and put to death. Thus, he became Isaiah's "suffering servant" personified (Is. 53:1–12) whose death is the sacrifice for the sins of the world. Jesus's death by crucifixion—a degrading punishment reserved mostly for slaves—marks for Christians the most important death in the world. Its painfulness, humiliation, and utter un-naturalness are among those features that Christians have emphasized in order to make sense of their own sufferings.

But, this death is not the end of the story. What follows death in Christianity is not bereavement, but resurrection. According to the accounts in the Gospels of the New Testament, three days after his death, Jesus was raised by God to new and transcendent life. His tomb is empty, he appears living to his disciples, and this triumph over death is greeted as a sign of his vindication. God has reversed what humans inflicted, and just as Jesus died and was raised, so all people can share in the promise of new and eternal life in Christ. As Jesus says in the Gospel of John, "Whoever hears my word and believes him who sent me has eternal life . . . he has crossed over from death to life" (Jn 5:24). Therefore, the story about Jesus is also a story of our own relation with death and life.

The implication behind this is that ordinary human life is entangled in sin, in need of salvation from this slavery, and is thus a kind of living death. Christians proclaim the need for repentance and "new birth," a means of rescue from this universal state. To be saved, to share in God's promise, one must accept Jesus as the Savior, and share in his death and new life symbolically through baptism, the Christian rite of initiation. From the time of the New Testament, it appears that this message had meaning as people in late Hellenistic times struggled with their anxiety over death. The Christian message continued to focus on this even as the peoples of northern Europe were eventually converted after the collapse of the Western Roman Empire. Christianity presents itself as the solution to death and its universal existential threat.

Another theme of great importance linked to the death of Jesus is its voluntary, sacrificial quality. Jesus "died for our sins," a sacrificial "lamb of God" whose death ends the need for continuing temple offerings. These expressions are found throughout the New Testament and into the later writings by leaders of the ancient church. It is important that Jesus knew what would happen to him, and accepted that to follow God's plan meant to undergo a gruesome death. Here, Jesus has served as a role model of patient willingness to suffer, among countless generations of his followers. Christians early on valued the figure of the martyr, the one who follows Jesus literally into death, and this has continued into the present. The 20th century has been dubbed "the century of martyrs" because of the many thousands of deaths endured for the sake of Christ. In the eyes of Karl Rahner, the distinguished 20th-century Roman Catholic theologian, the model for all Christian death should be the martyr, for whom death is truly a "free act" rather than a biological fate.

In the central Christian hope, "eternal life" and "resurrection" are promised to all those who share in Christ's suffering and death. These terms refer to life in intimacy with God first and foremost; their other meaning points toward transfigured nontemporary existence beyond this life and its ending in death. While there are modern debates over whether "resurrection" is the same as "immortality," for the vast majority of Christians the hope for life beyond death, sharing in God's heavenly realm, has been an accepted element in their faith. The imagery for this—and almost everyone agrees that it is *imagery,* not literal depiction of a transcendent state—ranges from scenes of heavenly worship from the Biblical Book of Revelation, Dante's Mystic Rose at the close of the third volume of *Divine Comedy,* to more small-scale and domestic hopes for family reunions.

These beliefs are enacted and made present for Christians in the yearly festivals of Holy Week: the Thursday of the Last Supper, Good Friday the day of Jesus's death, and Easter. More regularly, Christians celebrate the Lord's Supper (Holy Communion, the Eucharist) which marks Jesus's own farewell to his disciples, with the injunction to "proclaim the Lord's death until he comes." And, as already mentioned, baptism into Christ's death and resurrection is one of the universal rites shared by all Christians, although practiced in several different ways. These help forge and maintain the connections between Jesus's own dying and death, and those of his followers, through the history of the church.

Lucy Bregman

See also: Catholicism; Protestantism.

Further Reading

Alighieri, Dante. *The Paradiso* Volume 3 of *The Divine Comedy.* Translated by John Ciardi. New York: New American Library, 1961/c1320.

Rahner, Karl. *On the Theology of Death.* Edinburgh, London: Nelson, 1961.

Verhey, Allen. *The Christian Art of Dying: Learning from Jesus.* Grand Rapids, MI: Eerdmans, 2011.

CLONING

Cloning refers to the process of generating genetically identical copies of life forms, whether DNA fragments, genes, cells, or whole organisms such as plants, animals, or human beings. Although known primarily as a 20th-century biotechnology, "cloning" has long existed, both naturally and artificially. Asexual reproduction, which occurs via cell division (i.e., mitosis) and where offspring arise from a single parent (through processes such as budding, sporulation, fragmentation, and regeneration), is a natural form of cloning that is found in certain plants, microorganisms, and creatures such as sea anemones, starfish, flatworms, and some lizards. Twinning, or polyembryony (the development of two or more embryos from a single fertilized egg), is another example of natural cloning that is associated with sexual reproduction. Twinning occurs when a fertilized egg (a zygote) attempts to develop into a multicellular embryo through cell division. Instead of remaining part of the same embryo, however, these cells separate completely and begin to grow into full, but genetically identical organisms of their own. Thus, natural human clones exist in the form of identical twins.

Cloning also can be accomplished artificially. Three primary methods of artificial cloning include molecular cloning, embryonic cloning, and nuclear transplantation.

In molecular cloning, a host organism (usually a single cell bacterium) is used to replicate human DNA sequences and genes. This provides scientists with unlimited copies of genetic material that can be used for basic research and the development of medical treatments.

Embryonic cloning is also sometimes referred to as therapeutic cloning. Similar to twinning, in embryonic cloning stem cells are extracted from young embryos (blastocysts, which are fertilized eggs about five days old). Because stem cells are unspecialized cells with the ability to develop into any type of cell, therapeutic cloning offers the potential for advances in regenerative medicine, including the manufacture of genetically compatible replacement cells and tissues for people in need of new organs or suffering from degenerative diseases. Bioethical concerns exist regarding therapeutic cloning, however, primarily because the harvesting of stem cells from blastocysts destroys the embryo.

Nuclear transplantation was first proposed by German embryologist Hans Spemann in his 1938 book, *Embryonic Development and Induction,* which was based on animal experiments he conducted throughout the early 1900s. In nuclear transplantation, the nucleus of a host cell is replaced with the nucleus from a donor cell. Because the nucleus contains the complete genetic material of an organism (except for mitochondrial DNA, which exists outside of the nucleus), the host cell becomes a clone of the donor.

Reproductive cloning, or the duplication of existing organisms, is often associated with somatic cell nuclear transfer (SCNT). This involves replacing the nucleus of an egg (an oocyte) with that taken from a body (somatic) cell of an adult. The new cell, akin to a fertilized egg in that it possesses a complete set of genes, is implanted in a surrogate and allowed to develop and grow. The ensuing offspring is a clone or a twin (save for mitochondrial DNA) of the adult.

Perhaps, the most famous case of a successful SCNT clone is Dolly, a sheep cloned in the mid-1990s by Ian Wilmut and colleagues at the Roslin Institute in Scotland using the nucleus of a mammary cell from one sheep and an oocyte from another. A third sheep was employed as a surrogate that carried Dolly to term. Dolly's existence was announced to the world on February 27, 1997. Prior to Dolly, other animals had been cloned, including frogs, fish, and mice. Since Dolly, cattle, camels, goats, deer, horses, mules, pigs, monkeys, cats, and dogs, among others, have been added to the list.

In 2003, a Québec-based sect known as the Raëlians claimed it had cloned five human beings. Clonaid, a Bahamas-based company founded in 1997 by Raëlians leader and former race-car driver Claude Vorilhon (aka Raël), alleged that the first cloned baby, "Eve," was born on December 26, 2002, to a Florida woman and that four more cloned children had been born in the following six weeks. There was and continues to be no evidence for the validity of these claims.

In response to advances in cloning technologies and (potential) attempts to clone a human being, state governments and international agencies have drafted and/or passed laws or declarations limiting or banning cloning. Existing anti-cloning laws vary, some of which ban cloning outright, bar reproductive but not

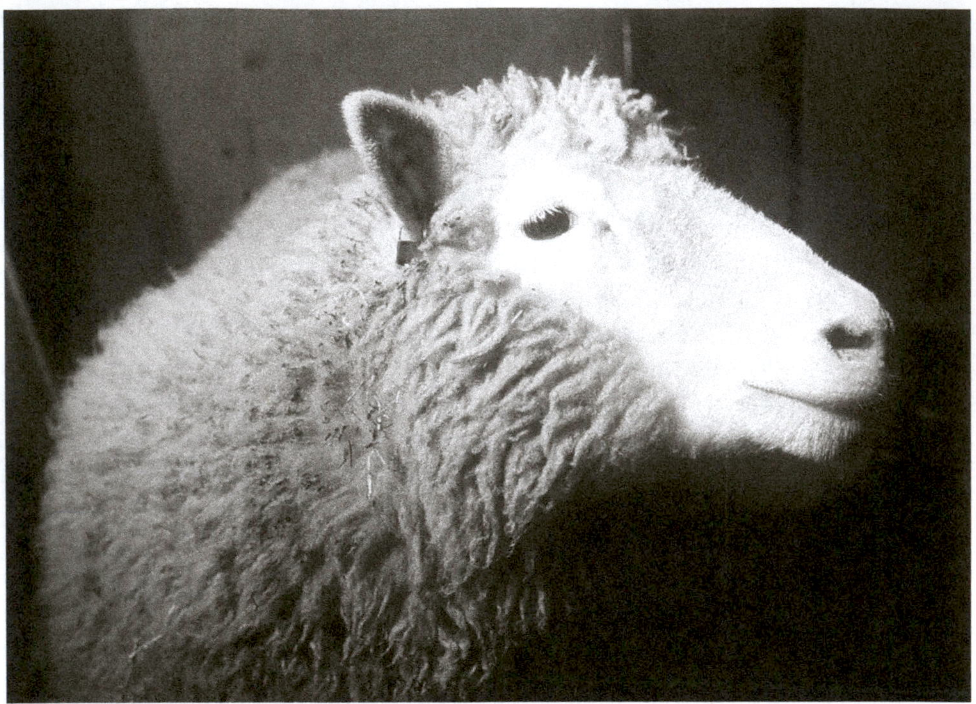

Dolly, shown here in March 1996, was the first mammal to be cloned from an adult somatic cell, using somatic cell nuclear transfer or SCNT. she was cloned by Ian Wilmut and colleagues at the Roslin Institute in Scotland. (Stephen Ferry/Liaison/Getty)

therapeutic cloning, regulate cloning, and/or prohibit the use of public funding for cloning. In 2005, the UN General Assembly approved the United Nations Declaration on Human Cloning.

While the ethics of both therapeutic and reproductive cloning remain important subjects in science, medicine, and the law, the power to replicate genes, cells, and even entire individual beings allows the technique of cloning to be seen as a potential defense against death and even a form of immortality.

Leigh Rich

Further Reading

Committee on Science. *Scientific and Medical Aspects of Human Reproductive Cloning.* Washington, DC: National Academies Press, 2002.

Lim, Hwa A. *Multiplicity Yours: Cloning, Stem Cell Research, and Regenerative Medicine.* River Edge, NJ: World Scientific, 2006.

Maienschein, Jane. *Whose View of Life? Embryos, Cloning, and Stem Cells.* Cambridge, MA: Harvard University Press, 2003.

Wilmut, Ian., A. E. Schnieke, J. McWhir, A.J. Kind, and K.H.S. Campbell. "Viable Offspring Derived from Fetal and Adult Mammalian Cells." *Nature,* 385(6619) (1997): 810–13.

CONDOLENCE (AND CONDOLENCE BOOKS)

Condolences are verbal utterances, usually expressed in writing, intended to convey sympathy and comfort to the bereaved following the death of a loved one. Condolences can be expressed in person (typically at a funeral service, visitation, or wake) or can take an epistolary form in the style of letters and bereavement cards. In the Jewish tradition, condolences are customarily paid in person to the bereaved family, who are visited at home by mourners during a week-long period of *shiva* (see **Judaism**). Whether expressed verbally or in writing, the intention of condolences is the same: to share in the pain of loss and provide solace, solidarity, and support to the bereaved.

Given in speech, condolences may typically involve expressions such as "I am sorry for your loss," often followed by a shared regret at how the deceased will be missed, and/or concern for the well-being of the bereaved. Expressed in writing, condolences may typically include phrases such as "You are in our thoughts and prayers" or "We are thinking about you at this difficult time," and are often accompanied by a fond reminiscence of the deceased that conveys how sorely the person will be missed and/or how they impacted the life of the person paying their condolences. It is not uncommon in written condolences for the writer to invoke an inspirational passage taken from literature or scripture, such as the 23rd Psalm, which is often referred to as a "psalm of providence," and was used by President George W. Bush in his televised address to the American people following the terrorist attacks of September 11, 2001.

In a culture in which, in the face of loss, our words may seem shallow and worn-out, where finding the right words and how to write them can be difficult, such ready-made "scripts" can be useful in helping us convey "hard-to-reach" emotions. Putting our innermost feelings into words, into a written narrative or reminiscence about the deceased, can, however, help us and others begin to make sense of, and come to terms with, loss. Condolences that convey fond memories of the deceased, ways in which they enriched the lives of those with whom they came into contact, and acknowledge efforts to keep the deceased's memory alive—either in thoughts or in deeds—can be especially comforting to the bereaved, who may retain condolence letters and cards for years to come.

The writing of letters of condolence, which can be traced to Roman times, has a long history that reached its apogee during Victorian times, one of the most literate periods in human history when—besides speech—letter writing was the principal mode of communication. It was during this time, before the invention of the telephone, that condolence cards and black-edged stationary became most popular. The long tradition of condolence can also be found in the linguistic origins (or etymology) of the term, which is derived from the Latin roots *com* (meaning together) and *dolere* (meaning to grieve or suffer pain).

Condolence Books

Toward the end of the 20th, and the beginning of the 21st century, a new tradition of signing public books of condolence became popular following large-scale disasters and the deaths of celebrities and public figures. The best-known example of this in recent years followed the death of Diana, Princess of Wales, in 1997, where people in London and around the world waited in line, often for several hours, to write their condolences. Available in both paper and electronic form, the signing of condolence books were part of a panoply of public mourning events that, for some observers, signaled the end of the taboo surrounding death and dying in modern societies (see **Public Mourning; Taboo**).

What was most striking about the messages contained in the condolence books signed following the death of Princess Diana (and to a lesser extent following other public disasters), was that, unlike in traditional condolence letters, the overwhelming majority were not addressed to the bereaved family but to the deceased themselves. Here, messages routinely spoke directly to Diana, often expressing admiration and affection for her as a role model who had touched the life of the writer in a deeply personal way. In condolence books signed following public disasters where the deceased were known personally, and in a face-to-face capacity by message writers, condolence messages often address the deceased directly, expressing a desire to "meet again in a better place" in ways suggestive not only of heaven as a human-centered (anthropocentric) place but of the "continuing bonds" that exist between the deceased and bereaved (see **Continuing Bonds**). In this way, not only do messages in condolence books allow the bereaved to render the deceased temporarily present, but they also allow the bereaved to say in writing, and in death, what they perhaps could not say to the deceased in speech and in life.

New Technologies

Even more recently, the advent of new forms of interpersonal communication technologies, such as e-mail and social media like Twitter and Facebook, has meant that the avenues for expressing condolences have been extended beyond traditional face-to-face speech, letter writing, and the telephone. This has caused anxiety among some people, who are unsure whether these new mediums are an appropriate and acceptable way of expressing condolences. In short, the general rule of social etiquette underpinning these evolving technologies seems to be that it is okay to offer condolences using these mediums if the bereaved first announced their loss using them.

In ways that are perhaps even more pronounced than public books of condolence, recent research suggests that online forms of condolence in social networking sites (SNS) such as Facebook routinely address the dead directly as social actors and *as if* they are listening. One explanation for this is that online communication in social networking sites—unlike either the telephone or face-to-face interaction—is asynchronous (happening at different times) and does not require the copresence of the other. Unlike in face-to-face or telephone conversation, communication in social networking sites does not necessarily demand a response, meaning that communication with the dead is no different from communication with the living. Cyberspace too, like heaven, is an ethereal place that cannot be physically seen but only imagined.

Michael Brennan

See also: Facebook.

Further Reading

Brennan, Michael. "Condolence Books: Language and Meaning in the Mourning for Hillsborough and Diana." *Death Studies,* 32(4) (2008): 326–51.

Zunin, L. M. and Hilary Stanton Zunin. *The Art of Condolence: What to Write, What to Say, What to Do at a Time of Loss.* New York: HarperCollins, 1992.

CONFUCIANISM

Confucianism is a philosophy associated with Confucius, a Chinese philosopher who lived from 551 to 479 BC. There is some debate as to whether Confucianism is a religion as well as a philosophy (it shares many characteristics with religion, but is not organized like religions usually are, nor is there a belief in a personal God). It is nonetheless a system of belief that has proven to be very influential not only in China, but also far beyond.

Unlike most philosophies, which tend to be written in a systematic form, Confucius's work is to be found in a set of sayings known as *The Analects.* These largely revolve around the key concept of "ren," which can be translated as "benevolence." Grayling (2008) argues that efforts to cultivate benevolence need to involve not only acting rightly, justly, and compassionately toward other people, but also ensuring that we ourselves avoid being arrogant, unfair, ingratiating, or tyrannical.

Confucius emphasized the importance of education and scholarship as part of this commitment to ren. It is through such study that the moral value of benevolence can be realized. People have the potential to build their moral character through study and learning and thus self-improvement.

There was, however, an element of elitism in Confucius's thinking. For example, he felt that ordinary people, because they did not study, would not understand the path to be followed and therefore had to be led (compare this with the much later views of Kierkegaard and Nietzsche) (see **Existentialism**).

There is also a strong element of conservatism in Confucianism, in so far as Confucius emphasized the importance of "li," a set of prescribed norms. He expected people to be quite submissive to accepted social norms or "etiquette" in the name of maintaining social order. This reflects the traditional emphasis on collectivities as compared with the more usual Western emphasis on individuals. There is a significant irony here, in the sense that, while there is a collective dimension to the philosophy, it remains largely an individualistic (or "atomistic") approach, in so far as the emphasis is on social improvement through individual moral actions. There is little or no scope for improving society by attempting to change it.

It seems to be the case that any problems lay with individuals and their moral virtues (or lack of), and not with the nature or composition of society.

Consistent with this atomism and conservatism, Confucianism also reflects an emphasis on conformity for the sake of moral virtues such as benevolence, and thereby places relatively little emphasis on the value of diversity, innovation, or social transformation.

In relation to death and dying, there is no specific Confucian conception of an afterlife, and so no sense that dying is a beginning as well as an ending. However, Chan et al. (2006) point out that the Confucian view of death is that, while we do not know life, we cannot know death. They go on to argue that, while many people have claimed that Confucius avoided facing death directly, others have said that what Confucius meant was: if we handle things in life properly, the problem of death will also be solved. This means that the Confucian way of inquiring into death is through life. According to Confucius, ren is a moral standard, a rule of living. Ren is characterized by "continuation" and "never-ending." If we live a life of ren, our mortality will be transcendent, and the spirit will be preserved. From a spiritual point of view, Chan et al. (2006) point out, we transcend into "immortality." Confucianism does not conceive of death as something horrible provided that one dies meaningfully. A "good death" involves having lived a moral life and dying for the preservation of the virtues.

Confucianism therefore offers an interesting perspective on death and dying, which broadens Western perspectives.

Neil Thompson

Further Reading

Chan, W.C.H., Tse, H.S., and T.H.Y. Chan. "What Is Good Death? Bridging the Gap between Research and Intervention." In *Death, Dying and Bereavement: A Hong Kong Chinese Experience,* edited by Cecilia Lai Wan Chan, and Amy Yin Man Chow (pp. 127–35). Hong Kong: Hong Kong University Press, 2006.

Grayling, A. C. Preface to *The Analects,* by Confucius. London, Folio, 2008.

Overmyer, Daniel. "Acceptance in Context: Death and Traditional China." In *Death and Eastern Thought,* edited by Frederick H. Holck (pp. 198–225). Nashville, TN: Abingdon Press, 1974.

CONTINUING BONDS

When a person dies, her physical life is over, but her effect on the lives of those who survive her lives on. For most of the 20th century, psychiatrists and psychologists thought the purpose of grief is the reconstruction of an autonomous individual who, in large measure, leaves the deceased behind and forms new attachments. Therefore, if a bereaved person reported that they sensed the presence of the dead, thought the dead were communicating with them, or thought the dead were still actively helping them, mental health professionals diagnosed those people as having pathological grief. Data, however, show that the dead continue as partners in our inner conversation, as examples of how we should live, as advisors in our important decisions, and as reminders of the important times when we were with them. That is, the bonds or attachments we have with significant people in our lives continue in a changed form after those people die.

In many cultures, people believe that the dead literally continue to exist in our world; spirits or ghosts may get angry at the living if the living ignore them, or do not perform the proper rituals to ensure the passage of the dead to the next world or the next life (see also **Ancestor Worship**). In the contemporary developed world, we are more likely to say that the dead live on in our memories or in parts of them that we find in ourselves.

Continuing bonds in contemporary developed societies may be experienced in the following ways:

1. Linking objects: Linking objects are objects connected with the person's death and life that link and evoke the presence of the dead. Some linking objects are temporary, used only in the first year or so. During that time, they often move from being experienced as external objects, to ones that are internalized within the self. For example, for several months after her child died, a mother reported a stuffed animal "was like a crutch for me." One day as she cleaned, she put it away and found she didn't miss it. By then, she said, the images of the child were "ingrained into my mind so well I didn't need to look at a symbol of his life to remember him." Other linking objects are more permanent; for example, the grave where people come regularly over the years to be with, and feel close to, those who have died.

2. Prayer and ritual: Religions in most cultures include elements that link the living with the dead: graves in the churchyard, flowers on the altar, and lanterns signaling the dead to return for a yearly visit. Many people feel connected with someone who has died when they feel close to God. A woman whose two daughters were killed in the same accident, and who attended Catholic Mass every day, reported that she sensed her daughters' presence at the moment the Host was elevated. Grief often includes experiences that feel spiritual, but are not directly connected with any religion. After a night of dreams of a crying baby, one bereaved mother reported that she awoke to rainbow colors on the ceiling and then discovered it was sunlight refracting off the glass of the framed photograph of her child. She reported that she felt blessed all day long. On another occasion, following a party for her sister's children, she found a butterfly inside the window and was convinced that it was her child attending the party. Although others might interpret these events more scientifically, for this woman, these moments remind her that she is still bonded to her child, and that her love for her child is stronger than death.

3. Memories: If a death has been traumatic or unexpected, memories are at first very painful. A bereaved mother, for example, reported how she believed that when the pain of grief following her daughter's death had finally subsided, that so too would her bond with her daughter. Only later did she begin remembering the good times they spent together more than the months she spent in the hospital with her daughter. The mother subsequently reported how now, when she feels in low spirits, she feels better and is comforted by looking at her daughter's photographs.

4. Enriched Identification: In psychological terms, and in the process of identification, a significant person who has died is integrated into one's representation of the self in such a way that it is very difficult to distinguish the two. The most common way, perhaps, of identifying is by transferring a particular role within the family to a family member of the next generation. One woman, for example, reported that after her mother died, she put away the plastic dishes and began using her mother's china. The dead also live on as role models of how to live now; for example, a loving grandfather can be a model of how to be a good parent. When faced with difficult decisions, people might ask what advice a deceased person would give, or what that person would do. A person who faced death bravely and with grace can be an inspiration and model for facing life's other hard realities.

Are Continuing Bonds "Real"?

In the contemporary world, we tend to define what is "real" as that which can be empirically proved by the scientific method. When something seems as real to us as the sense that a dead person is communicating with us, we want to think that the reality is scientifically provable. In the early 1840s, when people experienced the spirits of the dead, some thought it was like the recently invented telegraph because the messages transmitted over the wire from the next town seemed as amazing to them as messages from beyond the grave. Despite many attempts to prove that communications with the dead are scientifically real, no such studies have met the standard demanded by empirical science.

Communication with the dead, then, cannot be reduced to experimental science. But what the dead say is often important, and what we have to say to them is often deeply meaningful. They have lived and made an impact on our lives. A high school student, for example, whose mother had died 10 years earlier, chose a prom dress she thought her mother would like. People important to us who have died remain with us in parts of our lives, reminding us of who we are and how we should act. Those fundamental questions about life do not admit to scientific answers; but they are often the real questions of living, and the dead can be a real part of the answers we find to the meaning of our lives, and how we are to act in our relationship with others and our environment.

Dennis Klass

Further Reading

Braude, A. *Radical Spirits: Spiritualism and Women's Rights in Nineteenth-Century America.* Boston: Beacon Press, 1989.

Finucane, R. C. *Ghosts: Appearances of the Dead and Cultural Transformation.* Amherst, NY: Prometheus Books, 1996.

Klass, D. *The Spiritual Lives of Bereaved Parents.* Philadelphia: Brunner/Mazel, 1999.

Klass, D., P. R. Silverman, and S. L. Nickman. *Continuing Bonds: New Understandings of Grief.* Washington, DC: Taylor & Francis, 1996.

Stoeber, Michael and Hugo Meynell (eds.). *Critical Reflections on the Paranormal.* Albany, NY: State University of New York Press, 1996.

Walter, T. "A New Model of Grief: Bereavement and Biography." *Mortality,* 1(1) (1996): 7–25.

CORONER/MEDICAL EXAMINER

When an individual dies suddenly, especially under suspicious circumstances, the case falls under the jurisdiction of the local medicolegal death investigator's (MDI's) office. Depending upon the location, this may be a coroner, medical examiner, or rarely, a justice of the peace. The specific North American duty of official governmental investigation into questionable deaths originated directly from the Dark Ages' Pre-Norman English office of the Crowner (corrupted from the Latin *custosplacitorum coronae* or keeper of pleas of the Crown). A common misperception is that the office originated in 1194's *Articles of Eyre*. In fact, the existence of the office (but not the duties) can be traced to the era at the turn of the 10th century (ca. AD 871–910). The reintroduction of the office, in what eventually morphed into its modern form, was necessitated due to the depletion of England's treasury in ransoming King Richard from Vienna. Hubert Walker, Archbishop of Canterbury and Chief Justiciar (Prime Minister), needed to find new revenue streams and, based solely on Article 20 (cited in toto) of the September 1194 Eyre:

> In every county of the King's realm shall be elected three knights and one clerk, to keep the pleas of the Crown.

The Archbishop of Canterbury oversaw a re-empowerment of the institution. In order for the knight be elected coroner, he had to be a freeman of sufficient means to resist potential corruption. Toward that end, the office was unpaid. The specific concern was the general level of financial misconduct rampant at that time in the office of the Sheriff. A legacy of the taint of official corruption remains in the otherwise inexplicable unique power of the coroner to arrest the sheriff.

Although the medieval coroner's duties were many (as enumerated under King Edward I in 1278's *Officium Coronatis*), including involvement in granting sanctuary and treasure from shipwrecks, etc., first and foremost, the coroner was an administrator who was responsible for record keeping of complex codes regarding fines and penalties having to do with deceased bodies, including homicides and suicides. The *de facto* taxation of the populace hinged on the coroner's detailed accounting for all potential witnesses and properties associated with a cadaver and the steep levies if elaborate and serpentine rules were not strictly followed by the citizenry. Indeed, failure to report, initially investigate, and guard a "found" decedent was a major offense, leading some to ignore or conceal such abandoned bodies for fear of financial accountability. The coroner was charged with conducting an inquest into suspicious deaths; the process consisted of physically examining the remains and empanelling a group of locals to determine the nature of the death. The coroner conducted pseudo-medical examinations, despite no formal training or requirement, which included documentation of the extent and nature of traumatic injuries, including the occurrence of rape.

Circuit traveling *Justices in Eyre* actually heard the pleas held by the coroner at formal sittings or *Assize* courts, and rendered verdicts (often after multiyear intervals required to complete a single circuit). Eventually, the Office of the Justice of the Peace gained prestige, becoming the local administrator (even acting as judge

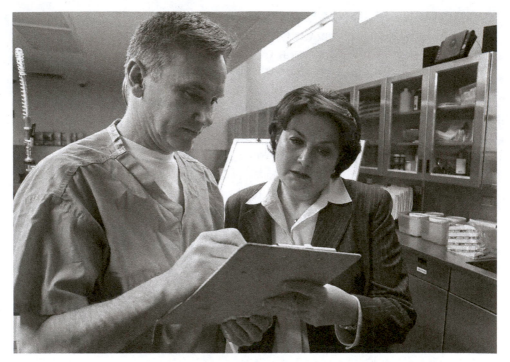

The Douglas County, Colorado Coroner looks over notes on an autopsy with a doctor in the county morgue in Castle Rock, Colorado, 2013. Colorado's 63 coroners are mostly elected, no medical degree required, and they operate under laws written in the days when Western coroners did little more than collect bodies after frontier shootouts. Colorado's coroners have been working for months with law enforcement and district attorneys to update death investigations statewide. (AP Photo/Ed Andrieski)

in minor legal matters) and, as such, the scope of Coronial powers diminished to include only medicolegal death investigation by approximately 1500.

The frugality of the Coronial system and the lack of sufficient resource investment are exemplified by the fact that the coroner had to rely on personal medicolegal investigative skills until the mid-19th century, when first allowed to employ a medical expert. As a British creation, the coroner's appearance followed the global dissemination of English ideology and governance, including to the colonies in the United States.

The first statutory physician MDI was created in Maryland in 1860. Massachusetts created the office of "Medical Examiner" in 1877, eliminating that jurisdiction's coroners. New York City established the first major American Medical Examiner Department in 1918. An obvious advantage to such systems remains the requisite medical knowledge of the practitioners, especially as contrasted with the lack of uniform basic standards for lay coroners. Despite numerous national studies (National Research Council 1928, 1932, 1968, and 2009; Institute of Medicine 2003; and National Association of Counties 1985) pointing out the benefits of a physician-led medicolegal death investigation system, the present medicolegal death investigation remains stagnated, with roughly half of the 3,130 county equivalents (constituting approximately 2,342 separate death investigation systems) represented by a coroner and the rest by a physician medical examiner. A lone exception is Texas, where a lay justice of peace may assume the duties of a coroner.

A 1954 Model Postmortem Examinations Act proposed by Forensic Pathology professionals, remains conceptual only. The more populous areas tend to be served by a medical examiner and the remainder by a coroner, a fact largely attributed to economy of scale, because—at least in the short term—a physician-led system tends to be more expensive. Assertions that costs might be reduced by centralization and/or regionalization remain largely unaccepted and unproven. Federal interest from both the executive and legislative branches has been directed toward improving medicolegal death investigation, but issues in driving improvement forward include altering the statutory (often constitutional) office of the coroner. Without a significant catalyst to upset the present equilibrium, there appears, at least in the short term, no uniform means of assuring best practices in each jurisdiction.

While the duties of medicolegal death investigation are largely identical, no two states have exactly the same system. The official, be it medical examiner or coroner, is charged with investigating cases of sudden, unexpected, and/or unnatural death and/or injury. This would include cases where the deceased has no physician of record, in-custody fatalities, potential public health threats, etc. Although the charged duties are identical, the differences between the general qualifications requisite to hold either office are dramatic. A coroner is generally an elected official *without* specific requirement for any form of medical or ancillary training to stand for office (although a handful of states require the candidate to be a physician, none require the doctor to be a specialist in the relevant field of forensic pathology). Some jurisdictions do require short overview courses as a marker of at least a modicum of fundamental knowledge. In many, if not most, areas the position amounts to a part-time job.

As a political office, the need to address public sentiment (especially when dealing with potentially unpopular rulings and in a litigious society) is always in the background in such systems. As a nonphysician, a lay coroner is unable to personally conduct autopsy examinations and so must hire a physician (not necessarily a forensic pathologist) to perform this fundamental task. In stark contrast, a medical examiner is an appointed physician, ideally a board-certified sub-specialist in forensic pathology. Both systems require a staff of medicolegal death investigators in order to fulfill all the duties of the job. Education and certification of staff, especially lay investigators, is actively encouraged in either system as a means of ensuring a standardized level of performance.

James Claude Upshaw Downs

See also: Cause of Death.

Further Reading

Miletich, J.J. and T.L. Lindstrom. *An Introduction to the Work of a Medical Examiner: From Death Scene to Autopsy Suite.* Santa Barbara, CA: Praeger, 2010.

Upshaw Downs, J. C. "Coroner and Medical Examiner." In *Handbook of Death and Dying, Volume II: The Response to Death,* edited by Clifton D. Bryant (pp. 909–16). Thousand Oaks, CA: Sage, 2003.

CREMAINS

Cremains (or *ashes*) are the cremated remains of a corpse disposed of through the modern process of cremation (see **Cremation**). Unlike in more traditional forms of cremation, such as the funeral pyre characteristic of Indian society, the intense heat produced by modern cremation reduces the body to small fragments of larger bones, which are then placed within a "cremulator" so as to reduce them to the granular fragments commonly referred to as "ashes." Contrary to popular belief, these cremains do not resemble the fine ashes created from burned wood or paper, but instead look and feel more like course coral sands. Weighing somewhere between approximately four and nine pounds, cremains have a whitish rather than gray complexion due to the calcium in a person's bones.

Following cremation, the bereaved are presented with a range of options as to what to do with their loved one's cremains. These include burial; placing them in an urn so that they can be kept in the family home, an urn garden, or in a colmbarium niche; or the scattering of cremains over land or at sea. For many, keeping a loved one's cremains nearby in the family home provides a source of comfort and is a constant reminder of their continued presence (see also **Continuing Bonds**). For others, the scattering of cremains at a site of natural beauty or cherished physical place once enjoyed by the deceased, such as a beloved sports stadium, is a preferred option. An alternative to the scattering of cremains in a public place, which in most Western societies is regulated and restricted by local authorities, is the burial of cremains on a family property, which are not governed by the same legal restrictions and procedures governing the disposal of a dead body.

One potential issue created by the scattering of a person's cremains, especially if scattered at sea or in a forest or wood with no visible marker as to their exact whereabouts, is the difficulty the bereaved may have in relocating them as a site to visit. While there is some concern that those whose cremains are scattered may go unmemorialized, thereby affecting the survivor's ability to grieve, there appear to be no such difficulties of remembering the dead among ethnic groups, such as Hindus, for whom cremation is the traditional mode of bodily disposal. For those who desire a physical reminder to memorialize their dead, memorial gardens (providing a nameplate of the deceased) and books of remembrance held at a cemetery or columbarium, offer a permanent material reminder of the deceased.

The term "cremains" tends to reflect cultural differences not only in spoken English but also in the funerary practices and sensibilities surrounding death, dying, and bereavement, and is reserved for North American rather British English, where "ashes" continues to be employed to refer to cremated remains. In her book *The American Way of Death,* English social critic, Jessica Mitford, thought that terms like cremains were euphemisms that helped conceal the reality of death, reflective of a wider culture of American death denial (see **Death Denial; Euphemisms**).

In recent years, innovations in memorial practices characteristic of the revival of long-forgotten traditions surrounding death and dying have included the incorporation of cremains into keepsake jewelry. One such example of *momento mori* practices involves the placing of cremains in pendants that can be hung from necklaces and worn by several family members. Other practices include the creation of a memorial diamond from a loved one's cremains and the underwater entombment of a person's cremains in an artificial eternal reef (see also **Memento Mori; Memorial Tattoos**). Others have gone further still by arranging to have their loved one's cremains flown into outer space.

Michael Brennan

Further Reading

Mitford, Jessica. *The American Way of Death.* New York: Simon and Schuster, 1963.

CREMATION

Cremation describes the incineration of the human corpse, usually in the ritual context of a funeral, often followed by a secondary ritual with the cremated remains. Depending upon weight, modern cremation reduces a body to 4–8 lb or 1.8–3.6 kg of ashes in 60–90 minutes at a temperature of approximately 800–1000°C. The ashes, remains, or "cremains," as they are usually called in the United States (see **Cremains**), are buried, placed in urns, sometimes in buildings called columbaria, or at sites of personal significance. Commercial innovations even generate jewelry from ashes.

Historical Background

Cremation occurs from the Neolithic period, around 7,000 years ago, throughout the Bronze Age and into historical and modern times. Premodern cremations on open-air pyres often led to ashes collected in urns for burial or location in funerary mounds. Homer's classical epics of approximately the eighth century BC describe cremation honoring heroic warriors, with friends' ashes even placed together in a single golden urn under funeral mounds (*Iliad,* Book XX111, 1–264, and *Odyssey,* XXIV: 110–80). Some pre-Roman, Etruscan remains were contained in urns shaped as small houses that might contain images believed to protect the deceased from evil or help them attain immortality. Cremation often occurs alongside inhumation or earth burial of the entire corpse. During the second century AD, except for Roman Emperors whose cremation symbolized transformation into deities, a major switch to burial took place in the Mediterranean world, though we are unsure why. In the fourth century, after Emperor Constantine converted to Christianity, he opposed cremation and encouraged burial.

Cultural Variation

Traditionally, African societies have practiced burial, opposing cremation as a disrespectful treatment of the dead, an outlook often found when ancestors play a significant part in cultural life, as in ancient Israel and modern Judaism, and perhaps also in Mormonism today. India, by contrast, is the country best known for open-pyre cremation and associated belief concerning the transmigration and potential reincarnation of the life force or soul. This enters the skull of the developing fetus in the womb, a "hot" place that "cooks" a person into a human being. Likewise, the funeral pyre becomes the hot place that takes the body apart again with the eldest son traditionally cracking the corpse's skull allowing that soul to depart for other dimensions of existence. The pyre smoke rises to the heavens before falling again as part of life-giving rain with ashes placed in sacred river water. This scheme makes sense of cycles of existence, including reincarnation, driven by ideas of merit or karma (see also **Reincarnation**). Hinduism, Buddhism, and Sikhism, originating from subcontinental India, all used cremation for their dead. Outside India, Hindus and Sikhs have often been enabled to continue adapted cremation practices in modern crematoria. In the United Kingdom, for example, even Parsees, descendants of Zoroastrians who settled in India where they exposed corpses in Towers of Silence for vultures to consume, and for whom fire was a sacred phenomenon that should not be desecrated by cremation, adopted cremation in electric cremators.

Modern Cremation

Western-focused cremation was not prompted by eastern karmic cycles, but by a combination of 19th-century engineering, scientific and innovatory thinking, often driven by urbanization and the Industrial Revolution. Sometimes, cremation was influenced by an antireligious sentiment, most especially by Freemasons in Italy but not by Northern European Freemasons, who easily combined cremation with their more frequent Protestant Christianity. Modern cremation incinerates the corpse within specially engineered equipment, rather than upon immediately constructed pyres. It originates in 19th-century innovative and free-thinking individuals, and newly created associations of professionals committed to improvements in medical, health, hygiene, and social welfare matters against the background of unhygienic and overfilled city cemeteries. Popular ideas of the disease-creating power of miasma, a dangerous atmosphere spawned in graveyards, reinforced the view of cremation as a hygiene-health opportunity. The later 19th century also witnessed potential problems between religion and science, not only over evolutionary theory and Biblical Creation, but also in the pragmatic encounter of corpses, health, town planning, and ideas of human destiny through resurrection.

International Comparisons: Italy, United Kingdom, and United States

Italy was especially important in the development of modern cremation. In 1857, Ferdinando Coletti, Padua University's professor of pharmacy, argued for cremation, seeing no basic ideological objection to it. The 1870s witnessed a variety of experiments in cremation with the World Fair in Vienna in 1873, for example, exhibiting a model cremator by the Italian Ludovico Brunetti which, among other things, stimulated Sir Henry Thompson, surgeon to Queen Victoria, to gather a group of influential people to establish the Cremation Society of England in 1874. They produced a declaration disapproving of burial and, until some better method might one day be found, supported cremation as the best means of rapidly resolving the body "into its component elements, by a process that cannot offend the living."

Another doctor, William Price, an eccentric Welshman, cremated his infant son, named Iesu Grist (Welsh for Jesus Christ), in the open air in 1884. His arrest for this disturbing incineration led to a legal trial and the first British judgment that deemed cremation not to be illegal as long as it did not disturb the public peace. However, it would not be until 1902 that fuller U.K. legislation was enacted. In Italy, the rich industrialist Alberto Keller was cremated in Milan in January 1876 in the very first purpose built "crematorium." It was on this very day that the first Cremation Society in Italy was established. Others would follow, with 14 Italian crematoria existing by 1886. The cremation of well-known people often had significant social influence in numerous countries. The period from the 1870s to 1880s marked the turning point for modern cremation, with support groups in many countries discussing cremation as an alternative to burial, and influencing legal changes.

In the United States, rapid population growth in the 19th century due to immigration from Europe led to concern over urban planning and sanitary welfare, while the American Civil War encouraged families to embalm dead soldiers and bring them home for burial (see also **Embalming**). This helped the United States shape funeral directing and shifted the focus from cremation to more elaborate caskets, displayed bodies, and concrete graves. However, the United States also had its own advocates for cremation, for example, Dr. Francis Julius LeMoyne of Washington Pennsylvania built his own cremation facility as early as 1876. American women, too, played an important role in associations and societies supportive of cremation, as did their British counterparts. These women, such as Julia Ward Howe and Elizabeth Cady Stanton, became national figures during the 19th century for their advocacy not only of women's rights but also of cremation as an aspect of sanitation reform. America did not, however, find a widespread affinity with cremation for most of the 20th century, as did, for example, the United Kingdom and Scandinavia. This was probably also due to a general Protestant and Catholic preference for burial in the United States.

In the first decade of the 21st century, another innovation called Resomation was invented by a Scottish engineer, Sandy Sullivan, as a method of reducing the body to ash through alkaline chemical dissolving in pressurized tanks (see also **Green Burials**). Time will tell if this method is publicly adopted and popularized. If it is, then "crematoria" might become mortality centers with both igneous (resembling or relating to fire) and aqueous (resembling or relating to water) methods of bodily resolution. Other cremation-related issues that sometimes attract public acceptance and opposition include the use of spare heat issuing from cremation to warm crematorium or other social facilities.

Religious Opposition

Christianity's traditional burial practice, derived from Judaism (amidst a wider Mediterranean culture familiar with cremation), was rooted in Biblical accounts of Jesus receiving tomb burial. Accordingly, early Christians used either inhumation (placing the corpse in the soil) or tomb burial (where bodies were placed in underground tunnels, as in the catacombs at Rome). Inhumation predominated with the earth grave symbolizing the place of rest or being "asleep" until the Resurrection of the dead in the last days. The symbolic coherence between death, burial, and resurrection allowed believers to identify with Jesus Christ. Cremation confused these conventions.

Italy became a particular focus for the emergence of modern cremation, with innovators leading the way by engineering machines capable of cremating bodies, and Freemasons challenging Catholic opposition to cremation (in teaching and ritual practice) by constructing "cremation temples" in Turin. To build such competing ritual space was deeply significant, and accordingly, a church Declaration of 1886 (*De Humana Corpora Cremendi*) forbade Catholics from engaging in cremation. It noted the negative influence of those of "dubious faith" involved in Masonic groups and described cremation as a pagan custom that was detestable and impious. So while many Protestant-influenced countries slowly adopted cremation and developed appropriate legislation over the closing decades of the 19th to the early decades of the 20th century, Catholics remained opposed until 1963 when cremation was formally allowed as long as it was not associated with anti-Catholic motivation. Still, as Table 1 shows, some Catholic-based countries were relatively slow to adopt the practice and, even by 2010, cremation rates often served as a rough index of Catholic or Protestant regional heritage. The Orthodox Greek and Russian Churches firmly oppose cremation because of the theological and liturgical emphasis on resurrection. Judaism, too, especially more orthodox groups, tend to oppose cremation, with some seeing burial as the basis for resurrection. Islam, too, follows this perspective with strong doctrinal belief in burial and resurrection.

These cremation rates reflect ideas on social change and the cultural-religious traditions of their respective countries, as well as, potentially, also serving as some index of secularization (the diminishing influence of religion in society and public life).

Even Christians accepting resurrection beliefs often think it would be as easy for God to create a resurrected being from scattered ashes as from entirely decayed grave remains. Indeed, many contemporary Christians seem to think of ultimate destiny in terms of their soul leaving their body at death and going on into a divine; for these, cremation becomes its own powerful form of symbolism of the body as something left behind by the departing soul.

Table 1 Selected Cremation Rates

	1970	1980	1990	2000	2010
Canada	6	19	33	48	58
China	–	–	–	46	49
France	0.28	1	6	17	30
Ireland	–	–	3	6	11
Italy	0.19	–	1	5	13
Japan	–	91	97	99	99
Spain	–	–	3	14	21
Sweden	38	51	61	70	77
UK	53	64	70	72	73
USA	4	10	17	25	40

Source: Davies and Mates (2005): 450–456, and *Pharos International* (2011): 24–25.

Economics and Ideology

Financial factors are also important for cremation, since facilities for the process cost money to build and run, with the issue of profitability always being significant in capitalist and free-market economies. It is likely that funeral directors may sometimes see the provision of elaborate funeral rites, preparation of bodies, and graves, along with memorial architecture, as more profitable in the long term than cremation. In other societies, such as those under Communist regimes, economics take a different form, with cremation being used as a vehicle of social change. During the 20th-century era of the USSR, the Soviet authorities introduced cremation as a form of ritual competition with the Russian Orthodox Church, something that has only been partially successful in the longer term, and especially, in the post-USSR history of Russia. Marking one distinctive aspect of Revolution, the People's Republic of China announced in 1956 that cremation would replace an age-old use of burial, and marked a key aspect of Revolution.

Cremation, then, focuses a myriad of cultural issues, from hygiene and town planning, through ideological politics, to religious beliefs about human destiny, and shows how death studies frequently open very revealing windows into social worlds.

Douglas J. Davies

See also: Body Disposal.

Further Reading

Davies, Douglas J. *Cremation Today and Tomorrow.* Nottingham: Alcuin/GROW Books, 1990.

Davies, Douglas J. and Lewis H. Mates (eds.). *Encyclopedia of Cremation.* Aldershot: Ashgate, 2005.
Homer. *Iliad.* Translated and with an Introduction by Martin Hammond. London: Penguin Books, 1987.
Homer. *Odyssey.* With an 'Introduction' by Peter V. Jones. London: Penguin Books, 1991.
Jupp, Peter C. *From Dust to Ashes: Cremation and the British Way of Death.* Basingstoke: Palgrave Macmillan, 2006.
Parry, Jonathan. *Death in Banaras.* Cambridge: Cambridge University Press, 1994.
Prothero, Stephen. *Purified by Fire: A History of Cremation in America.* Berkeley: University of California Press, 2001.

CRYONICS

Cryonics (from the Greek κρύος meaning intensely cold) is the scientific study and practice of using extremely low temperatures to induce a state of "cryobiosis" that temporarily slows or halts a life form's metabolic processes to death-like levels for the purposes of preservation and later resuscitation. Cryobiosis is also sometimes referred to as "cryostasis," "biostasis," or "suspended animation," and is a form of "cryptobiosis," a more general category of biological mechanisms that enable organisms to survive extreme environmental conditions such as drought, food scarcity, oxygen deprivation, or excessive temperatures or salinity (i.e., the salt content in a body of water). Cryptobiosis, including cryobiosis, occurs naturally among some organisms, particularly those that are single celled. (Hibernation is a similar, though not as extreme, type of metabolic depression.) For most multicellular organisms, including human beings, cryobiosis does not occur naturally but may be induced through laboratory techniques.

Today, cryonics is frequently associated with the "banking" of human body parts and the "freezing" of human beings. Cryonics has played an important role in the creation of immortal cell lines for medical research and the long-term storage of human gametes (spermatozoa and oocytesor eggs) and embryos for use in assisted reproduction technologies (ART). Often, the term "cryonics" is used specifically to refer to the practice of preserving the bodies or heads of human beings, who have been pronounced legally dead, with the intention of later reviving them and extending life once medical technologies advance.

Robert C. W. Ettinger is commonly considered the "father of cryonics." An American college math and physics teacher, his 1962 book *The Prospect of Immortality* (published in 1964) made popular the science of cryonics as a possible life-preserving and life-prolonging technique for human beings. The history of cryonics, however, dates back at least to the 1600s, when scientists began exploring the preservative effects of cold temperatures on organisms and bodily tissues. During the 17th, 18th, and 19th centuries, scientists studied the possibilities of freezing and later reanimating life forms such as rotifers, eelworms, frogs, fish, butterfly pupae, caterpillars, salamanders, bats, and human sperm. Many of these experiments proved successful. Nevertheless, the discipline of cryobiology, particularly in relation to human beings, did not formally arise until the 20th century. One of the obstacles to successful cryobiosis is the damage supercooling causes to the structure of cells, primarily due to ice-crystal formation as the water in tissue freezes. Research conducted in the 1900s demonstrated that dehydrating cells or organisms prior to freezing, or adding protective chemicals such as glycerol that lower the freezing point of water, can prevent ice-crystal formation and mitigate cellular injury. The process of vitrification, or the use of such "antifreeze" cryoprotectants that enable solidification to occur without freezing, revolutionized cryobiology and the science of long-term tissue storage or "banking."

Since cryobiosis slows or halts metabolic processes, this prevents aging and decay and allows biological materials to be stored long term for later use. This technology has become an essential tool in both medical research and practice, including pathology, organ and tissue transplantation, ART, and cord blood banking.

Some proponents of cryonics, however, focus on its speculative promise for life extension; that is, the cryopreservation of human beings (or the brains of human beings) until a time when scientific advances in regenerative medicine such as stem cell research, genetic engineering, cloning, and nanotechnologies offer treatments (both for the initial ailments and any damage caused during cryobiosis).

During the mid-20th century, several cryonics organizations were formed. The first was Evan Cooper's Life Extension Society in 1963. Like Ettinger, Cooper was a proponent of cryonics as a form of human life-prolongation and the author of a commercially unpublished text, *Immortality: Physically, Scientifically, Now,* written in 1962. The Cryonics Society of New York (CSNY) emerged in 1965, followed by similar societies in Michigan and California. These four groups no longer exist. The American Cryonics Society (originally named the Bay Area Cryonics Society) was established in 1969. Members from this group formed the California-based company, Trans Time, in 1972. In this same year, the Alcor Society for Solid State Hypothermia was created, although its name was changed in 1977 to the Alcor Life Extension Foundation and it was relocated in the early 1990s from California to Scottsdale, Arizona. In 1980, an original member of the CSNY began another organization, also called the Life Extension Foundation, in Fort Lauderdale, Florida, although today it focuses more on nutritional supplements.

Although, to date, several human beings have been cryopreserved, none has been resuscitated. The first successful cryopreservation of a human being occurred in California in 1967, when scientists associated with the Cryonics Society of California froze 73-year-old psychology professor and cancer patient James Bedford. Since the early 1980s, Bedford's body has been housed at the Alcor Life Extension Foundation in Arizona. Arguably, the most famous person to be cryogenically preserved is Hall of Fame baseball player Ted Williams, whose head was frozen by Alcor in 2002.

The small town of Nederland, Colorado, also boasts of a now-famous cryonics resident: a Norwegian grandfather who was originally cryopreserved by Trans Time from 1989 to 1993 but has since been maintained by family members in a shed. This has sparked an annual town event known as Frozen Dead Guy Days. Ettinger himself, who died on July 23, 2011, has been cryopreserved at the Cryonics Institute.

Leigh Rich

See also: Immortality.

Further Reading

Cantor, Norman L. *After We Die: The Life and Times of the Human Cadaver.* Washington, DC: Georgetown University Press, 2010.

Ettinger, Robert C. W. *The Prospect of Immortality.* Garden City, NY: Doubleday, 1964.

Griffith, Daniel V. "Donaldson v. Van de Kamp." *Issues in Law & Medicine,* 8(1) (1992): 105–9.

Gruman, Gerald Joseph. *A History of Ideas about the Prolongation of Life.* New York: Springer, 2003.

Romain, Tiffany. "Extreme Life Extension: Investing in Cryonics for the Long, Long Term." *Medical Anthropology,* 29(2) (2010): 194–215.

Shaw, David. "Cryoethics: Seeking Life after Death." *Bioethics,* 23(9) (2009): 515–21.

Sheskin, Arlene. *Cryonics: A Sociology of Death and Bereavement.* New York: Irvington Publishers, 1979.

Turner, Bryan S. "Longevity Ancient and Modern." *Society,* 46(3) (2009): 255–61.

CULTS

There is no agreed-upon definition of the word "cult," although it typically refers to a minority religious group, possibly with a charismatic leader, whose beliefs and practices are at variance from that of mainstream society and culture. Events involving the deaths of members of a relatively small number of religious minority groups in the 1990s led to media headlines labeling them as "suicide" or "doomsday cults." Since then the word "cult" has become heavily polluted in the public imagination, academics in the sociology of religion have preferred the more value-neutral term "new religious movement" (NRM), since it avoids the value judgments implicit in the term "cult." Both the moral panic created by the media and the anti-cult movement that developed in response to the perceived threat posed by these groups, have served to create a disproportionate and generalized anxiety about NRMs in the minds of the general public.

Media reports of apocalyptic violence were frequently exaggerated and distorted, claiming that "evil cults" were headed by "manipulative" and "deranged" leaders who "brainwashed" their converts. As a result, the general public and some analysts assumed that *all* NRMs were dangerous and violent and should be controlled or even prohibited, even though the majority are peaceful and law-abiding. The anticult movement developed with the simple goal of protecting potential converts from, in their opinion, being coerced into joining cults.

Apocalypse Now: Doomsday Cults

The Jonestown massacre, in November 1978, in which 918 members of the Peoples Temple were killed or completed suicide in Guyana, was swiftly used as a prime example of a destructive "doomsday cult" by the media and anticult movement. In the three decades that followed, a series of similarly catastrophic events contributed to general anxiety about the threat posed by NRMs. These events included: the 90 members of the Branch Davidians, a Seventh-day Adventist sect, who, in 1993, died in Waco, Texas, as a result of a standoff with the United States Bureau of Alcohol, Tobacco and Firearms; the 74 members of the Order of the Solar Temple, who between 1994 and 1997 were found dead in a series of ritualized murders or suicides in Quebec, Switzerland, and France; the Japanese group, Aum Shinrikyo, who carried out murders of individuals and two Sarin gas attacks (one in the city of Matsumoto in 1994, followed by another on the Tokyo underground in 1995), in which 12 individuals died and around 5,500 commuters were injured; the 38 members of Heaven's Gate, a so-called UFO cult based in California, who, in 1997 completed suicide after their leader convinced them that a spaceship hidden behind the Hale-Bopp comet would rescue members from the impending destruction of the earth; and the approximately 780 members of The Movement for the Restoration of the Ten Commandments of God, a Catholic splinter group based in Uganda, who in early 2000, died in a series of murder suicides. While concern about the well-being of people who join more extreme NRMs, and the potential threat these pose to society, is not without foundation, there is some concern in academic circles that this threat has been exaggerated. Thus, placed in perspective, the events reported above, and others like them, represent less than 5 percent of NRMs, known to the British information center *Inform*, which have been associated with violent acts.

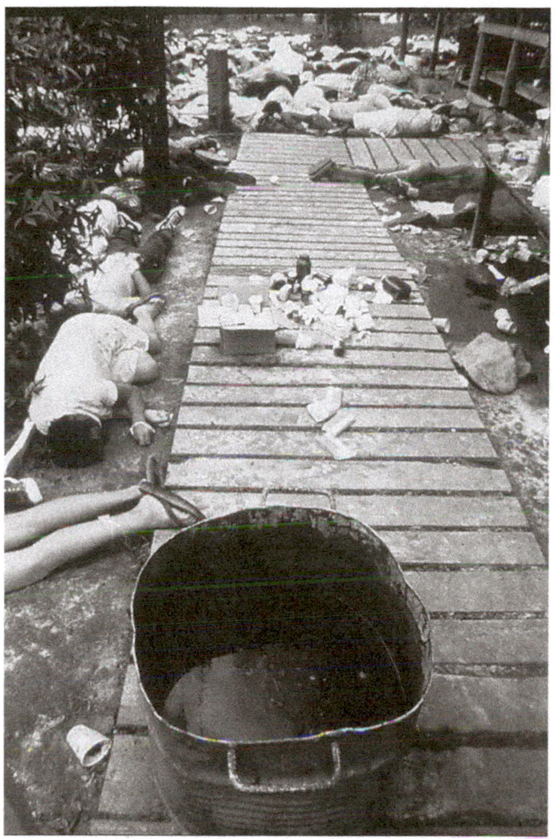

Vat and scattered bodies at Jonestown, November 1978. (AP/Wide World Photos)

Defining Features of Millennial Groups

Apocalyptic elements tend to be one common feature at the core of the beliefs of NRMs that have turned violent. One strand of millennial literature is frequently based on the Book of Revelation, predicting that Christ's rule on earth will come to an end after 1,000 years, culminating in the final judgment and the destruction of evil. Millennialism can also refer to a belief in the imminent end of the world and the development of a millennial kingdom. So-called millennial groups, therefore, often display a dualistic worldview, which can lead to predications of a cataclysmic end of the world. Catastrophic millennialism is routinely characterized by a pessimistic outlook, whereas progressive millennialism is defined by a more optimistic perspective on humankind; yet the risk of violence may increase in groups that have given up hope for the salvation of non-members.

NRMs can be precarious in nature if they have a charismatic leader who, by definition, is perceived as having exceptional powers and/or of being in direct contact with God, since he routinely has to renew his charismatic status by engaging in "legitimation work" in order to retain his authority. The lack of opportunities for legitimation can create a "crisis of charismatic authority," which in turn increases the risk of volatility and violence (which appeared to be the case with Jim Jones and The Peoples Temple at Jonestown). Frequently, this increased risk results from the breakdown of charismatic leadership rather than from the charismatic leadership itself. Leaders of some NRMs can, nevertheless, exert high levels of control over the group and its individual members.

Other factors that appear to predispose some NRMs to violence can be categorized as "totalizing" or "authoritarian." World-rejecting NRMs, a term first described by Roy Wallis, display processes of psychological splitting, physical and/or ideological distancing from larger society, and processes of resocialization, which can lead to a state that Edgar W. Mills has termed "super commitment," in which the individual displays unquestioning obedience to the organization to which he or she belongs. This is more likely to develop if a group's isolation has eradicated members' exposure to values and norms differing from those of the group.

Millennial groups have also been classified as fragile, assaulted, and revolutionary. So-called fragile catastrophic millennial groups initiate violence in an attempt to preserve their millennial goal, examples of which are the Peoples Temple, Aum Shinrikyo, The Order of the Solar Temple, and Heaven's Gate. Assaulted millennial groups are characterized by having been attacked by law enforcement agents who regarded them as dangerous, an example of which would be the Branch Davidians at Waco, involving deviance amplification, labeling, and misinterpretation of actions by law enforcement agencies. Revolutionary millennial movements have an inherent predisposition for violence, since they want to overthrow what they consider to be the illicit and "evil" government, an example being the Montana Freemen, an armed group who were involved in an FBI siege in 1996.

In the 21st century, the increase of terrorism and of suicide martyrs who are willing to die to achieve their millennial goals has opened up new areas for research. So too have the cult deaths connected to beliefs in possession, or resulting from practices concerning health care, such as the claims made by some leaders that their practices can cure cancer, making children that are believed to be possessed fast for days, or refusing medical treatment on religious grounds.

Silke Steidinger

See also: Apocalypse.

Further Reading

Barker, E. "In God's Name. Practicing Unconditional Love to the Death." In *Exercising Power: The Role of Religions in Concord and Conflict,* edited by T. Ahlbäck and B. Dahla (pp. 11–25). Åbo: Donner Institute, 2007.

Introvigne, M. "'There is No Place for Us to Go but Up': New Religious Movements and Violence." *Social Compass,* 49(2) (2002): 213–24.
Tabor, J. T. and E. V. Gallagher. *Why Waco?* Berkeley and Los Angeles: University of California Press, 1995.
Thompson, D. *The End of Time: Faith and Fear in the Shadow of the Millennium.* London: Sinclair-Stevenson, 1996.
Wallis, R. (ed.). *Millennialism and Charisma.* Belfast: The Queen's University Belfast, 1982.
Walliss, J. "Charisma, Volatility and Violence." In *Exercising Power: The Role of Religions in Concord and Conflict,* edited by T. Ahlbäck and B. Dahla (pp. 11–25). Åbo: Donner Institute, 2007.
Walliss, J. "Understanding Contemporary Millenarian Violence." *Religion Compass,* 1(4) (2007): 498–511.
Wessinger, C. *How the Millennium Comes Violently.* New York: Seven Bridges Press, 2000.
Wright, S. *Armageddon in Waco: Critical Perspectives on the Branch Davidian Conflict.* Chicago: University of Chicago Press, 1995.

CURSES

The origins of the word curse can be found in Old English (*curs*), where the word was used to describe a verbal utterance invoking a magical or supernatural power capable of inflicting death, disease, or misfortune on a person or thing. Throughout recorded history, curses have been seen to provide two main functions: (1) to invoke the dead, demons, or spirits against the living; or (2) to protect the dead from the living or the living from the dead (also known as *necromancy*). The history of curses, and of cursing, can also be found within religious discourse and oral cultures governed predominantly by magical, superstitious, or religious beliefs. In this context, curses, together with blessings, represent "verbal formulae" that are capable of exercising power over the individual(s) to whom they are directed. Within the Judeo-Christian tradition, the Biblical plagues visited upon Egypt in Exodus (12:2) are perhaps the best known example of a curse intended to cause harm. It is this event in Biblical history—as an expression of God's wrath—that was intended to persuade Pharaoh to release the Hebrew slaves from bondage, triggering the exodus of the Jewish people. This event also conveys the power of the spoken word to affect material change; that is, as a symbolic force capable of producing physical outcomes. Evidence provided by archaeologists and anthropologists suggests, however, that curses were widespread in earlier periods of history—from ancient Egypt and Rome, to Scandinavia and medieval Britain—in ways that extended beyond religious experience and belief. Even in modern secular societies, in which the influence of religious doctrine has declined, the continued legacy of curses and potency of verbal utterances to inflict harm can be found in laws aimed at regulating and preventing slander, blasphemy, and insult.

Michael Brennan

Further Reading

Gager, John G. *Curse Tablets and Binding Spells from the Ancient World.* Oxford and New York: Oxford University Press, 1999.

Goody, Jack. *The Logic of Writing and the Organization of Society.* Cambridge: Cambridge University Press, 1996.

Sayer, Duncan. "Curses and Hexes." In *Encyclopedia of Death and the Human Experience,* edited by Clifton D. Bryant and Dennis L. Peck (pp. 248–49). Thousand Oaks, CA: Sage, 2009.

CYBERSPACE

The Internet is the engine behind the technological revolution that has transformed ways in which people across the globe communicate with one another, from their personal relationships to their business deals. This has also been true for the ways in which people have dealt with matters concerning dying, death, and bereavement (the experience of loss). Using communication technology has led to new ways of thinking about death. For example, the Internet can be used to find social support in times of upheaval due to death; to seek out death-related information (such as finding out how to build your own casket via Google); and to commemorate the dead through virtual memorials and online tributes. These changes have been so profound that a new term, "thanatechnology," has been coined to refer to the uses of the Internet and related communication technology for dealing with issues connected to thanatology (the study of death and dying).

Forms of Thanatechnology

Classifying the different formats of thanatechnology is difficult because of its rapidly changing nature. Several years ago, most communication technology occurred through the use of personal computers. However, by 2011, the number of people using wireless technology via handheld devices has increased exponentially, facilitating the ease by which the Internet can be used to communicate and receive information about death and dying. Wireless technology facilitates global communication that previously was not possible because many nations lacked the infrastructure to support "older" devices that relied on plugged-in connections. Now, for example, mobile devices make it relatively easy to witness a funeral in Kenya, armed conflict in the Middle East, and videoconference with family members who are ministering to a dying loved one in Europe. Currently, the ways in which technology is used for death-related concerns primarily take on the following formats:

1. Social Networking

Instant communications via social networking sites (SNS) such as Facebook and Twitter provide the means for people (i.e., "friends") to share information and remain connected. E-mail may also serve in this capacity, as do blogs, a form of an online journal (the term "blog" is a new word created by blending the two words web and log). Social networking may be a significant source of up-to-date information about people and provide forums for posting ideas, current activities, and feelings. Minutes after an individual's death, the news can be communicated across the globe. It can be an advantage to have ready access to this information, but also quite upsetting to those who might be "blindsided" when such information is unexpected and delivered in an impersonal way.

2. Websites as Sources of Information about Death and Dying

These are web pages that may be stored on a server and can offer a wide variety of functions, from the selling of goods to providing valuable, as well as bogus, information. Part of what it means to become digitally literate entails learning how to navigate the World Wide Web for reliable sources of information. Such can be the case when seeking information about thanatological concerns. Entering the keywords "death and dying" in the Google search box brings up 225,000 sites. Even more striking is that a search using the words "bereavement and grief" yields some 11 million links. Many of these sources provide material on a variety of death-related topics, ranging from the signs and symptoms of grief, through selecting a hospice, to variation in cross-cultural funeral practices. Finally, the number of webinars (web-based seminars), classes, and online courses on death, dying, and bereavement geared chiefly to higher and continuing education is proliferating on the Internet and is accessible to a very wide audience. [One of the largest providers of webinars and online educational programs in this field is the Association of Death Education and Counseling, see **ADEC (Association for Death Education and Counseling)**.] U.S. professors now can teach an online course on death and dying to students in many different continents. Consequently, the Internet has become increasingly accepted as a source of information, and it should thus come as no surprise that ever more people are using it to get the death education that they never received in school or at home.

Online Support Groups and Other Therapeutic Modalities

In North America, seeking professional assistance and organized support groups for coping with a death-related loss has gained increased acceptance. Now, such help can also be found on the Internet. Support groups can take on a variety of forms based upon who leads the group (e.g., a licensed therapist or peer), the purpose of the group, its membership, and its structure. Some of these include groups for the survivors of suicide (see **Suicide Prevention and Postvention**), widows, those who have experienced the death of a child, and for people grieving over the death of a pet (see **Pets**). In addition, live chats and videoconferencing via venues such as Skype make it possible to have a personal consultation or bereavement counseling with a professional hundreds of miles away (see also **Grief Counseling**).

Virtual Commemorations

The Internet is also used to commemorate the dead. Beginning in 1995, Web cemeteries were created to honor the dead, to visit a place where a deceased loved one is memorialized, and to record tributes. For those who are homebound or far away from a cemetery, grieving over the loss of a person who has not been interred (as when the body is missing), or who find real cemeteries disturbing, such locations offer a way to individualize and continue a relationship with the deceased (see also **Continuing Bonds**).

3. Interactive and Dynamic Digital Experiences

Games and interactive Internet-based media such as "Second Life" offer infinite ways for people to encounter death and dying. It is now possible to participate in an online funeral with an Avatar (a virtual representation of the self) and the Avatars of many others, who may be anywhere in the world. This has even occurred in a real-time format to honor the death of a beloved "gamer." Although they frequently include murder and mayhem, computer-based games may also present a way for the player to confront the notion that life is time bound and limited, as in the game "Heavy Rain" where the player's choices may lead to the death of a protagonist. Such virtual experiences may be particularly appealing to adolescents and young adults who may be confronting the prospect of their own mortality as a very real possibility for the first time (see **Video Games**).

Another experientially based aspect of the thanatechnological revolution allows those who are dispersed across the globe (e.g., those serving in the military) to participate in a funeral of a loved one through the use of a Webcam.

Consequences of Thanatechnology

Much of modern living has been greatly affected by our "brave new world" of computer-mediated communications. So too has modern dying. Some of the major effects involve the following:

- ***Easy access to information about death and dying***
  Individuals are no longer passive recipients of medical advice and diagnoses. It is fairly simple to type in a series of symptoms and access information about possible illnesses and treatments. At its best, this common practice enables patients and their families to be better informed as they consult with their physicians about the treatments of life-threatening diseases. At its worst, misinformation regarding particular conditions and their treatment can have potentially fatal implications (see also **Disease**). End-of-life decision-making may also be enhanced by what is provided on the web. One can submit an online request to become an organ donor. It is now also possible to download advanced directives (designating another to make medical, legal, and financial decisions should a person become incapacitated or incapable of making decisions by themselves), fill out the forms online, and e-mail the completed forms to the relevant parties (see **Advance Directives**). Easy access to this information and the submission of these forms will hopefully lead to more people taking advantage of these options.
- ***Promotion of awareness of cultural diversity***
  The Internet has the potential to enhance our understanding of the multitude of ways in which death and dying, and the rituals and practices surrounding them, are group specific and subject to cultural variation. The sharing of web-based information, including the use of audio and video media, can thus raise awareness of cultural diversity in the meanings, attitudes, and practices surrounding death, dying, and

bereavement; reminding us that there is anything but a "one-size-fits-all" approach to human mortality. In the United States, for example, a number of states have seen the growth of refugees from countries in Africa and Asia. One such group, the Hmong (originally from Laos), has many members who still practice shamanistic rituals at the time of death that involve chanting, playing instruments, and the use of symbolic objects. Since humans are visual creatures, being able to watch such rituals can enhance cultural understanding, and hopefully tolerance of differences.

- ***Compressed time frame in which information is accessed and transmitted***
  Learning about the death of significant others, public figures, and the loss of life due to public tragedies or natural disasters is almost instantaneous today. Not only this, but a detailed record of a person's life in the form of an obituary (see **Obituary**)—especially in the case of celebrities and public figures—is today available for public consumption in online newspapers and news sites within minutes of a person's death.
- ***Shared community for isolated bereaved***
  Social permission to grieve is sometimes denied to the bereaved for a variety of reasons. Homosexual couples may not be able to openly express profound sorrow over the loss of a partner in a homophobic culture where such relationships are not recognized (see **Grief**). The significance of the grief over the loss of a friend, pet, or celebrity may also not be fully acknowledged by family or friends. The Internet, however, provides places for people who are suffering from such losses (the disenfranchised) to find the social support that they may lack in "real life." In addition, a number of individuals (males in particular) are hesitant to overtly express their grief in face-to-face encounters, or may have work/family schedules that make it very difficult to attend support groups or meet with people in similar circumstances. In these cases, the ease with which one can communicate with others over loss and grief at any time, and in the privacy of one's home, can be invaluable.

Controversies and Issues

An irony of thanatechnology (and social media in general) is that it has the power not only to simultaneously bring people together but also to distance them from one another. Sometimes, consolation and understanding of death and dying are best done in real places with actual physical hugs and eye contact. People gather together in times of public tragedy, hold hands during a funeral, and find solace around the deathbed of a loved one (see **Deathbed Scene**). Digitizing death and dying makes it easier to avoid such physical interactions even when it is possible to physically engage in them. A drive-through funeral, where the body can be viewed on a monitor and a message of sympathy expressed online is a good example of this. In addition, people on the "have-not" side of the *digital divide* (the relative lack of access to the latest computer-based technologies among low-income groups, racial and ethnic minorities, people in rural areas, and those in developing nations) have limited access to information about end-of-life issues, participation in family and community discussions, and social support during times of loss. Perhaps, this situation creates a new group of disenfranchised grievers.

The way in which death is viewed and understood may also take on new meanings as immortality may be now be achieved in a digital sense (see also **Immortality**).

The images and voices of loved ones may thus be preserved in perpetuity in cyberspace. It may also be possible to interact with a virtual image of a loved one even after he or she has died. How does this affect the grieving process and the meanings attributed to death? Currently, there are no definitive answers, either in a theoretical or empirical sense, to such questions.

A new form of ethics and social etiquette ("netiquette") must therefore be considered, particularly from professional counselors and therapists who must include additional safeguards to protect the online identities of their clients in a cyberworld where information can go "viral" at the click of a mouse.

Despite these caveats and concerns, it would be foolhardy to dismiss the significance and impact of technology on our "death systems" (the ways in which society enables people to mediate their understanding of death and dying) as we try to integrate death into our modern, technologically evolving ways of living.

Illene Cupit

Further Reading

deVries, Brian and Judy Rutherford. "Memorializing Loved Ones on the World Wide Web." *Omega,* 49(1) (2004): 5–26.

Fieler, Bruce. "Mourning in a Digital Age." *New York Times,* January 13, 2012. http://www.nytimes.com/2012/01/15/fashion/mourning-in-the-age-of-facebook.html?_r=1&adxnnl=1&pagewanted=all&adxnnlx=1329512480-Nf1kizuneX5bqlRaMVvk/A

Kasket, Elaine (ed.). "Death and Dying in Digital Age." *Bereavement Care,* Special Issue, 31(1) 2012.

Roberts, Pamela, and Lourdes A. Vidal. "Perpetual Care in Cyberspace: A Portrait of Memorials on the Web." *Omega: Journal of Death and Dying,* 40(4) (2000): 159–71.

Sofka, Carla J. "Social Support 'Internetworks,' Caskets for Sale, and More: Thanatology and the Information Superhighway." *Death Studies,* 21(6) (1997): 553–74.

Sofka, Carla. J., Illene Noppe Cupit, and Kathleen R. Gilbert (eds.). *Dying, Death, and Grief in an Online Universe: For Counselors and Educators.* New York: Springer, 2012.

D

DANCE OF DEATH

The *Dance of Death* (*danse macabre*) is a short theatrical performance (masque) intended to convey essential truths about human existence; namely, that death is inevitable and universal, the "great leveler" that comes to everyone regardless of their wealth, status, or standing in the social hierarchy. It was most widespread in Europe during the late 13th and early 14th century, at a time when the public imagination was gripped with thoughts of death as a result of the Bubonic Plague, which claimed the lives of one-fourth of the population of Europe between 1347 and 1351. Although originally a play, the *Dance of Death* was later represented in poetry, music, and the visual arts (in paintings, murals, woodcuttings, and engravings). In paintings that appeared on cemetery walls, in mortuary chapels, charnel houses, and sometimes churches, death is often personified as a skeleton and messenger of God, leading the living away from this earthly existence to a life beyond the grave.

Set in a graveyard or cemetery, the plot evolves from a monk preaching about the inevitability of death. This is followed by a group of skeletal figures who, emerging from a charnel house, invite their first victim (usually an emperor or pope) to accompany them to purgatory. Despite the refusal of the invitation, the victim is led away. Following this, a second messenger approaches a cardinal or prince, who is similarly led away, followed by others representing all sections of society. The performance concludes with a second sermon emphasizing that death is a fate shared by all and that everyone should therefore prepare for judgment.

Down the centuries, representations of the *Dance of Death* have changed, from early depictions of death as an entirely natural event, to later portrayals that characterize death as a violent and unwelcome rupture between the living and the dead. Further representations include an erotic element in which death is likened to the momentary break in consciousness provided during sexual intercourse by orgasm (see also **Sex and Death**). Contemporary echoes of the *Dance of Death* can be found in musical interpretations, such as Camille Saint-Saëns's *Danse Macabre,* and in the symbolism of cultural festivals and holidays such as Halloween and the Day of the Dead.

Michael Brennan

See also: Charnel Houses; Day of the Dead.

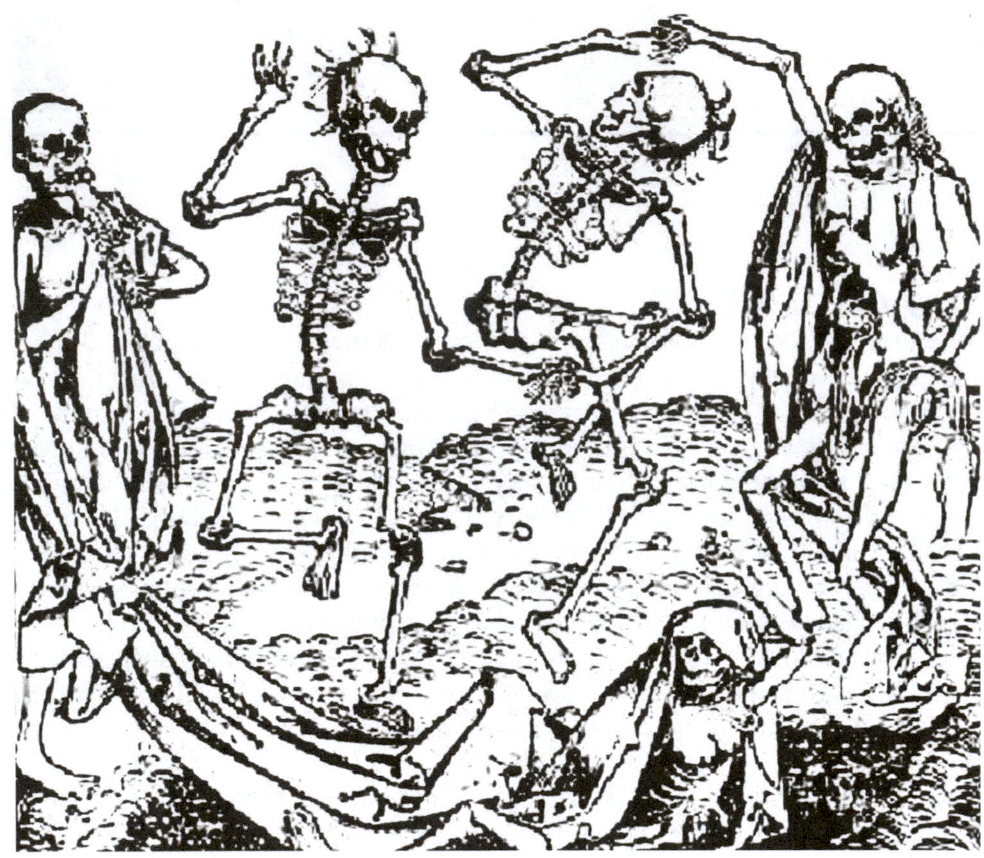

The Dance of Death, German woodcut by Michael Wolgemut for the *Nuremburg Chronicle* (1493). (Dover Pictorial Archives)

Further Reading

Eichenberg, Fritz. *Dance of Death: A Graphic Commentary on the Danse Macabre through the Centuries.* New York: Abbeville, 1983.

Gallery, Steven. "Dance of Death." In *Encyclopedia of Death and Dying*, edited by Glennys Howarth and Oliver Leaman (pp. 134–35). London: Routledge, 2001.

DARK TOURISM

The term "dark tourism" (sometimes referred to as "grief tourism" or "thanotourism") refers to the intriguing phenomenon by which sites of death and disaster become transformed into sites of popular tourist attraction. Most striking is the apparent incongruence between tourism (as a leisure pursuit associated with pleasure and enjoyment) and sites that were once host to grisly events involving pain, suffering, violence, and death. This incongruence is further amplified, and sits uncomfortably for some, by the fact that these sites have become commercial ventures on which death and suffering have themselves been turned into a commodity. The definition of dark tourism first coined by researchers John Lennon and Malcolm

Foley in 1996 has since been extended to include sites that are not only scenes of death and disaster, but also exhibitions that commemorate tragedy in which death and suffering are *re-created* (through artifacts, films, and simulations) as their core theme. Notable examples of dark tourism include Ground Zero in New York City; Arlington National Cemetery in Washington D.C; Alcatraz Prison in San Francisco; the Auschwitz concentration camp in Poland; and Elvis Presley's former Graceland home in Memphis, Tennessee.

Typologies of Dark Tourism

In order to understand death and dying at sites of dark tourism, attempts at presenting a comprehensive typology have resorted to classification of sites according to popularity, theme, or functionality. For example, the five most popular categories of dark tourism include the following:

- Holocaust tourism: travel to sites linked to the Holocaust, such as Nazi death camps in Eastern Europe (especially Auschwitz, which has its own visitor center); to Anne Frank's house in Amsterdam; or to Holocaust museums around the world (such as the United States Holocaust Memorial Museum in Washington, D.C).
- Battlefield tourism: visits to areas where significant battles were fought, including Gettysburg, Pearl Harbor, and Normandy (sites of battles involving the mass fatalities of World Wars I and II).
- Cemetery tourism: this represents the more gothic side of tourism that surfaced in the early 19th century, including sites such as Pere Lachaise cemetery in Paris (last resting place of former *The Doors* singer Jim Morrison); Arlington National Cemetery; and La Recoleta cemetery in Buenos Aries, Argentina (burial site of Eva Perón, Argentina's first-lady from 1946 until her death in 1952).
- Slavery-Heritage tourism (also known as "roots tourism"): this type of tourism extends throughout Africa, to villages such as Jufree in Gambia and Elmina Castle in Ghana, but has also included sites in the southern United States. It typically takes the form of visits and guided tours to former slave plantations, including the slave owner's mansions, slave quarters, and the remains of plantation buildings. Visitors, many of whom are African Americans, are encouraged to imagine the experiences of their ancestors through sensory stimulation of sight, smell, and touch.
- Prison tourism: institutions such as San Francisco's Alcatraz and Singapore's Changi Prison attract thousands of visitors a year because of their architecture and infamy. Many former prisons (including Karosta Prison in Latvia) now permit tourists to sample the experience of being a prisoner by spending several hours or even a full night behind bars in a simulated experience of prison life.

Shades of Dark Tourism

Attempts have been made to distinguish between different levels or degrees of dark tourism based on a site's proximity to death and dying. Some have argued that sites on which death and dying occurred can be distinguished in their intensity from sites that are simply memorials to death and disaster but in which death and disaster did not take place. For example, some argue that the "placeness" (and the feelings of deep emotional significance and attachment conjured by it) associated with a site such as Ground Zero—where thousands of lives were lost—is a place much "darker," and of greater emotional intensity, than a museum or memorial to death and disaster located in a space far removed from the actual site where death occurred (such as the collection of artifacts recovered following 9/11 that were temporarily displayed in the Smithsonian Museum of American History in Washington, D.C. to mark the 10th anniversary of the 9/11 attacks). Others, however, have rejected this distinction, arguing that the intensity of such an experience can be just as great, even if located thousands of miles from the site of death and disaster (think, for example, of Holocaust museums in Israel, such as Yad Vashem in Jerusalem).

The Significance of Dark Tourism

Growing public interest in "dark" sites as a lucrative source of tourist revenue and niche area within the broader field of mass tourism has sparked academic interest among scholars spanning the interdisciplinary domains of sociology, tourism, cultural studies, history, psychology, memory, and death studies. One way of making sense of dark tourism is as modern-day pilgrimage. Using this historical lens, what may seem as a uniquely modern and morbidly curious fatal attraction to sites of death and disaster can, however, be understood as an activity with a long and established provenance and thereby as an entirely normal (and not particularly recent) phenomenon after all.

Pilgrimage can be understood in this light as one of the earliest forms of tourism and is often associated with the death of significant individuals or groups in ways that are central to ethno-religious identity. The cultural-ideological significance of these sites is such that they transcend the particular individuals killed within them, providing a mythical function within the collective memory of particular groups. Take, for example, the ancient hilltop fortress of Masada in the Judean Desert overlooking the Dead Sea, which, as witness to the mass suicide of 960 Jews who chose death over surrender to the invading Roman army in AD 73, has, for some, become a potent source of Jewish national identity.

The media too may well have an important role to play in the spread of knowledge about sites that are sources of dark tourism; for it is often via the media in the first place that affective connections are forged with distant celebrities, whose sudden and unexpected deaths prompt the spontaneous outpouring of public mourning (see **Public Mourning**). As a corollary of public mourning, sites of fatal road traffic accidents (such as Pont de l'Alma in Paris, the scene of Princess Diana's death in 1997) or fatalities, such as the book depository in downtown Dallas, Texas (the site of President John F. Kennedy's (JFK's) assassination in 1963), themselves become tourist attractions (the former book depository is today a museum to the life of JFK and the fatal events of November 22, 1963). These sites, especially carefully choreographed museums, can also function as "transferential spaces" in which, as Alison Landsberg (2004, 113) puts it, drawing upon the notion of prosthetic memory, "people are invited to enter into experiential relationships to events through which they themselves did not live."

Together with recent popular interest in genealogy and the seeming desire to connect with one's ancestral roots, we can see how the media help to facilitate the vicarious experiences (of memory and grieving) that form part of the basis of dark tourism. Indeed, once we suspend the assumption that tourism is exclusively connected with the pursuit of pleasure and happiness, we can begin to see that dark tourism may also provide the potential to not only commemorate various losses but also begin to grieve them in ways that are also central to healing wounds from the recent and distant past.

Erin Dermody and Michael Brennan

See also: Body Worlds Exhibition; Holocaust.

Further Reading

http://www.dark-tourism.org.uk

Landsberg, A. *Prosthetic Memory: The Transformation of Remembrance in the Age of Mass Culture.* New York: Columbia University Press, 2004.

Lennon, John and Malcolm Foley. *Dark Tourism: The Attraction of Death and Disaster.* London: Thomson, 2006.

Sharpley, Richard and Philip R. Stone (eds.). *The Darker Side of Travel: The Theory and Practice of Dark Tourism.* Bristol: Channel View Publications, 2009.

DATABASES

The reporting of death and its circumstances is an important public health function that has been revolutionized by the advent of information technology. This has furthered the development of databases that contain large amounts of information about death. These databases are maintained by public local, state, and federal agencies as well as by private organizations. In the United States, individual states use the standard death certificate to report deaths. The standard death certificate includes details about the decedent (the person who has died) and the circumstances of their death, including the underlying cause. Preliminary data for 2010 indicates that there were 2,465,936 deaths resulting in a considerable amount of information needing to be collected and reported.

In the United States, there is no publicly available national database of death certificates. Instead, individual states have their own death certificate databases and rules governing the accessibility and confidentiality of death records. There are other types of death databases, including the Social Security Administration Death Master File (SSA-DMF), which contains the decedent's social security number, date of birth, date of death, state of residence, zip code of last residence, as well as zip code of where the last payment was received. The SSA-DMF, which contains death information for every individual with a social security number, is the only national-level death file that is publicly available. In addition to these death databases, others are maintained by public and private organizations including the Departments of Defense and Veterans Affairs, U.S. Census Bureau, state historical societies, the Church of Jesus Christ of Latter-day Saints, and genealogy organizations.

How Databases Are Used

There are several uses of death databases, the first of which includes a key function of tracking the vital status (i.e., whether a person is dead or alive) of individuals and groups. It is important to know the circumstances of death for an individual, but it is also valuable to be aware of national trends regarding the circumstances and underlying cause of death and how they vary according to the characteristics of the deceased.

Second, death databases have critical administrative uses. Knowing an individual's vital status is necessary for government and private agencies that administer income and health support programs such as Social Security, Medicare, unemployment insurance, pension, health, and life insurance programs. Accurate and comprehensive databases help prevent abuse and fraud and are needed to ensure that deceased individuals are not receiving benefits that are supposed to stop at death.

Third, there is today considerable popular interest in genealogy (tracing family histories and lines of descent), and with the burgeoning of the Internet there are many websites that offer both search services and software for constructing genealogies. An indispensable element of these services is the ability to search for deceased relatives. The SSA-DMF is the key component of any death records search, but there are other historical resources such as the U.S. Census and archival state death records that include death information. Many of these records are "paper only," but the number in electronic format is increasing.

Fourth, death databases are used by researchers, for whose studies, vital status is a key variable. This is especially true for investigations that have hundreds of thousands of subjects, thereby making it impractical to contact individual subjects or their families directly. The National Death Index (NDI) is a vital status search service available only to researchers and contains select elements of the death certificate. It is viewed as the "gold standard" for death reporting.

Concerns about Databases

Users of death databases, including genealogists, must be concerned about the completeness and accuracy of all databases, especially the SSA-DMF. When compared with the NDI, the SSA-DMF has performed favorably, but there may be underreporting of younger decedents, as they are less likely to have received Social Security benefits. Also, the SSA learns about deaths from many sources, including relatives and state vital statistics offices, some of which do not report to the SSA because of concerns over privacy.

Access to many current death databases is limited due to privacy rules, but advances in information technology offer great promise for developing historical death databases. Significant work is being done, but resources are needed to locate and digitize historical records and to construct electronic databases. Such databases will be of value to those individuals and organizations who want to better understand the "when" and "how" of death in the past as well as in the present.

Charles Maynard

Further Reading

Centers for Disease Control and Prevention. *National Vital Statistics Reports,* 60(4) (2012), Death: Preliminary Data for 2012. http://www.cdc.gov/nchs/data/nvsr/nvsr60/nvsr60_04.pdf

Cowper, D. C., J. D. Kubal, C. Maynard, and D. M. Hynes. "A Primer and Comparative Review of Major U.S. Mortality Databases." *Annals of Epidemiology,* 12 (2001): 462–68.

DAY OF THE DEAD

While uniquely expressed in different locales depending upon the particular culture, the Day of the Dead is most commonly celebrated as an annual multiday event between October 31 and November 2. As such, the holiday is often known as Days of the Dead, but frequently it is also referred to as All Saints Day. Presently, it is celebrated in Latin America; within Latino communities in the United States, Canada, and Europe; and in other regions of the world previously colonized by Spain (such as the Philippines). The origins of the holiday are disputed, with some scholars contending that it is pre-Columbian in origin, while others arguing that present-day practices were established in the 17th century.

Nowhere is the holiday more elaborately celebrated or renowned than in Mexico, where it is called *Los Días de los Muertos* (Days of the Dead). In Mexico, Days of the Dead practices include the public mocking of death. Humorous pageantry and parades satirize the solemnity of death in everyday life. Images of death, notably skeletons and skulls (*calaveras*), are made out of sugar candy and are festively portrayed as living beings going about daily tasks. Political cartoons poke fun at high-ranking officials, depicting them as skeletons and giving the holiday an atmosphere much like Carnival. Through these customs, the holiday is intended not only to honor the lives of the deceased, but also to alleviate the fear of death in the living.

Celebrants believe that the spirits of their dead loved ones return to them during the holiday. Upon this return, people welcome the spirits home by erecting altars to honor them. These altars are sometimes set up in people's homes, but it is also common for family members to prepare these altars on top of their loved ones' gravestones in cemeteries. During the Days of the Dead, gravestones are routinely washed, tidied up, and decorated with candies, beloved foods and beverages, photos, candles, and flowers. Families also spend weeks before the celebration baking sweet bread in different shapes, such as babies and ladders, to help spirits in the journey from one world to the next. In the Andes, home altars are often enclosed with tree branches with a designated entry for visiting spirits. Groups of children visit the homes of family members and friends where they recite Catholic prayers in front of the altars in honor of the deceased. Like Halloween trick-or-treaters, they often receive sweets or sweet breads for their efforts.

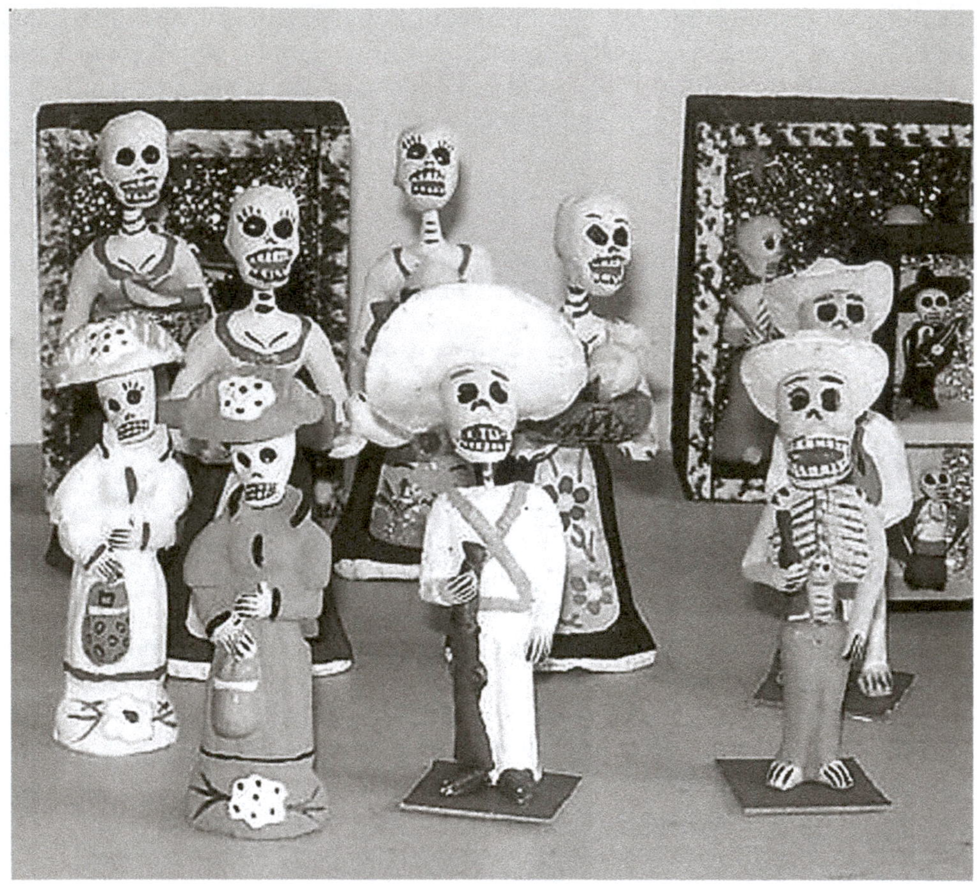

The Day of the Dead celebrations in Mexico have their roots in pre-Columbian Aztec and other native festivals memorializing departed loved ones. Modern traditions include the use of entertaining skeleton figurines to represent the hobbies and occupations of the deceased, whereas the Aztec and Mesoamerican portrayals were serious. (Judy King/http://www.mexico-insights.com)

Due to increased political, economic, and cultural connections within the Western Hemisphere, Day of the Dead celebrations have become widespread throughout the United States. Many people of Mexican or Latino descent find that the holiday ties them to their cultural heritage, while some people from Anglo-Saxon backgrounds participate because it allows them an outlet to talk about the life and death of their loved ones in a culture which, for most of the 20th century, repressed all expression of feelings engendered by loss (see **Death Denial**). Moreover, in a politicized environment where immigration has been highly scrutinized, many Latinos living in the United States use Day of the Dead practices as a vehicle of public political expression, asserting an ethnic identity that has often been maligned and "othered" in mainstream culture.

Christine Hippert

Further Reading

Brandes, Stanley. *Skulls to the Living, Bread to the Dead: Day of the Dead in Mexico and Beyond.* Malden, MA: Blackwell Publishing, 2007.

Marchi, Regina M. *Day of the Dead in the USA: The Migration and Transformation of a Cultural Phenomenon.* New Bruswick, NJ: Rutgers University Press, 2009.

DEATH ANXIETY

Attitudes toward death and dying have long been the focus of scholarly endeavors, though largely from a religious and philosophical perspective. The focused psychological study of attitudes toward death and dying, however, only began in the 1950s, and has gained considerable momentum since. Reflecting the core themes of the "death awareness movement" (see **Death Awareness Movement**), early research focused on the fear and anxiety precipitated by thoughts of death. Research was conducted with relevant groups, such as elders and physicians, producing results which suggest that the discomfort with death stemmed from a combination of individual factors (such as unconscious avoidance of personal mortality) and cultural attitudes (such as the denial of death) (see **Death Denial**). Although contemporary literature within the field of death and bereavement studies continues to focus on anxiety about death and dying, it has also grown to include the study of a broader range of attitudes toward death in different cultural settings. The result is a literature that has become more methodologically sophisticated, more topically diverse, and more practical in its applications.

The Problem of Measurement

Philosophers have long debated questions of whether the fear of death is intrinsic to human beings; the extent, if at all, to which this fear relates to anxieties about a painful process of dying; and concerns about what happens to us after death, especially the terror induced by the thought of nonexistence. Building upon these insights, psychologists have sought to devise rigorous scientific measures of attitudes toward death that not only permit the systematic study of such attitudes, but also move beyond metaphysical speculation by providing evidence-based knowledge about them. Early research on attitudes toward death used straightforward interviews, measures of fantasy (such as asking research participants to draw an image of death that was then evaluated for emotional tone), and projective tests (such as having participants tell stories about ambiguous death-related pictures). Few of these variables, however, were carefully assessed for their reliability or validity as scientific measures. By the mid-1970s, research on attitudes toward death became more rigorous, with questionnaires carefully constructed and designed to assess global death anxiety, threat, and fear. In the years that followed, instruments were developed to measure more subtle aspects of negative attitudes toward death, such as concerns about bodily deterioration, fear of premature death, anxiety about a painful and/or protracted dying, fear of nothingness or divine punishment, and concerns regarding the impact of one's own death on loved ones. Beyond these measures of anxiety, recent investigators have added scales to study death obsession (the tendency to ruminate about death and dying) and death depression (a sense of despair and resignation about mortality), as well as to assess reasons for death anxiety (such as death putting an end to our plans and objectives, disrupting our religious duties, or separating us from loved ones). Finally, researchers have begun to recognize that attitudes toward death are not limited to a negative preoccupation with mortality, but may also involve active behavioral avoidance, neutral acceptance of death as a part of life, as well as the active embracing of death as a form of release from a painful world or as positive anticipation of an afterlife as reward. Consequently, researchers are now better placed to study how people actively process the reality of death in human life.

Correlates of Death Anxiety

In the past few decades, literally thousands of studies of death anxiety have been conducted. The findings of these studies have identified some reliable trends as well as some ambiguous patterns. Some findings are predictable: physical and mental illness are both associated with greater anxiety about personal mortality. Others are contradictory or ambiguous, such as the inconsistent relationship between religious beliefs and the fear of death, with greater religious conviction predicting more intense anxieties in some studies and less intense fear in others. Finally, some findings are counterintuitive or remain largely unexplained. For example, as a group, elderly people are not more fearful of death than their younger counterparts, despite their greater statistical proximity to death, though they may show greater fears regarding what could happen in an afterlife. For whatever reason, women commonly acknowledge greater discomfort with death than men (particularly in terms of what death implies for bodily deterioration), a finding that tends to hold across ethnic and cross-cultural comparisons. Often, studies of the correlates of death anxiety have very practical application, such as the finding that hospice patients facing the end of life have increased fears of dying when they suffer more life regrets about what they did and did not do and when they feel unsupported by others. Such findings suggest the need to intervene with families at the end of life to review and validate people's life stories and facilitate forgiveness and support during this critical period.

Experimental Studies

Correlational and group-comparison studies are informative; however, only studies that control some variables, while manipulating or changing others, can determine the causes of death attitudes, per se. One example of this experimental approach concerns *terror management,* the psychological process by which people unconsciously moderate their fears of death through engaging in behaviors that enhance their self-esteem or reinforce their identification with cultural worldviews that serve as a kind of "buffer" against personal mortality (see **Terror Management Theory**). In a typical study, participants would first be subjected to either a *mortality salience* manipulation (such as watch a film on traffic fatalities or read material that highlights the frailty or vulnerability of the human body, or being asked to complete their own death certificate), or be assigned a neutral task (such as to describe their living room). Participants would then immediately engage in an unrelated task to distract them from consciously focusing on their feelings or thoughts, such as responding to a series of mathematical problems. Finally, they would be assessed in order to evaluate whether or not they manifest any of the attitudes or behaviors associated with attempts to guard against death anxiety, such as evaluating their performance more favorably relative to that of others or adopting more conservative political standpoints. Findings from terror management studies demonstrate that encounters with death can trigger a wide variety of social attitudes and behaviors, from recommending more severe penalties for drug offenders to prejudice against people who are culturally different, the latter of which indirectly reinforces mainstream cultural beliefs at the expense of others. Further, some of the findings are paradoxical: college students may be more prone to practice unprotected sex following a sex-education presentation on HIV/AIDS, and young men whose self-esteem is reinforced by aggressive driving may indeed drive more recklessly having been exposed to a curriculum on motor vehicle accidents, as if to boast their personal invulnerability. Findings such as these may help us to understand societal responses to events like terrorism, which can spark significant shifts toward conservative social and political attitudes and associated behaviors, ranging from greater religious participation to support for armed retribution against parties or nations perceived to be responsible.

Future Directions

With new measures and many real-world concerns motivating it, it is likely that the scope of research on death attitudes will continue to grow. For example, the study of attitudes toward death among children and adolescents that makes creative use of artistic and narrative methods. This may include the drawing of pictures of death as a personified figure, which are then analyzed to reveal developmental trends in boys versus girls. Another example would be the increasing diversity of populations studied, which extend well beyond the actual base of this research among American college students to include school children, health care workers, and medical patients throughout the world, both East and West. Future research holds the promise of elucidating trends in attitudes toward death in ways that transcend a single culture (such as the tendency for death imagery to become less violent and more abstract with greater maturity), as well as findings of specific relevance to a particular culture (such as the recognition of fears distinctively associated with bodily torture in the grave (*Azab Al-Kabr*) by people in the Islamic world, or increased separation worries regarding the death of a loved one among ethnic Chinese).

Robert A. Neimeyer and Ahmed M. Abdel-Khalek

Further Reading

Abdel-Khalek, Ahmed M. "Why Do We Fear Death? The Construction and Validation of the Reasons for Death Fear Scale." *Death Studies,* 26(8) (2002): 669–80.

Neimeyer, Robert A. (ed.). *Death Anxiety Handbook.* New York: Taylor & Francis, 1994.

Neimeyer, Robert A., Joachim Wittowski, and Richard P. Moser. "Psychosocial Research on Death Attitudes: An Overview and Evaluation." *Death Studies,* 28(4) (2004): 309–40.

Neimeyer, Robert A., Joseph M. Currier, Adrian Tomer, and Emily Samuel. "Confronting Suffering and Death at the End of Life: The Impact of Religiosity, Psychosocial Factors, and Life Regret among Hospice Patients." *Death Studies,* 35(9) (2011): 777–800.

Neimeyer, Robert A., Richard P. Moser, and Joachim Wittkowski. "Assessing Attitudes toward Dying and Death: Psychometric Considerations." *Omega,* 47(1) (2003): 45–76.

DEATH AWARENESS MOVEMENT

The death awareness movement is unlike other social movements to the extent that it is not a singular association but is made up of a diverse collection of individuals, groups, and organizations. Despite differences in emphasis and approach, what unites these sometimes disparate groupings is a shared ethos in the primacy, inevitability, and naturalness of human mortality as well as a shared belief in the potential risk posed to social relationships and psychological well-being if issues of death, dying, and bereavement are not addressed or engaged with in a fully transparent, honest, and mature fashion. The individuals and organizations that comprise the death awareness movement span a wide range of areas: from death educators and counselors, through self-help societies (such as The Compassionate Friends), to academic journals, research centers, and professional organizations (such as the Association for Death Education and Counseling) (see **ADEC (Association for Death Education and Counseling)**).

The origins of this movement, a movement rooted in thanatology (see **Thanatology**), can be traced to the late 1950s and the fledgling, if heterodox, academic interest in the topic of death and dying first stimulated by the symposium organized by Herman Feifel in Chicago in 1956. It was the publication, three years later, in 1959, by Feifel of *The Meaning of Death,* a collection of essays resulting from the symposium, that helped give impetus to the interdisciplinary study of death and dying in an academic arena that had, hitherto, been unreservedly cool on the idea of mortality becoming part of the formal curriculum of higher education.

By the 1960s, a group of individuals arguing in favor of a patient-centered, "whole-person" approach to care of the terminally ill had emerged outside of academia, providing a challenge to medical hubris, while at the same time issuing a clarion call for greater public awareness of the issues confronting the dying person and those caring for them. Spearheaded in England by Cicely Saunders—a clinically trained nurse, social worker, and physician—the modern hospice movement (see **Hospice Movement**) envisioned a form of care quite unlike anything that had gone before it, incorporating pain management and relief, spirituality, and greater choice and flexibility, in ways reflective of the dying individual's personality. The ideals of the hospice movement, consistent with those of the death awareness movement, were first realized in the opening of St. Christopher's hospice in London, England, in 1967. These ideals, although realized somewhat differently, were quickly spread to other parts of the Western world: to the United States by advocates of hospice care such as Elisabeth Kübler-Ross and William Lamers (where hospice was envisioned less as an institution than an ideal that could be realized in the patient's own home), and to Canada by Balfour Mount (where hospice was incorporated within the same physical structures of conventional hospital care).

The synergy created by these developments in academia as well as clinical practice helped sustain and grow the momentum of the death awareness movement so that, by the 1970s and beyond, ideas that had once appeared iconoclastic and somewhat *left field* had begun to permeate mainstream thinking. A reflection of the mainstreaming of these ideals can today be found in television documentaries and dramas whose explicit focus is death, dying, and bereavement (such as the PBS documentary *The Undertaking,* about Lynch and Sons family undertakers in Michigan, and HBO's highly acclaimed drama *Six Feet Under,* whose real-life inspiration was said to be the Lynch family firm); in the public debate about assisted dying and end-of-life care; and in the tremendous growth in academic and popular literature, academic courses, conferences, and research centers devoted to the study of dying, death, and bereavement.

The death awareness movement, however, has not been without its detractors, some of whom have accused it of creating a fetish and cult of death. Recent criticism has accused the institutional elements of the movement, such as the Association for Death Education and Counseling (ADEC), of profiting from other people's misery by promoting outdated models of grief and the need for clinical intervention in the treatment of grief, against a backdrop of evidence purportedly demonstrating the dubious efficacy of grief counseling for most people.

Michael Brennan

See also: ADEC (Association for Death Education and Counseling); Death Education; Grief Counseling; Hospice Movement; Right-to-Die Movement; Thanatology.

Further Reading

Davies Konigsberg, Ruth. *The Truth about Grief: The Myth of Its Five Stages and the New Science of Loss.* New York: Simon and Schuster, 2011.

Doka, Kenneth, J. "The Death Awareness Movement: Description, History, and Analysis." In *Handbook of Death and Dying, Volume 1,* edited by Clifton D. Bryant (pp. 50–56). Thousand Oaks, CA: Sage, 2003.

Neimeyer, Robert A. "The (Half) Truth about Grief." *Illness, Crisis & Loss,* 20(4) (2012): 389–95.

DEATH CERTIFICATION

Death certification is a process whereby the circumstances and mechanism of a victim's demise are officially codified and certified by the county clerk. The process is designed to serve two fundamental purposes: proving that a particular death occurred and how it was accomplished. The former is primarily for the benefit of the surviving next of kin, in that it provides information essential for tending to related matters such as settling the decedent's affairs, including probate, insurance paperwork, governmental and other benefits, and so on. The latter is of benefit to the state (Department of Vital Statistics) for purposes of providing statistical information by a jurisdiction's board of health showing overall population causes and manners of death. Such information may then be used in targeting governmental strategies to handle specific recognized and/or potential threats to the citizens' health and longevity. By following trends in such data, epidemiologists may recognize unusual patterns or anomalies that point to subjects meriting further scrutiny. For example, a cluster of pneumonia-related deaths may be the harbinger of an impending viral epidemic which might be minimalized or at least allow preparations to be made for the coming calamity. Population studies might similarly allow detection of an unusual number of deaths from heat-associated causes, signaling the impact of a heat wave and prevent further deaths by allowing governmental agencies to inform and educate the populace about potential dangers and possible preventive strategies.

Most death certificates are filled out by the attending physician of record, that is, the last doctor who treated the patient. For a document with such obvious and far-reaching significance, the qualifications required to complete the process are surprisingly minimal. Intuitively, one would assume that a physician would always sign the death certificate. Such is not the case, as Coroners are usually (but not always) elected politicians and in most jurisdictions typically have no requirement for any medical expertise at all, let alone the medical study of death. Regardless, in cases of sudden, unnatural, unexpected death and/or injury, the law usually requires the case be reported to the appropriate medicolegal investigator (MDI) authority (typically the County Coroner or Medical Examiner). Since most deaths start outside a hospital, it might be quite some time since a person was medically evaluated, meaning no personal physician with specific knowledge of the victim would be able to certify the death. Thus, an otherwise unsuspicious death might also be referred to the local MDI.

The physical design of the death certificate varies slightly, on a state-by-state basis, but it generally contains demographic data about the individual (date of birth, date and time of death, residence address, marital status, etc.), place of death, whether or not an autopsy was performed, means of body disposition (burial or cremation), and manner and cause of death. Manner of death is a short-hand means of categorizing the circumstances surrounding death, usually into one of five categories: natural, accident, suicide, homicide, or undetermined. Cause of death is a summation of how the death physically occurred, such as coronary artery disease (causing a heart attack), hypertension, or gunshot wound, to mention a few. The certificate provides several subheadings under the "cause of death" with the immediately lethal event heading the list, followed by several repeated "due to" clauses with additional spaces to allow the creation of a logical sequence of events explaining how the cause came to be. The sequence is most easily completed as a series of questions linked by the query "why did this occur?" For example, such a chain might be "ruptured myocardial infarction" due to "myocardial hypoxia" due to "arteriosclerotic coronary vascular disease" (ASCVD). The last line is also referred to as the proximate or initiating cause of death, in that it started the overall process. The certificate also provides a section allowing for entry of "other significant condition(s)" described as disease(s) contributing to death but not included in the former section (section 1), which might reasonably include hypercholesterolemia and diabetes mellitus in the cited example. Abbreviations such as ASCVD are discouraged, even though in common usage, in effort to maximize understandability and uniformity.

As a specialist in the medical analysis of death, the forensic pathologist (or medical examiner) is singularly and uniquely qualified to correctly certify the true underlying medical cause of death, ideally informed by a physical examination of the body, including autopsy. The public health significance of such official documentation would seem to mandate such a standard of excellence. Regrettably, such is often not the case. Most physicians are not specialists in the medicine of death but rather are appropriately concerned with saving life and might tend to see the completion of the document as an additional burden and/or a reminder of an unsuccessful outcome, particularly if not well familiar with a patient's recent health status and terminal events. Little actual time is devoted in medical school to the process of accurate death certification. As such, simple errors may creep into the document, such as inversion of underlying causes such that the proximate cause is listed at the top. More significant errors occur if an attending doctor, believing a patient to be in good health, assumes the death had to have occurred from a single catastrophic event and incorrectly generically assigns the cause as pulmonary embolism rather than performing a careful review of the available medicolegal investigative data.

Surprisingly, nonphysician elected coroners are empowered by law to certify death as part of the duties of the office, thus nonmedical practitioners routinely certify the medical parameters of the death certificate *by design* as the result of the surviving Dark Ages Office of the Coroner. Not surprisingly, information gleaned from death certificates may be viewed with skepticism, as there is no assurance of any level of standardization with regard to any medical information (even if an autopsy is performed, the result can be ignored, modified, or editorialized upon by whomever is legally charged with completing the certificate). Even if an attending physician does certify the death based upon personal knowledge of the patient, studies have consistently shown a major discrepancy (upward of 20 percent) between such a clinical determination and that made by an autopsy pathologist actually conducting an independent medical examination. The danger is that critical public health information may be erroneously determined based on personal preference of the certifier rather than objective evidence, as for example, if one routinely assigns a generic cause of death as hypertension or heart disease without conducting sufficient investigation to support such a conclusion. Similarly, if unqualified or underqualified practitioners incorrectly certify deaths, serious public health threats such as infectious diseases and even homicides, may go undetected.

James Claude Upshaw Downs

See also: Cause of Death; Coroner/Medical Examiner.

Further Reading

DiMaio, V.J. and D. DiMaio. *Forensic Pathology: Practical Aspects of Criminal and Forensic Investigations,* 2nd edition. Boca Raton, FL: CRC Press, 2001.

Hanzlick, R., J.C. Hunsaker, and G.J. Davis. A Guide for Manner of Death Classification. National Association of Medical Examiners, 2002.

Hoyert, D.L. and J. Xu. Deaths: Preliminary Data for 2011. National Vital Statistics Reports, 61(6) (2012). U.S. Department of Health and Human Services, Centers for Disease Control and Prevention, National Center for Health Statistics, National Vital Statistics System. http://www.cdc.gov/nchs/data/nvsr/nvsr61/nvsr61_06.pdf

National Center for Health Statistics. Physicians' Handbook on Medical Certification of Death, 2003 Revision, Department of Health and Human Services. National Center for Health Statistics, Centers for Disease Control and Prevention National Center for Health Statistics, Hyattsville, MD. http://www.cdc.gov/nchs/data/misc/hb_cod.pdf

National Center for Health Statistics. Vital Health and Statistics: Education Reporting and Classification on Death Certificates in the United States, 2(151) (2010). Hyattsville, MD: U.S. Department of Health and Human Services, Centers for Disease Control and Prevention. http://www.cdc.gov/nchs/data/series/sr_02/sr02_151.pdf

Spitz, W.U. and D.J. Spitz. *Spitz and Fisher's Medicolegal Investigation of Death: Guidelines for the Application of Pathology to Crime Investigation,* 4th edition. Springfield, IL: Charles C. Thomas, 2006.

DEATH DENIAL

Human beings know they will die, and, according to existential philosophers, psychoanalysts, and other psychodynamically oriented behavioral scientists, it is the knowledge of one's own mortality which produces a fear of death that would paralyze humans were it not possible to repress such awareness. It is the repression of the fear of death, and thus the "denial of death," which has been identified by scholars in these fields of study as the fundamental motive at the core of human thought and action. Death denial, like the concept of denial more generally, has its origins in the work of Sigmund Freud, the founder of psychoanalysis (see **Freud, Sigmund**) and refers to the defense mechanism by which a person attempts to deal with a traumatic perception by denying its reality.

As the unconscious refusal to accept reality, aspects of denial can be found in the grieving behavior following the death of those we love (bereavement), as well as in the reaction to the news of one's own impending death. In his classic 1917 essay "Mourning and Melancholia," Freud illustrated how the loss of a love object is never willingly abandoned but is always met with an (un)conscious resistance that involves a "turning away from reality" and a "clinging to the object through the medium of a hallucinatory wishful psychosis." In her study of terminally ill patients, Elisabeth Kübler-Ross noted that the first of the five stages through which the dying patient passes is that of denial. In this stage, Kübler-Ross described a situation in which, the dying patient, when confronted with the news of his or her own mortality would react with a sense of shock, numbness, and disbelief; a denial that manifested itself as "no, not me!"

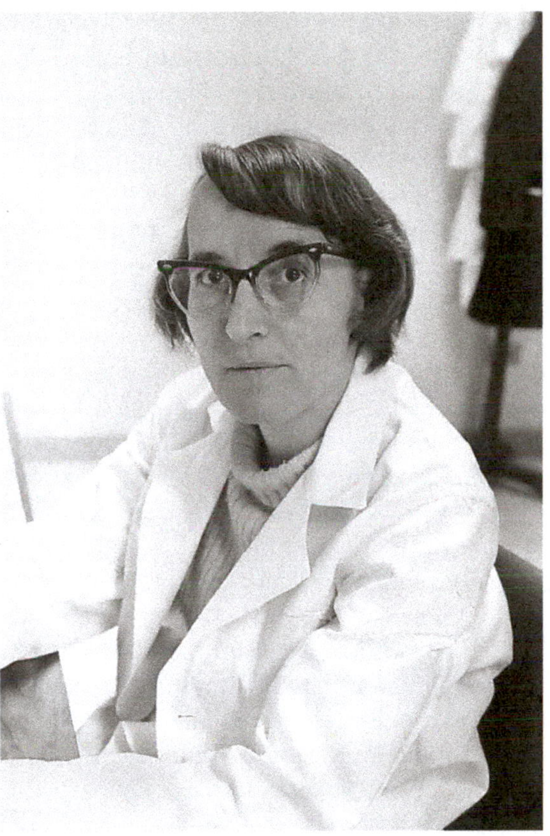

American psychiatrist Elisabeth Kübler-Ross, 1970. (AP/Wide World Photos)

Robert Kastenbaum has suggested that we think of death denial along a continuum that extends from complete denial of death to complete acceptance. Kastenbaum has argued that few individuals engage in complete denial or acceptance, that partial denial is the more normal response, and that denial can prove adaptive if it is not overused. Further, fears elicited by an awareness of one's own mortality are not uniform across all people. Thus, some people's fear may not be of death itself but of the *process* of dying (for instance, in pain, isolated, and without dignity), while other people may fear the loss of relationships and how their death will adversely affect their loved ones.

Sociologists and anthropologists refer to a culture's death ethos—its composite stance or position on death—as providing a sense of order and meaning that serves as a societal bulwark against the potential chaos and meaninglessness heralded by death. Commensurately, a society's death ethos influences the individual's stance toward death. In his influential book *The Denial of Death*, cultural anthropologist Ernest Becker extended this notion of a death ethos through his assertions that successful cultures provide usable frameworks that enable individuals to fend off the fear of death. These frameworks provide plausible narratives to deny death's ultimate significance. Two examples of such frameworks would be the Buddhist assessment that existence is an illusion of suffering overcome when one becomes enlightened and enters *nirvana;* and the Christian assessment that existence is transformed by the life, death, and resurrection of Jesus Christ and the promise of everlasting life to followers of the faith.

Kastenbaum has further delineated a societal response to handling the reality of death by describing what he refers to as "the death system." For the most part, this system keeps death away from impinging upon most people's everyday existence, and hence from conscious awareness. The death system thus functions in four key ways: (1) by preventing, where humanly possible, death from happening—thus, we have medical research to cure fatal maladies; (2) by taking care of, and sequestering from public life, dead bodies—thus, we have the funeral industry, cemeteries, and crematoriums; (3) by providing frameworks for reflecting upon the meaning of death—thus, we have religious systems of beliefs and philosophical approaches for making sense of human mortality; and (4) by sanctioning, in some countries, state executions—thus providing explicit guidelines about how people convicted of capital crimes may be put to death.

The works of Ernest Becker and existentialist philosopher and writer Albert Camus have illustrated how all cultures develop myths about heroic responses in the face of death, elevating to prominence individuals whose courageous actions make them heroes by creating meaning in the face of chaos and absurdity. Similarly, in his book *The Hero with a Thousand Faces,* American mythologist Joseph Campbell details how the myth of the hero permeates all human cultures, primitive and modern, and how, in all cases, these hero myths emphasize individual accomplishment in the face of ultimate threat.

This mythic expression of the hero defying death raises the question of whether the hero is repressing the fear of death, and the answer seems obvious: rather than denying death, the hero is openly, consciously addressing this threat to his or her existence. The myth of the hero, whatever form it takes, exemplifies what Becker meant in his seminal book about successful cultures developing frameworks to fend off the terror of extinction.

Within contemporary society, the biomedical model of health care, with its focus on curative repair, has made death the ultimate enemy. The denial of death emerges in medical centers when a life-threatening illness defies effective treatment or cure; and doctors and nurses scatter to other parts of the hospital. And yet in the midst of such institutionalized death denial—which encompasses the fear of death and the fleeing from its reminders—there exists a hospice movement which openly acknowledges that a terminally ill person is dying. Here, particular emphasis is placed on the importance of keeping in mind that the individual is a living human being, with efforts made to enable the person to achieve a "good death" through attempts to alleviate the multidimensional manifestations of pain (see also **Hospice Movement; Palliative Care**). It is thus possible to perceive the modern hospice movement as providing a specialized form of what Becker identified as a cultural framework for enabling people to deal openly with death and dying.

Terror Management Theory (TMT) is a burgeoning area of psychology that builds upon Ernest Becker's notion of death denial. TMT maintains that humans defend themselves against conscious awareness of death (mortality salience) because death presents a formidable challenge to a person's ultimate sense of self-worth. Death, in effect, offends a person's self-esteem, rendering the individual impotent. Thus, for TMT, the denial of death is a matter of the person fending off the end of existence, which, as absolute nothingness, represents ultimate meaninglessness. TMT researchers use various approaches to understand how an awareness of one's own mortality affects people and their behavior. For instance, researchers may have some participants read sentences that compel them to briefly ponder their own mortality, while other participants (the control group) read sentences with no discussion of their own mortality. Both groups are then given a set of non-death-related statements to evaluate. TMT researchers insist that exposure to mortality-laden sentences produces significantly different answers to other sentences that are read subsequently. In response to a series of open-ended questions following exposure to one's own mortality, research has demonstrated that participants are, for example, more likely to: recommend harsher penalties for moral offenders; show preference for people who praise their country over those who criticize it; and physically distance themselves from foreigners.

Evidence does not support the sweeping assertion that human beings are always on guard against the fear of death. There are too many encounters with death to keep the awareness of it from consciousness, and these encounters do not result in psychic collapse or in a retreat from the awareness of mortality. Perhaps, it is more correct to say, following Kastenbaum, that societies and individuals engage in a partial denial of death; and there is evidence that some people reach a point when death no longer terrifies them.

David E. Balk

Further Reading

Becker, E. *The Denial of Death.* New York: The Free Press, 1973.

Hayslip, B. "Death Denial: Hiding and Camouflaging Death." In *Handbook of Death and Dying, Volume One: The Presence of Death,* edited by Clifton D. Bryant (pp. 34–42). Thousand Oaks, CA: Sage, 2003.

Kastenbaum, R. *Death, Society, and Human Experience,* 7th edition. Boston: Allyn and Bacon, 2001.

Solomon, S., J. Greenberg, and T. Pyszczynski. "Terror Management Theory of Self-Esteem." In *Handbook of Social and Clinical Psychology: The Health Perspective,* edited by C. R. Snyder and D. R. Forsyth (pp. 21–40). Elmsford, NY: Pergamon Press, 1991.

DEATH EDUCATION

A plethora of topics can be grouped under the umbrella term "death education." These topics are broad in scope, including areas spanning attitudes toward death, dying, and bereavement; funeral and mortuary practice; and hospice, palliative care, and end-of-life issues. These topics are studied from a multidisciplinary perspective that includes sociology, psychology, history, anthropology, biomedicine, philosophy, social work, and theology. Within writings on death education it is common to find these topics organized into a framework of *formal* and *informal* death education.

Informal Death Education

Informal death education takes place within the context of "teachable moments" that emerge from the experiences of day-to-day life. Impromptu moments, such as finding a dead insect on the street, provide opportunities for death education that typically involve interactions between parents and children. Such interactions may be conversations, while others may take the form of children simply observing how parents and other family members cope with death-related matters (see **Children**)

Efforts to bridge these opportunities for informal death education with more structured approaches include the use of media, such as books, television, and a host of online resources, each of which present useful opportunities for parents to discuss death with their children. Other instances of informal death education involve mostly adults. Examples include instances in which one is compelled to inquire about advance directives, writing a will, planning a funeral, or learning one has a terminal illness. A minister's reflections on the meaning of life when conducting a funeral, provides another common example of informal death education. These moments include both explicit and tacit messages that inform participants of what is expected when death is near.

Formal Death Education

There are today a wide variety of workshops, courses, and webinars (online seminars) organized to provide death education. One writer, Samuel Blumenthal, has asserted that, at the end of the 20th century, formal death education was occurring in nearly every public school in the United States. This statement stands in stark opposition to Illene Cupit, President of the Association for Death Education and Counseling (ADEC), and her assessment that death education classes are still relatively rare in middle and high school. When offered in public schools, formal death education at the elementary and secondary level has aroused fierce opposition from political conservatives and from fundamentalist Christians. People concerned about death education that targets children and adolescents commonly assert that death education should occur only in the home and express fears that death education may involve the teaching of values that may be contrary to those held by parents.

Many colleges and universities in the United States offer courses on death, dying, and bereavement. These courses range from undergraduate surveys of thanatology to integrated graduate curricula leading to Master's degrees or advanced certificates. Many colleges and universities offer these courses in fully asynchronous online mode. Because physicians and nurses will more likely come into contact with death than most other members of society, some medical and nursing programs offer education for communicating empathically about death.

Formal approaches to death education are guided by explicitly stated learning objectives. These learning objectives comprise both *cognitive* outcomes (for instance, "the student will understand how people in different cultures organize funerals" or "the student will analyze and evaluate arguments about physician-assisted suicide") and *affective* outcomes (for instance, "the student will voluntarily seek out material about coping with loss and grief" or "the student will listen attentively to diverse points of view about death").

Charles Corr and his colleagues identify six goals in formal death education:

1. Enriching the lives of students
2. Informing people about options available when dealing with death
3. Preparing students to act as engaged citizens on social issues pertinent to death and dying
4. Offering a framework for people whose professional careers center on thanatology
5. Strengthening competency to communicate about death, dying, and bereavement
6. Examining how attitudes toward death-related matters interplay with development across the life span

Formal death education opportunities are also available outside the college campus. These educational offerings may, for instance, occur as part of a series of lectures in a community organization (such as the YMCA) or as training for volunteers working with the dying and the bereaved (such as those provided by hospice programs for their staff and volunteers).

Leading figures in formal death education emphasize that, at its core, such education emphasizes life and living. This focus on living mirrors the emphasis of hospice: that dying individuals are first and foremost living human beings (see **Hospice Movement; Palliative Care**). Death education also mirrors another core element of the philosophy underpinning hospice, namely, the holistic dimension of human existence. Thus, formal death education, focusing on celebrating the value of human life, looks at the various dimensions in which human life is expressed and experienced: the physical, the behavioral, the emotional, the cognitive, the interpersonal, and the spiritual.

The number of peer-reviewed journals which focus on thanatology has increased to meet scholars' and practitioners' burgeoning interest in death, dying, and bereavement. An incomplete list of English language peer-reviewed journals focused on thanatology is given in Table 1, along with the country where the journal is published. The table is organized in descending order based on how long the journal has been in operation.

There are concerns over the knowledge, skill level, and preparation of people who come to the assistance of people who are traumatized or bereaved. These concerns have prompted ADEC to design and administer an exam assessing a person's basic understanding of core issues in thanatology. ADEC has also published a key text, *Handbook of Thanatology,* now in its second edition, setting out the essential body of knowledge for the study of death, dying, and bereavement.

David E. Balk

Table 1 English Language Thanatology Journals

Name of Journal	Country Where Published	Year Started
Omega: Journal of Death and Dying	United States	1970
Suicide and Life-Threatening Behavior	United States	1970
Death Studies	United States	1977
Bereavement Care	United Kingdom	1981
Illness, Crisis, and Loss	United States	1991
Mortality	United Kingdom	1996
Grief Matters	Australia	1997

Further Reading

Balk, D., Wogrin, C., Thornton, G., and D. Meagher (eds.). *Handbook of Thanatology: The Essential Body of Knowledge for the Study of Death, Dying, and Bereavement,* 2nd edition. New York: Routledge, 2013.

Bertman. S. L. *Facing Death: Images, Insights, and Interventions.* New York: Hemisphere, 1996.

Corr, C. A. and D. M. Corr. "Death Education." In *Handbook of Death and Dying. Volume 1: The Presence of Death*, edited by C. D. Bryant (pp. 292–301). Thousand Oaks, CA: Sage, 2003.

Corr, C. A., C. M. Nabe, and D. M. Corr. *Death and Dying, Life and Living,* 6th edition. Belmont, CA: Wadsworth, 2009.

Marks, S. C. and S. L. Bertman. "Experiences with Learning about Death and Dying in the Undergraduate Anatomy Curriculum." *Journal of Medical Education,* 55 (1980): 48–52.

Noppe, I. C. "Death Education." In *Encyclopedia of Death and the Human Experience,* edited by C. D. Bryant, and D. L. Peck (pp. 316–18). Thousand Oaks, CA: Sage, 2009.

Sofka, C. J. "Ethical and Legal Issues and Death Education." In *Handbook of Thanatology: The Essential Body of Knowledge for the Study of Death, Dying, and Bereavement,* edited by D. Balk, C. Wogrin, G. Thornton, and D. Meagher (pp. 355–67). New York: Routledge, 2007.

DEATH MASK

A death mask is a wax, plaster, or clay cast taken of a dead person's face soon after death. This cast is used to make a reproduction of the face of the deceased to provide a memento for bereaved survivors or to create a portrait of the dead person. Death masks also function as *memento mori,* from the Latin phrase "Remember, you must die," a reminder to the living that death awaits us all, that we are mortal, similar to the message of the death's head, or human skull, found on early gravestones (see **Memento Mori**).

History

The making of a death mask is an ancient practice, going back to early Egyptian and Roman cultures. Notable historical figures for whom death masks were created include Julius Caesar, William Shakespeare, Napoleon Bonaparte, George Washington, Abraham Lincoln, and John Dillinger, to name just a few. In some cases, the "death" mask was, strictly speaking, a life mask, created while the person was still alive.

In ancient Egypt, where mummification of the body was an important part of the funeral process, a special element of death rites was the creation of a sculpted mask that would be placed on the face of the dead person. The best known example of this is the mask prepared for Tutankhamen, the youthful Egyptian king who died around 1352 BCE.

In European culture, by the Middle Ages, a shift had occurred from the use of sculpted masks to the creation of actual death masks. These were typically of royalty and nobility, as well as of other eminent persons, such as poets and philosophers. Examples of this latter category include Dante, Pascal, and Voltaire.

With the death of Isaac Newton (1643–1727), the creation of a death mask, formerly an honor reserved for members of royalty and the nobility, was extended to an ordinary citizen, a testimony to his human genius as well as the changing social values of the Enlightenment.

Effigies and Postmortem Photography

The death mask is related to the effigy, a representation or image of a person. Although an effigy may be created for either an alive or a dead person, historically the term refers to a more or less life-like model, composed of wicker and waxwork, which could be used ceremonially, primarily to honor dead kings. Although a simple death mask is created during the making of an effigy, this mask is simply a technical aid in the modeling process.

Death masks also bear similarity to postmortem photography. Both death masks and postmortem photographs have been used for identification purposes, as well as for the making of mementos or portraits (see **Photography**).

Resusci Anne

A fascinating story about death masks concerns Resusci Anne, or CPR Annie, a model used since the beginning of cardiopulmonary resuscitation (CPR) training in the 1960s and still the most popular CPR manikin face.

The designer of Resusci Anne is Asmund Laerdal, a Norwegian toy maker, who had also devised artificial wounds for use in military training. When his friend, Dr. Peter Safer, the father of CPR, asked him to design a device for the new CPR training, Laerdal agreed to participate.

Laerdal decided that the best way to learn resuscitation would be to practice on a manikin; all that was needed was the perfect face. While visiting his parents, Laerdal noticed a mask of a woman's face on their wall. This image was actually a death mask known as "L'Inconnu de la Seine," which means "the unknown woman of the Seine."

This mask is of a beautiful young woman who apparently died by suicide in the river Seine in Paris around the late 1880s. After she was pulled out of the river, workers at the Paris Morgue were struck by her beauty and decided to memorialize it by creating a death mask. Over time, as reproductions of the death mask became available, people, captivated by her beauty and her unknown identity, began to display the mask as art in homes across Europe. Her beguiling smile has been compared to the enigmatic smile of Mona Lisa, whose portrait was painted by Italian Renaissance artist and polymath, Leonardo da Vinci.

Now, because of her death mask, the unknown beautiful young woman who drowned is symbolically resuscitated, again and again, in CPR classes around the world.

Albert Lee Strickland

Further Reading

Benkard, Ernst. *Undying Faces: A Collection of Death Masks.* Translated by Margaret M. Green. New York: W. W. Norton, 1929. http://www.undyingfaces.com

DEATH NOTIFICATION

Death notification involves communicating the news to an individual that a loved one has died. Understandably, such notification will leave survivors in a state of shock, experiencing all of the intense emotions that sudden death elicits: denial, anger, and anxiety. Hearing bad news leaves people feeling powerless, defenseless, and vulnerable. Honest and compassionate communication about the death can enable survivors to understand the death, and gain some measure of control and even comfort in knowing what happened, how it happened, and why it happened. It is for these reasons that death notification should be done sensitively and with much care. Failing to do so can leave a lasting emotional scar that may never heal. While it may seem logical, being brutally honest is often seen as being insensitive. Likewise, trying to "spare someone's feelings" by being dishonest is likely to elicit a great deal of anger and shock, in that one has been lied to.

The process of notifying someone that a loved one has died is an inherently difficult task. Indeed, firefighters, emergency personnel, nurses, doctors, police officers, military personnel, and others who are often in a position to break news of death are often left to rely on their own skills. It is because these personal skills alone are often inadequate that many personnel are trained in breaking such news in a supportive and empathic manner. This training may also include learning how to manage the emotional impact that communicating such distressing news can have on the notifier. Many such deaths are by their very nature, traumatic. People may die in war, in a motor vehicle accident, have been murdered, or have drowned. Often, next of kin are far away, adding to the shock that they feel when learning about a family member's death. As a general rule, those who are most likely to be impacted by the death should be informed first, and the individual who notifies these people should, unless circumstances prevent it, do so in person. When information is provided over the phone, the individual should be careful about providing too much information all at once and to schedule a meeting with the family as soon as possible as a follow-up. This is important because little may be known about the family's circumstances and their emotional responses to the death.

For death notification to be most effective, yet compassionate and sensitive, the following guidelines should be observed: (1) ask family members what they already know about the situation; (2) based upon what they do know, provide a brief, but accurate description of the events that led up to the person's death; (3) give information about efforts made to save the person's life; (4) conclude with a statement about the person's death; and (5) provide a brief explanation about the likely cause of death. This approach to notification is termed the "sequential notification technique." This technique allows the individual to prepare the family fully for the news of death, allowing for what is said to be coordinated with the family's emotional responses to it, which in effect gives them the time to anticipate and prepare themselves for the shock of bad news.

In the process of death notification, if a family requests to do so and have been prepared for what they might see, the family should be allowed to view the body. This should be done carefully, especially when the death was violent or disfiguring, as may be the case with murder, suicide, or death by fire. This is often an intrinsically painful process, and the people present (e.g., a coroner, chaplain, or medical examiner) should only show what survivors ask to see.

Bert Hayslip Jr.

Further Reading

DeSpedler, Lynne A., and Albert L. Strickland. *The Last Dance: Encountering Death and Dying,* 9th edition. Boston: McGraw-Hill, 2011.

Leach, R. Moroni. *Death Notification: A Practical Guide to the Process.* Hinesburg, VT: Upper Access, 1994.

Stewart, Alan E. and Janet Harris Lord. "The Death Notification Process: Recommendations for Practice, Training, and Research." In *Handbook of Death and Dying: Volume Two,* edited by Clifton D. Bryant (pp. 513–22). Thousand Oaks, CA: Sage, 2003.

DEATH OBSESSION

Death obsession is defined as repetitive thoughts or ruminations, persistent ideas, or intrusive images that are centered around death of the self or significant others. One can speculate about the existence, and extent, of individual differences in obsession about, and dominating thoughts of, death. The notion of death has a central role in the life of humans from the beginning of recorded history. One of the most distinguishing characteristics of human beings is their ability to grasp the concept of a future, and the inevitability of death. Concern for death can be traced back to ancient Egypt. The Harper's Song in the tomb of the ancient Egyptian King, Intef, succinctly puts the human relationship to death as follows:

None come from there
To tell of their state
To calm our hearts
Until we go where they have gone

Despite this universal cultural focus on death, little psychological attention was paid to attitudes toward death until the aftermath of World War II. It was then that thanatology (the study of death and dying) emerged as a legitimate domain of scientific inquiry. Most psychological research on death-related topics has been dominated by studies of death anxiety. However, some researchers have begun asking whether anxiety is the only significant emotion that people experience in relation to death.

Death Depression

In the 1990s, a group of researchers introduced the concept of death depression and constructed a scale to measure it. Death depression can be defined as the sadness or sober reflection associated with one's own death, the death of significant others, and the concept of death more generally. A correlation has been identified between depression and death. Clinicians have reported their impression that there is a particular stage and a strong element of depression that occurs during the process of dying. Many researchers have also demonstrated a close relationship between death, depression, and bereavement. Depression and its relationship with death is the fourth stage of Elisabeth Kübler-Ross's famous five stages of dying (see **Kübler-Ross, Elisabeth**). Furthermore, existential philosophers identified a similar phenomenon in the overwhelming sense of despair, meaninglessness, and absurdity in connection with human finitude (see **Existentialism**).

Death Obsession

It was not until 1998 that a third component in death distress was identified: death obsession. This element was intended to complement areas of research that have investigated death anxiety and death depression.

In modern literature, there are a number of examples depicting the domination of death obsession in the lives and novels of creative men and women. As has been noted by psychoanalysts, the Czech writer Franz Kafka (1883–1924) displayed his obsession with death, and the process of dying, in his novels, stories, and autobiographical works. Virginia Woolf (1882–1941), the British novelist and critic, never resolved her obsession with the cumulative, untimely deaths of her parents and older siblings and, in her writings, engaged in a perpetual mourning of these and other psychological losses for most of her life. Woolf eventually completed suicide. The British poet Philip Larkin (1922–1985) wrote an *aubade* (a poem appropriate to the dawn or early morning that usually speaks of happiness and love). Larkin's poem, however, is anything but happy, as it too reflects an obsession with death.

The writings of Sigmund Freud are chiefly concerned with the twin topics of sex and death, topics which, in the 19th and 20th centuries respectively, were highly taboo (see **Freud, Sigmund**). In particular, Freud asserted that underlying concerns with these topics dominated the unconscious thoughts of all humans, often in ways that determined and served as a guide to human action. By examining references to death, whether implicit or explicit, in various aspects of culture (including novels, theater, music, film, and television), we can begin to see that most people, to varying degrees, are routinely, if unconsciously, preoccupied with thoughts of death and dying.

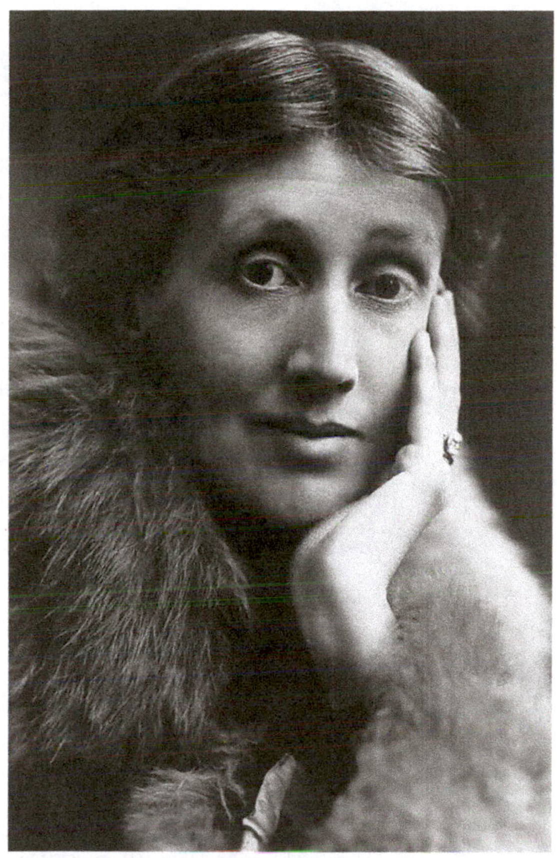

Themes of death and mourning pervade the work of British feminist writer Virginia Woolf, one of the most important writers of the early 20th century, reflecting an underlying preoccupation with death and its meaning for life. (Library of Congress)

Assessment of Death Obsession

Apart from analyzing literary documents, diaries, and autobiographies, psychologists have used the Death Obsession Scale as the major tool of assessment. This scale has good psychometric characteristics, producing valid and reliable findings in a variety of different countries. Arabic and British studies using this scale have identified three factors: (1) death rumination, (2) death domination, and (3) death idea repetition. These factors are reflected in the following sample items included in surveys administered to research participants:

- The idea that I will die dominates me.
- I fail to dismiss the notion of death from my mind.
- I find myself rushing to think about death.
- The recurrence of the idea of death annoys me.

Correlates of Death Obsession

In its relatively short history, a number of studies have found a correlation between death obsession and the following variables: death anxiety, death depression, obsession-compulsion, general anxiety, general depression, neuroticism, and religious orientation. It has also been found that female and male anxiety-disorder patients exhibit higher mean scores on death obsession than the following groups: normal (nonclinical) participants, patients suffering from schizophrenia, and addicts of various kinds. Other studies have found that college students, both male and female, from Arab countries (Egypt, Kuwait, Lebanon, and Syria) had higher mean death obsession scores than did their Western counterparts from Britain, Spain, and the United States.

Future Directions

Inasmuch as death obsession is a relatively new concept, there is a need to investigate its correlates with personality, especially with what psychologists regard as the five core personality traits (neuroticism, extraversion, openness to experience, agreeableness, and conscientiousness), as well as with factors that include, but are not limited to, individualism/collectivism; religiosity; thoughts of, and attempts at, suicide; and demographic variables such age, sex, and socioeconomic status.

Ahmed M. Abdel-Khalek

Further Readings

Abdel-Khalek, Ahmed M. "Death Obsession in Arabic and Western Countries." *Psychological Reports,* 97 (2005): 138–40.

Abdel-Khalek, Ahmed M. "The Structure and Measurement of Death Obsession." *Personality and Individual Differences,* 24 (1994): 159–65.

Abdel-Khalek, Ahmed M. and David Lester. "Death Obsession in Kuwaiti and American College Students." *Death Studies,* 27 (2003): 541–53.

Maltby, John and Liza Day. "The Reliability and Validity of the Death Obsession Scale among English University and Adult Populations." *Personality and Individual Differences,* 28(4) (2000): 695–700.

DEATHBED SCENE

The deathbed scene is the site of death, the place where dying occurs. It may be in the home, a hospital, a nursing home, a hospice facility, or some other location. Unlike the case with accidental and other sudden deaths, deaths that are characterized by the term "deathbed scene" are generally anticipated and occur in settings in which family members and caregivers are present.

Traditional Deathbed Scenes

"I see and know that my death is near": Thus did the dying person during the early Middle Ages acknowledge impending death, anticipated by natural signs or by inner certainty. The dying person offered his or her suffering to God with the expectation that everything would take place in a customary manner.

The elements and characteristics of the traditional deathbed scene were codified in writings on the art of dying called *ars moriendi* (see **Ars Moriendi**). The family, along with clergy, the doctor, and any other interested persons who were in attendance, had secondary roles in the deathbed scene. Attention was focused on the dying person. And that person's attention was, in turn, focused on those who were present at the deathbed scene.

Marked by a simple and solemn ceremony, dying occurred within the context of familiar practices. The principal participant was the dying person. Ideally, each person, especially family members and close friends, would be summoned to the bedside to be given a farewell, perhaps some advice, and a final blessing. Finally, the dying person turned his or her attention away from the earthly realm and toward the divine. Nothing more need be said: The dying person was prepared for death.

In the later Middle Ages, there were subtle changes in the deathbed scene. In addition to the presence of public participants, there now hovered an invisible army of celestial figures, angels, and demons, battling for possession of the dying person's soul. Death became the *speculum mortis,* the mirror in which the dying person could discover his or her destiny by tallying the moral balance sheet of his or her life. The moment of death became the supreme challenge and ultimate test of an entire lifetime.

In later centuries, with the rise of scientific rationalism, a secular hope for immortality and reunion with loved ones became more important than churchly images of heaven and hell (see **Heaven; Hell**). Religion became less prominent in the thoughts of the dying person and the grief of survivors. The focus changed from the dying person to his or her survivors (see **Ariès, Philippe**).

Modern Deathbed Scenes

By the turn of the 20th century, the deathbed scene was becoming a more private event. The emotional focus was narrowed to the immediate family. Medical technology, shifting disease patterns, professionalization, urbanization, and other demographic changes influenced the deathbed scene. Technology brought about a medicalization of dying and the deathbed scene, which moved from home to hospital. The deathbed scene became subject to the control of health care professionals (see **Medicalization**).

By the mid-20th century, the traditional rituals of dying had been overtaken by a technological process whereby death happens by a series of little steps, which tend to diminish the great dramatic act of death (see **Definitions of Death**). These little steps have been characterized as a process resulting in the dying person's "fading away."

The latest chapter of the modern story of dying is perhaps best termed *managed death.* Even when a prognosis of death has been accepted by medical staff and families, and when further treatments intended to cure have been put aside, there may nevertheless be a strong desire to manage the situation so that it comes out "right." Death becomes an efficiency issue. Scholars describe trajectories of dying, patterns of physical decline and dying that are intended to be useful for understanding patients' experiences as death approaches (see **Dying Trajectory**).

Dying persons are likely to find themselves surrounded by sophisticated machines, monitoring such biological functions as brain wave activity, heart rate, body temperature, respiration, blood pressure, pulse, and blood chemistry. Signaling changes in body function by light, sound, and computer printout, such devices often determine the nature of the deathbed scene. Family and friends may be distanced from the patient who is dying.

In the 21st century, the deathbed scene is certain to undergo further change, stimulated in part by initiatives in end-of-life care, such as hospice and palliative care (see **Hospice Movement; Palliative Care**), approaches that offer opportunities for dying persons and their families to find renewed meaning in the last acts of a human life.

Albert Lee Strickland

Further Reading

Kastenbaum, Robert. *The Psychology of Death* (especially chapter 7), 3rd edition. New York: Springer Publishing, 2000.

Kastenbaum, Robert and Claude Normand. "Deathbed Scenes as Imagined by the Young and Experienced by the Old." *Death Studies,* 14(3) (1990): 201–17.

Warton, John. *Death-Bed Scenes and Pastoral Conversations.* 3 Volumes, edited by his sons. London: John Murray, 1830. http://www.archive.org/stream/deathbedscenesa02woodgoog#page/n6/mode/2up

DEFINITIONS OF DEATH

Death of a person is the end of his or her life; and, although all living persons die, one's definition of life may influence when the exact end of life is reached. Two hundred and fifty years ago, in the first *Encyclopaedia Britannica,* death was defined as the separation of the soul and body. In more recent years, the end of life occurred when a person's heart stopped beating. Yet, with the technological advances of today's life support systems, a person's heart can go on beating despite the fact that a person cannot eat, think, or breathe on his own. An understanding of the *process* of death may therefore be aided by considering the stages of death, which include clinical, brain/cortical, and cellular death.

Clinical Death

In clinical death, the heartbeat stops. Oxygen carried by the blood no longer circulates throughout the body, and a bluish tint occurs (livor mortis). Nevertheless, a person can be revived in this stage of death. For example, immediate cardiopulmonary resuscitation (CPR), which involves mouth-to-mouth breathing and chest compressions, can bring a person back to life. To prevent irreversible brain damage, however, CPR should begin within about 4 minutes of when the heartbeat first stopped. To avoid brain death, CPR should begin within about 15 minutes of the last heartbeat. It is in this stage that people report near-death experiences (see **Near-Death Experiences**).

Brain Death

The next stage is that of brain death. A common procedure to test brain death is the electroencephalogram (EEG), which measures brain voltage. Even a person in a deep coma will show some electrical activity in the brain, but a dead brain will not. A flat line is shown on the EEG to indicate brain death. In addition to a flat EEG for at least 10 minutes, medical personnel use some of the following to signal brain death:

- Pupils of the eyes are fixed when a bright light is shone into them.
- No oculocephalic ("doll's eye") reflex, which means that the eyes remain fixed when the head is turned from side to side.
- Unresponsiveness to painful stimuli.
- Physician observes no movement for a continuous hour and no breathing after three minutes when removed from a respirator.

These determinations are checked twice, with most clinical authorities calling for six hours to elapse between the first and second determinations of brain death for adults. For children up to one year, as much as 24 hours is the recommended time.

The breakthrough for this concept of death occurred in 1968 when a committee of the Harvard Medical School proposed the nonreversible loss of brain activity should be the definition of death. A flat reading on the EEG and lack of blood circulation in the brain were added to the above four indications. This approach to defining death is known as "the Harvard criteria." This definition won acceptance by the American Medical Association and, in 1981, the definition was incorporated into a new Uniform Determination of Death Act, which gained nationwide application.

Akin to brain death is cortical death, also called a persistent vegetative state (PVS), which is a permanent brain dead condition. In this condition, severe brain damage, in which a person has progressed to a state of wakefulness without detectable awareness, occurs. A fairly recent, and much publicized, case of PVS involved Terri Schiavo who, in 1990, at age 26, collapsed at her home in St. Petersburg, Florida, and never recovered. She entered into a coma and was kept alive by technological advances of the time for three years before she was officially diagnosed as being in a PVS. Nevertheless, her "wakefulness" persuaded her parents that she could recover.

Schiavo's legal guardian was her husband, Michael, who, eight years after her original collapse, petitioned the state courts to remove her feeding tube. Her parents objected. A series of state and federal court actions ensued, with the case resulting in 14 appeals and petitions. Finally, her feeding tube was removed (for the third time), and she died 13 days later of dehydration on March 31, 2005. The Schiavo case raised ethical questions about the "right to die" (see **Right-to-Die Movement**) and prompted many people to make their end-of-life wishes known to their family members through an advanced directive; that is, a living will or a medical power of attorney (see **Advance Directives**).

Similar to brain death for determining the exactness of death is "eye death." As an unknown physician in the 1950s, Dr. Jack Kevorkian (see **Kevorkian, Jack**) who was later nicknamed "Dr. Death" for his work in helping people complete suicide, asked nurses to call him when a patient's death was impending. He wanted to be at the patient's side at the moment of death to peek into the eyes of the patient, because he believed that the condition of the eyes provided the most accurate basis for determining death. He assessed that, at the time of death, the eye had interruption of blood circulation, as well as paleness and a haziness of the cornea. Dr. Kevorkian asked other physicians to determine death like he had by examining their patients' eyes with an opthalmoscope. Few followed his suggestion, then or now. Determining death, predominately by a flat line of an EEG, prevailed.

Cellular Death

Cellular death refers to the gradual death of a cell after all metabolic activity has stopped at the point of a person's death. The rate of cellular death varies according to the type of tissue involved. For example, brain cells typically die 5 to 8 minutes after respiration stops, but kidney cells die after about seven hours. Hair and nail cells die after several days. Rigor mortis, the temporary stiffening of muscles (see **Rigor Mortis**), is associated with cellular death. In cellular death, no one can be brought back to life, unlike in the clinical stage of death. Eventually, all parts of the body decompose and leave behind only the teeth and skeleton.

Ways of Conceiving Death

Even with these distinct stages of death, questions may still remain, depending upon whether death is thought of as an event, a condition, or a state of nonexistence.

- **Death as an event:** Events happen. Regarding a death event, death cuts off life at a particular time. Moreover, time, place, and cause can be recorded on a death certificate.
- **Death as a condition:** In this usage, death is a nonreversible condition in which the person cannot carry out the vital functions of life. This usage of the word death is close to the first usage; that is, as an event.
- **Death as a state of nonexistence:** In this term, death is not conceived of as an event or condition but thoughts are instead geared toward what becomes of someone who has died. In other words, in this state, thoughts center on the form of existence after death.

It is important to realize that people do not always talk about death in the same way. Physicians typically focus on determining the instant at which life ends—the event or condition—while a grieving family member is often more concerned about the family member being gone; that is, being nonexistent. Adding to the potential confusion is that death may not happen all at once but gradually and in increments.

Death Redefined?

Someone who is breathing, talking, and walking around is clearly alive. In contrast, a body that is rotting obviously signifies death. *What* constitutes death has, therefore, always been quite clear; that is, the end of a life, with no mental, emotional, physical, or social functioning, the final stage of which is decomposition. But, regardless of attempts by attorneys, clergy, physicians, and philosophers, *when*, exactly, death is deemed to occur depends on medical technologies or a person's belief system or his or her culture. By and large, in the United States and other developed countries, brain death is accepted as the definition of death, even if the heart continues to beat by way of artificial means for some time afterward. Yet, in some countries, Japan, for example, brain death is not widely accepted. In the United Kingdom, it takes the independent judgment of two physicians before someone can be declared dead. In Islamic doctrine, death is not complete as long as the spirit continues in any part of the body. Among persons of the Hindu faith, birth, death, and rebirth (i.e., reincarnation) are cyclical, meaning persons are born to die but die to be reborn (see **Reincarnation**). Possibly, one day, as technological advances continue beyond what can presently be imagined, and are extended globally, death will have to be redefined and could be similar across cultures.

Dixie Dennis

Further Reading

Dennis, Dixie. *Living, Dying, Grieving.* Sudbury, MA: Jones and Bartlett Publishers, 2009.

Kastenbaum, Robert. *Death, Society, and Human Experience,* 10th edition. Boston: Allyn & Bacon, 2008.

DEVIL

A name used by Christians to denote the leader of evil spiritual beings who are adversaries of God and tempt humans. The devil is alternately known as *Satan, Lucifer, Beelzebul, Beliar,* or *Leviathan.*

The term devil is derived from the Greek word "διάβολος" (accuser or slanderer) and was adopted by early Christians who added the definite article (ό διάβλος) to transliterate the term Satan, meaning adversary in Hebrew. In the Hebrew Bible, the word *Satan* is used to describe humans, an angel, or a member of the heavenly court.

While belief in the existence of personified evil—identified in ancient and living religions as demons, devils, evil spirits, or even gods—it was only during the post-exilic era that Israel developed a sense of malevolent spiritual beings dwelling independent of God. Belief in the existence and influence of evil spirits was prominent during Jesus's lifetime; sickness and physical harm were blamed on malevolent forces, also deemed capable of struggling within the human soul and tempting people to do evil.

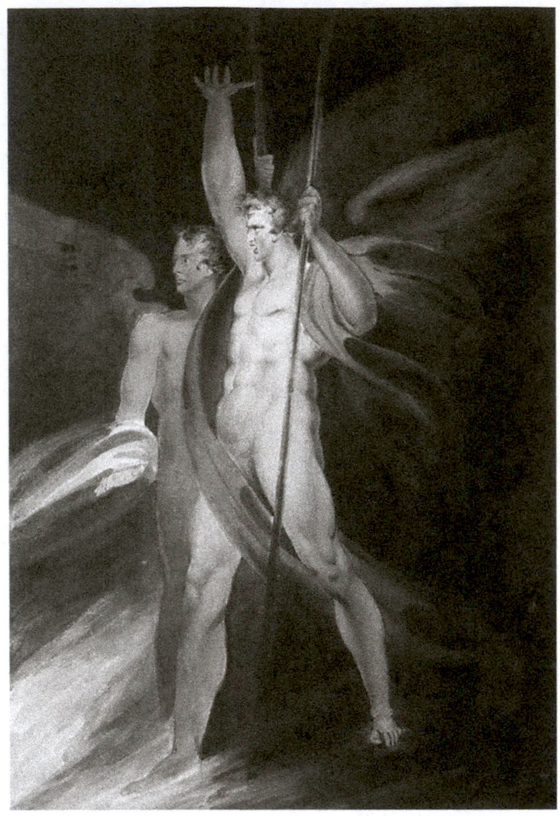

***Satan Exulting* by Richard Westall (1765–1836). Pencil and watercolor. (Christie's Images/Corbis)**

Jews and Christians of the first centuries CE believed that devils were the descendants of angels and human women. Christians later sensed that Satan was a prideful fallen angel who conscripted confederates and now worked to bring human souls to eternal torment, an idea also found in Islam. Since the time of Justin Martyr, the serpent that tempted Eve has been associated with Satan.

Christians retain a belief in the devil's malfeasance; the possibility of human possession and Satan's power to tempt people. Rejection of Satan is professed by Catholics prior to baptism. In modern cultures, mental illness is no longer associated with demonic possession, but is instead most often ascribed to the human subconscious.

Regina A. Boisclair

Further Reading

Kelly, Henry Ansgar. *Satan: A Biography.* Cambridge: Cambridge University Press, 2006.

Oldridge, Darren. *The Devil: A Very Short Introduction.* Oxford: Oxford University Press, 2012.

DIGNITAS

Dignitas is a not-for-profit organization based in Zurich, Switzerland, which provides assistance to people wishing to engage in voluntary euthanasia, providing the lethal drugs so that they may voluntarily choose to end their own life. Since it was founded in 1998 by human rights lawyer, Ludwig Minelli, Dignitas has helped more than 1,000 people from over 60 countries end their lives by suicide. Dignitas has taken advantage of Switzerland's unusually liberal laws on assisted suicide, whereby an individual cannot be prosecuted for helping a person to die unless there is a selfish intent (such as helping a relative to die to get his or her inheritance). Underpinned by a philosophy of self-determination, in which individuals should have sovereign right to decide whether or not to take their own life, Dignitas has courted controversy by helping people die who have expressed a repeated desire to end their lives, including those who are not terminally ill (such as 23-year-old Daniel James, who was paralyzed while playing rugby).

Dignitas operates a rigorous policy of screening people who contact them with a view to ending their own lives. This process, which involves a review by an independent physician of the case presented by the person for ending their own life, culminates in the creation of an affidavit, which is countersigned by independent witnesses and provides legally admissible proof that the person wishes to die. In cases where an individual is physically incapable of signing (such as those with advanced motor neuron disease or ALS), Dignitas makes a short video to document a person's desire to die, in which they are asked to confirm their identity and that the decision was made freely and without duress (see also **Informed Consent**).

On the day of a person's anticipated death, and minutes before a lethal overdose is voluntarily ingested, the individual is reminded that the overdose would kill him and he is asked if he still wishes to proceed, giving him the opportunity to change his mind. After drinking an antivomiting drug to prepare the stomach, the individual drinks a lethal cocktail of barbiturate (pentobarbital) that works by depressing the central nervous system, resulting first in drowsiness and eventually in respiratory arrest, usually within about half an hour. Although Dignitas is a nonprofit organization, it nevertheless charges a fee for the preparation and assistance of helping a person terminate her own life. Because the services of Dignitas are open to nonresidents of Switzerland, it attracts foreign nationals from countries where assisted suicide is not legally permitted, such as Germany, the United Kingdom, and France. It is for this reason that Dignitas has been seen as providing a haven for "suicide tourists." The work of Dignitas, and the journey of some of those seeking to end their lives by assisted suicide, is the focus of John Zaritsky's 2007 documentary film, *The Suicide Tourist*.

Michael Brennan

See also: Physician-Assisted Suicide.

Further Reading

The Suicide Tourist. Directed by John Zaritsky. Vancouver: Point Grey Pictures Inc., 2007.

DISASTERS

Disasters are defined as sudden, unpredictable, and uncontrollable events that wreak major destruction. The Federal Emergency Management Agency (FEMA) lists three categories of disasters: (1) natural disasters, such as hurricanes, floods, mudslides, and avalanches; (2) accidental disasters, such as fires, explosions, and motor vehicle accidents; and (3) human-made or technological disasters, such as industrial accidents and acts of terrorism. Disasters are environmental stressors, which, by their very nature, are capable of ripping apart communities and changing people's lives forever. The devastating results of a disaster are immeasurable in terms of physical injuries, loss of loved ones, and destruction of property. Sometimes, disasters, depending on the level of severity, can become national disasters. This occurred with Hurricane Katrina and the terrorist attack on New York and the Pentagon on September 11, 2001.

Seeking Information

Factual information about how a loved one died in a disaster becomes critically important for family and close friends. Survivors will want to know the specific details surrounding the death of a relative. However, it is unlikely that all of a survivor's questions will be answered and this may delay and/or compromise the grieving process. Some people affected by disaster may gain some comfort, and perhaps even a sense of "closure," from visiting the area where the disaster occurred and loved ones died. However, the length of time between the occurrence of a disaster in which a loved one died and the visiting of the disaster scene will differ among survivors.

Media

Media coverage of disasters can always be expected. However, the media has a tendency to sensationalize news. It may be painful and traumatizing for survivors to watch repeated airing of a disaster that has taken a loved one's life. Reporters may want to interview disaster survivors about their losses and reactions. Although it

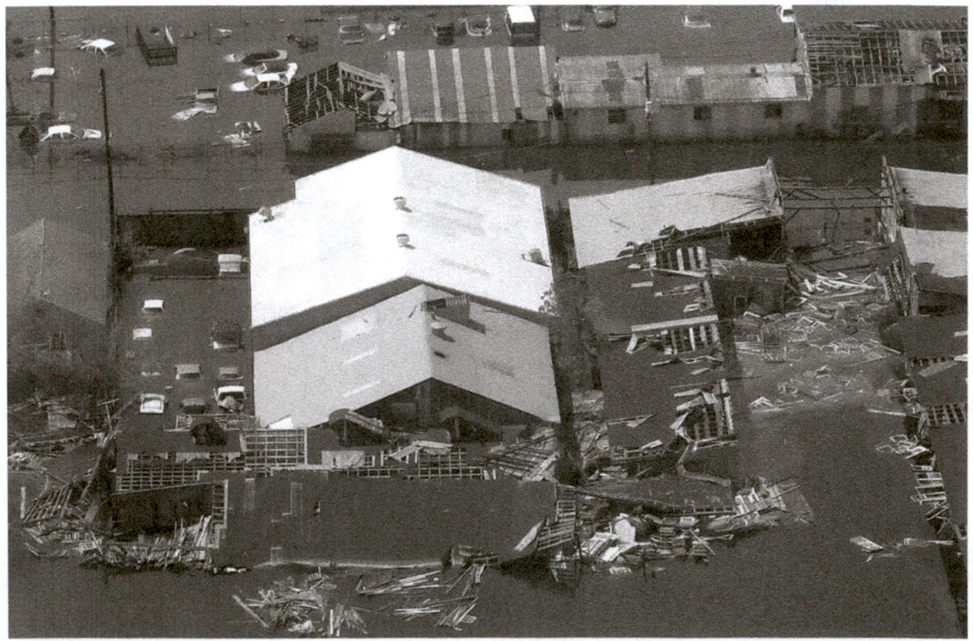

Aerial view of homes in New Orleans engulfed in floodwaters in the aftermath of Hurricane Katrina on September 4, 2005. (U.S. Department of Defense)

may be tempting to participate in radio or television interviews, some people who have spoken to the media have later come to regret it. Assessing one's motivation for talking to the media, and talking to someone else before agreeing to participate, may be wise.

Common Reactions to Death after a Disaster

The process of mourning the loss of a loved one after a disaster and healing emotional wounds takes time. A wide range of responses and reactions usually follow the loss of a loved one after a disaster. Recovery and healing are complicated and delayed by the stress associated with any related issues, such as lawsuits or criminal trials. Reactions may vary depending upon contextual factors that are related to the individual, the environment they inhabit, and the event itself. Expectable reactions can be categorized as emotional, cognitive, behavioral, and physical. If any of these reactions continue to be a problem more than a month after the disaster, it is important that the person seeks professional help. The following are some reactions that confront survivors.

Shock and Numbness: Immediately after learning about the death of a loved one in a disaster, some people feel profound numbness, often likened to "being in a fog." A sense of shock can render some individuals helpless and hopeless. Others may report denial, disbelief, and an inability to cope. When there is little or no warning before a disaster makes landfall, disbelief, bewilderment, and a refusal to accept the reality of the situation are likely to develop.

Chaotic Memories: When the shock subsides and numbness wears off, survivors' emotions can become chaotic. Disaster survivors sometimes describe themselves as being on a rollercoaster. Flashbacks of when the notification of the death of a loved one was delivered and/or the last time the loved one was seen may flood the minds of survivors. Feelings of restlessness and an inability to concentrate can also interfere with daily activities.

Depression: As the reality of the death of a loved one sinks in, depression may follow. Life may seem meaningless and tasks that were once enjoyable may become burdensome. Survivors may feel as if there is little point in living; they may lose interest in social activities and may avoid contact with others. Seeking the help of professionals becomes important during these times; and talking to someone who listens empathically can reduce feelings of sadness.

Guilt: Survivors often describe feelings of guilt for having survived a disaster and may feel that they do not deserve to live. Some people may feel responsible for the loss of a loved one or they may feel that they could have stopped the death from occurring. It is normal to speculate about what could have been done differently. Sometimes, feelings of guilt and self-blame are legitimate, especially when parents feel that they could have taken better precautions to protect their children. It is also not unusual for children to feel that they caused the disaster by their actions and thoughts.

Anger: Anger is a normal reaction that may develop after a disaster. It may be directed at the government, the emergency system, or an airline. After Hurricane Katrina, many residents of New Orleans were unhappy with the Federal Emergency Management

Agency (FEMA) for not doing enough to warn local residents to evacuate the city. Close family members and friends may also be blamed for not doing enough to protect the deceased. It is also common to be angry with God or a higher power for allowing the disaster to happen, and some people may even feel guilty about feeling angry. Anger diminishes with time and with the help of appropriate support.

Physical Reactions: Physical disturbances in sleep and appetite occur commonly. Some people may report having a poor appetite, and even when they are able to eat, they may experience nausea or stomach aches. Others may want to eat constantly, seeking comfort in junk food. Similarly, while some people may want to sleep a lot, others may have difficulty falling asleep. Dreams of the dead and hopes that they will walk through the door are also common. Some survivors experience spasms of grief and cry constantly, while in contrast, some people may find that tears are not possible because the hurt is so profound.

Mourning after disasters usually involves a whole community, since many people are affected at the same time. The commonality of the experience provides opportunities for sharing and increased understanding. However, it can also amplify one's own feelings of loss, as one observes the reaction of others in the community.

Stages of Mourning and Loss after a Disaster

Mourning is a physical expression of grief, which is influenced by cultural factors. Four key tasks have been identified by grief theorists, including (1) acceptance of the reality of the loss by coming to terms with the fact that the loved one will no longer be physically around (this acceptance eliminates denial of the death of a loved one); (2) grieving and its physical expressions (crying, yelling, or ruminating), which allow for a full experience of loss; (3) adjusting to an environment in which the deceased is "missing" (which can be challenging for survivors, as they have to find new ways of coping, and may have to adopt new roles in a loved one's absence); and (4) withdrawing emotional energy from the deceased and investing in new relationships. However, the latter can be experienced as a betrayal of the deceased and has been modified and revised by contemporary theorists of grief and bereavement (see **Bereavement**). Through supportive grief programs, survivors can, however, learn how to acknowledge and accept that, although the loved ones may no longer be here, they are not forgotten.

Funerals after a Disaster

Funerals serve several purposes. They provide rituals that give survivors opportunities to celebrate and honor the lives of those who have died. They also provide an important opportunity for mourners to receive social support from family, friends, and the wider community; as well as giving individuals permission to express their grief publicly, surrounded by those who love and care for them. Funerals are the symbolic acknowledgement of loss and this acknowledgement plays a central role in the healing and recovery of survivors, especially those who experience the loss as traumatic. Moreover, the religious rituals that are sometimes included in funerals provide survivors with opportunities for a sense of spiritual and psychological closure.

However, disasters that overwhelm local resources may very well compromise survivors' abilities to arrange funerals. This happened in New Orleans after Hurricane Katrina in 2005, where the traditional jazz funeral is a time-honored and distinguishing aspect of New Orleans' culture. Here, the funeral typically lasts a week, features jazz bands and parades, and draws big crowds. However, this tradition was interrupted when Hurricane Katrina fragmented many of the communities that make New Orleans funerals so extraordinary. The floods that claimed so many lives in New Orleans also forced the city's institutions that are responsible for managing death (such as funeral homes, churches, and cemeteries—part of what Robert Kastenbaum has described as the "death system") to close down. The sheer number of fatalities made the task of providing each deceased individual with a New Orleans-style burial almost impossible, and for thousands of survivors, the inability to provide loved ones with a traditional funeral filled them with guilt and complicated their grieving.

Support to Survivors

A disaster brings most family members closer together. However, it is not unusual for some family members to become physically and emotionally distant following the death of a relative. Communication is thus very important after a disaster and family members need to express their feelings and provide support to one another. When this is not possible, support has to be sought from those outside the family, such as from friends, voluntary agencies, or professional providers.

The Importance of Anniversaries

Recognizing and acknowledging feelings that may surface around the anniversary of a disaster and the death of a loved one is a crucial part of the recovery process. Efforts to remember this special time and to do something to acknowledge the significance of the anniversary can have a healing effect. Survivors should seek healthy ways to cope with the distress that emerges during this critical period by spending time with family and friends in order to share memories and feelings of loss.

Contemplative practices too, such as walking, meditating, praying, journaling, and scrap-booking can provide bereaved individuals with much needed solace during a challenging time in their lives. Crucially, in order to heal, survivors need to allow themselves enough time in which to do so.

Conclusion

Remembering the dead and acknowledging that they are no longer with us is very important for bereaved individuals following disasters. Funerals and other burial practices are important traditions to uphold, as these rituals may help people deal with traumatic grief by providing structure and stability, increasing feelings of personal power and control, and adding meaning to the experience of loss. Additionally, rituals create a sense of community and give bereaved individuals an opportunity to integrate their loss as they receive acknowledgement, support, and acceptance from people who care. Most survivors are able to heal and resume their lives, but this is a challenging and tumultuous process and each person is unique in terms of the amount of time they need to heal. Some may use their own experiences to engage in volunteer work by joining national relief organizations, like the American Red Cross, in order to offer support to those who experience similar losses after a disaster.

Priscilla Dass-Brailsford

Further Reading

Brennan, M. "Finding Meaning in Disaster," *ADEC Forum,* 37(2) (2011): 6–7.
Brennan, M. *Mourning and Disaster: Finding Meaning in the Mourning for Hillsborough and Diana.* Newcastle: Cambridge Scholars Publishing, 2008.
Dass-Brailsford, P. (ed.). *Crisis and Disaster Counseling: Lessons Learned from Hurricane Katrina and Other Disasters.* Thousand Oaks, CA: Sage, 2009.
Dass-Brailsford, P. *A Practical Approach to Trauma: Empowering Interventions.* Thousand Oaks, CA: Sage, 2007.
Zinner, E. S. and M. B. Williams (eds.). *When a Community Weeps: Case Studies in Group Survivorship.* Philadelphia, PA: Brunner and Mazel, 1999.

DISEASE

A disease is a disruption of the normal physical functioning of the human body causing a person to be ill or unwell. When someone is ill there are warning signs and symptoms that prompt the person to seek medical help. Some diseases such as colds and influenza are described as *acute* because of their rapid onset and resolution. In contrast, *chronic* diseases, such as heart or lung failure, usually progress slowly and may affect a person's functioning for several months and even years. Since 1900, there has been a major decline in deaths from acute infectious diseases such as pneumonia, influenza, and tuberculosis. The major causes of death today are heart failure, cancer, and respiratory diseases. While research continues to uncover causes of disease, it is now apparent that environmental factors play a key role. For example, people who were exposed to asbestos in the construction industry have been found to suffer from asbestosis (scarring of the lung tissue); asthma has been linked to traffic pollution; and lung cancer has been linked to tobacco use, both directly through smoking and indirectly, through passive smoking (either in the home or in workplaces such as bars and nightclubs). Excessive alcohol use in combination with smoking has been implicated in some forms of oral cancer.

While there are incurable diseases that ultimately lead to death (see **Terminal Illness and Care**), most diseases in the developed world today can be cured, prevented, or controlled. It is in less developed countries that certain diseases persist due to shortage of medical resources, including diagnostic technology, vaccinations, and treatment and medication. Socio-environmental factors also influence the incidence and severity of disease. These factors may include a lower standard of living with inadequate infection control, poor nutrition, and sanitation. Despite advances in medical research over the past century, there are still many diseases, including autoimmune conditions, certain types of cancer, and neurological conditions, for which there are no known causes or cures.

Management of Disease

Once a doctor diagnoses the condition for which help is being sought, treatment may consist of support and advice, prescribed medications (such as antibiotics for a bacterial infection), surgical procedures, counseling, or a combination of these. Sometimes, further investigation such as blood tests, X-rays, and medical imaging are needed to identify the particular causes and the extent of an illness, as well as to determine the most effective course of treatment. Referral by a family physician or general practitioner to a specialist in a particular branch of medicine can be arranged when the need arises. For example, when cancer is suspected, a referral will be made to an oncologist, or in the case of heart disease, a cardiologist will usually be consulted.

While not all chronic conditions are curable, they can often be well managed with a number of strategies and drug regimes. Diet and exercise, and complementary therapies such as meditation and relaxation, are also used by patients to mitigate the effects of both their illness and its treatment.

Chronic Disease in Old Age

As the population ages and medical technology continues to improve, there is an increasing (and growing) number of elderly people with multiple chronic illnesses, though these may be successfully managed in ways that prolong and improve the quality of life. Chronic illnesses may flare up into periodic acute episodes that may result in brief hospital admissions to relieve symptoms and to develop new treatment protocols. For example, an elderly person with a chronic heart condition might experience an acute episode with heart palpitations and high blood pressure, leading to the surgical insertion of a pacemaker to regulate the heartbeat. They may be subsequently discharged with medications that will help prevent similar episodes. Although death will be the inevitable outcome, the life of the older person is significantly prolonged and quality of life enhanced (see **Aging**)

Chronic Disease and Mortality

Diseases such as cancer and HIV/AIDS are increasingly being described as chronic rather than acute diseases. The mortality rates for these diseases have been considerably reduced over the past three decades. Where a diagnosis of HIV/AIDS was once thought of as a “death sentence,” the availability of antiviral drugs has transformed the disease into a well-controlled chronic condition which allows many affected patients a much higher quality of life and greater longevity than previously (see **HIV/AIDS**). Similarly, more than 80 percent of cancers today are curable and treatments are constantly being developed and improved. While chemotherapy and radiation treatments for some forms of cancer can still produce serious side effects such as nausea, hair loss, and lowered immunity, there are medications and complementary therapies that aim to enhance well-being and reduce the damaging effects of treatment.

Historically, acute illnesses and epidemics have always led to a higher incidence of death. However, the leading causes of death today have shifted from acute to chronic illnesses. According to the National Vital Statistics report of 2010, the three major causes of death in the United States were diseases of the heart, malignant neoplasm (cancer), and chronic lower respiratory diseases (e.g., emphysema and chronic bronchitis). Deaths from diseases of the heart and malignant neoplasm combined accounted for 47 percent of deaths in the United States in 2010. Other chronic illnesses resulting in death include cerebral vascular disease (strokes), Alzheimer's disease, kidney and liver failure, hypertension (high blood pressure), Parkinson's disease, respiratory diseases, and diabetes.

"Dr. Google" Phenomenon

Today, many people search the Internet to find answers and advice about symptoms of illness before going to a doctor and, in some instances, instead of or in addition to, seeking qualified help. Referred to as the "Dr. Google" phenomenon, this serves to illustrate the modern tendency for patients to take greater responsibility for their own health and illness without necessarily relying solely upon professional help. However, there may be some limitations in this use of the Internet, as serious illnesses could be misdiagnosed or necessary treatment delayed. On the other hand, the Internet and media offer useful educational resources in disease prevention (such as early detection of cancer), diabetes education, and in reducing the risk of heart disease and strokes.

Self-Help and Mutual Aid

Self-help groups that focus on a particular illness and Internet-based support groups are also more commonly used in today's society, and can offer helpful information and support to sufferers of a particular condition. Support groups can potentially reduce isolation by offering opportunities for sharing experiences of illness. They can help members gain more realistic perspectives on their situation and to maintain hope. The diagnosis of a serious illness can undermine a person's confidence and sense of self, and mutual aid can be an empowering experience that builds self-esteem and strengthens the individual's capacity to cope. With increased social mobility and work patterns, family and friends may not necessarily be the primary source of support. The Internet also provides a degree of protection and anonymity at times when a person suffering from an illness might feel most vulnerable.

Illness Narratives

There are numerous examples of illness narratives or stories about illness in the world of nonfiction today. When someone with cancer or another serious chronic condition records a personal account of her journey through illness, it not only provides an opportunity to document her own unique experience, but may also help others in similar circumstances to maintain a positive and hopeful outlook. In his classic book, *Anatomy of Illness as Perceived by the Patient,* American writer Norman Cousins argues that sick people should share in the responsibility for their illness and its treatment. He also refers to the natural recuperative powers of the body, and stresses the importance of recognizing the connection between body, mind, and spirit.

Irene Renzenbrink

Further Reading

Brody, H. *Stories of Sickness.* Oxford University Press, 2003.

Cousins, N. *Anatomy of an Illness as Perceived by the Patient.* New York: W. W. Norton & Co., 2005.

Murphy, S. L., J. Xu, and Kenneth D. Kochanek. "Deaths: Preliminary Data for 2010." *National Vital Statistics Report,* 60(4) (2012). Hyattsville, MD: National Center for Health Statistics. http://www.cdc.gov/nchs/data/nvsr/nvsr60/nvsr60_04.pdf

Peek, Chuck, W. and Kenzie Latham. "Acute and Chronic Diseases." In *Encyclopedia of Death and the Human Experience,* edited by Clifton D. Bryant and Dennis L. Peck (pp. 9–13). Thousand Oaks, CA: Sage, 2009.

DOMESTIC VIOLENCE

Domestic violence is the willful intimidation, assault, battery, sexual assault, or other abusive behavior perpetrated by one family member, household member, or intimate partner against another. Partners may be married or not married; heterosexual, gay, or lesbian; living together, separated, or dating. Domestic violence and emotional abuse are about power and control. Perpetrators of domestic violence have learned abusive, manipulative techniques and behaviors that allow them to dominate and control others and obtain the responses they desire. Feminists and others who research issues of domestic violence argue that they do not result from individual pathology or mental illness, but rather from the structure of a social order that condones the exercise of power of men and their control over women. Domestic violence victims may minimize the seriousness of incidents in order to cope, and often suffer in silence and isolation. Furthermore, because they fear the perpetrator and may be ashamed of their situation, victims may be reluctant to disclose the abuse to family, friends, work, the authorities, or victim-assistance professionals.

Battering is the leading cause of injury for women between the ages of 15 and 44. Recent surveys estimate women in the United States suffer 5 million violent assaults annually. Furthermore, it is estimated that up to one-third (22 to 35 percent) of women who go to the emergency room, do so because of injury or stress from living in an abusive situation. Recent data for 2010 from the National Intimate Partner and Sexual Violence Survey (NISVS) indicate that one in three women (32.9 percent) have experienced physical violence at the hands of an intimate partner during their lifetime, while the National Institute of Justice reports that somewhere between 1,000 and 1,600 women are killed each year as the result of domestic violence.

Domestic violence takes many forms and can happen frequently or occasionally. Acts of violence can be criminal and include physical assault (hitting, pushing, shoving, etc.), sexual abuse (unwanted or forced sexual activity), isolation (keeping a partner from contacting his or her family or friends), intimidation, and stalking. Psychological and financial abuse, while not considered criminal behaviors, are forms of abuse and can lead to criminal violence.

Victims of domestic violence can be of any age, sex, sexual orientation, race, culture, religion, education, employment, or marital status. Although both men and women can be abused, research finds that 85 percent of victims are women. Acts of domestic violence affect not only the individual being abused, but witnesses of the abuse, family members, coworkers, friends, and the community at large. In fact, research suggests that children who witness domestic violence are victims themselves and growing up amidst violence predisposes them to a multitude of social and physical problems.

Domestic violence often has subtle origins. What starts out as love, courtship, and concern, may turn into domination, forced adherence to rigid sex roles, and obsessive jealousy. Victims may stay with someone who is abusing them for various reasons, which include fear of the abuser; belief the abuser will change, believing that violence is "normal"; denial; love of the abuser; religious reasons; threats to harm the victim, loved ones, or pets; cultural beliefs; self-blame; feelings of hopelessness or helplessness; limited housing or financial options; isolation, embarrassment, or shame; cultural beliefs about marriage and family; low self-esteem; and pressure from friends or family to stay in the relationship.

Domestic violence has been present since the early days of recorded history, and was even sanctioned in English common law as late as the early 20th century. The women's movement in the 1970s, which sought to explore women's issues and advocate for women's rights, fostered a growing concern over the violent treatment of women in the home and sought to make these issues public. In response to this increase in public consciousness and acknowledgment of domestic violence as a crime, shelters and resources were established to provide emotional, financial, vocational, and sometimes legal assistance and support to domestic violence survivors and their children.

Melissa Sandefur

Further Reading

Black, M. C., K. C. Basile, M. J. Breiding, S. G. Smith, M. L. Walters, M. T. Merrick, J. Chen, and M. R. Stevens. The National Intimate Partner and Violence Survey (NISVS) 2010 Summary Report. Atlanta, GA: National Center for Injury Prevention and Control, Centers for Disease Control and Prevention, 2011. http://www.cdc.gov/ViolencePrevention/pdf/NISVS_Report2010-a.pdf

Catalano, Shannan M. *Criminal Victimization, 2005*. Washington, DC: Bureau of Justice Statistics, 2006.

Mariani, Cliff. *Domestic Violence Survival Guide*. Flushing, NY: Looseleaf Law Publications, Inc., 1996.

National Center for Victims of Crime: www.ncvc.org

National Center on Domestic and Sexual Violence: http://www.ncdsv.org

National Coalition Against Domestic Violence: www.ncadv.org

National Coalition of Anti-Violence Programs. *Lesbian, Gay, Bisexual and Transgender Domestic Violence: 2003 Supplement*. New York: National Coalition of Anti-Violence Programs, 2004.

National Council on Child Abuse and Family Violence: www.nccafv.org

National Institute of Justice Journal, 250 (2003) https://www.ncjrs.gov/pdffiles1/jr000250g.pdf

Statman, Jan Berliner. *The Battered Woman's Survival Guide: Breaking the Cycle*. Dallas, TX: Taylor Publishing Company, 1990.

Tjaden, Patricia and Nancy Thoennes. National Institute of Justice and the Centers of Disease Control and Prevention, "Extent, Nature and Consequences of Intimate Partner Violence: Findings from the National Violence Against Women Survey." (2000).

U.S. Department of Justice, Bureau of Justice Statistics, "Intimate Partner Violence in the United States," December 2006. https://www.ncjrs.gov/pdffiles1/nij/181867.pdf

U.S. Department of Justice, Bureau of Justice Statistics, "Family Violence Statistics," June 2005.

Walker, Lenore. *The Battered Woman*. New York, NY: Harper & Row Publishers, Inc., 1979.

White, Evelyn C. *Chain, Chain, Change: For Black Women in Abusive Relationships*. Seattle, WA: Seal Press, 1994.

DRUGS

A drug is a substance that has a physiological effect when ingested into the body. There are a multitude of different drugs in the world with various effects. The effects of these drugs are very different and vary in length and strength of "high."

How Are Drugs Consumed?

The most common way to ingest a drug is by oral intake. There are various methods to consume a drug, including intravenously, smoking, intranasal (snorting), or through the anus (plugging). The drug's level of effectiveness and the strength of that specific drug are impacted by the method by which the drug is ingested. A recent trend that is occurring is called "bombing" a drug, which consists of wrapping the drug in toilet paper or cigarette paper and then ingesting the drug. The paper will dissolve once it hits the stomach and a more intense effect of the drug will occur. Generally, the faster the onset of the drug, the shorter in duration that effect will last.

Diversity of Drugs

There are five legal classifications of drugs that incur various penalties if misused. Level I drugs have a high rate of abuse, no recognizable medical benefit, and generally lack safety. Drugs in this class include heroin, lysergic acid diethylamide (LSD), and marijuana. On the opposite end of the spectrum, level V drugs have a low rate of abuse, numerous medical benefits, and are typically safe to take. Examples of level V drugs include cough suppressants with low amounts of codeine, many antidiarrheal drugs, and some anticonvulsants.

Effective Dose/Lethal Dose

Each drug has an effective dose and a lethal dose. Effective dose is the amount of the drug that needs to be taken to reach the desired effect. Lethal dose is the amount of the drug that needs to be taken to prove fatal in the majority of the population. A drug's effective/lethal dose ratio shows how dangerous a drug is in terms of potential for overdose. Heroin has an effective/lethal dose ratio of 1:5; it takes one gram of heroin to get the desired "high," and it will take only five grams to kill the average person. The 1:5 ratio of heroin makes it one of the most deadly drugs with a high potential for overdose. Marijuana on the other hand has an effective/lethal dose ratio of 1:>1,000, showing that it is a drug that is very difficult to overdose on.

Age Range

The age range of drug users is quite wide and varies depending on state. Overall, drug use increases with age from ages 12 and 13, and peaks around age 20. After age 20, the drug use rate slowly declines with age. In 2008, the drug overdose death rate was highest among those aged 45–54. The lowest death rates due to drug overdose were among those aged 65 and older. Between 1999 and 2008, there has been an increase in drug overdose death rates among all age groups.

Withdrawal

Most drugs will cause withdrawal symptoms if addiction to that drug occurs. Drug withdrawals range from poor concentration on an emotional level to nausea and diarrhea on a physical level. The symptoms depend on the drug that was used and the duration of the drug use. Opiate withdrawals, for example, can produce vomiting and cramping and can last from one week up to one month. Recent research shows that caffeine withdrawal can cause symptoms that include headaches and fatigue, but may also cause symptoms that are similar to the flu with nausea and muscle pain.

Public Health Policy

Proactive measures are being taken through the implementation policy intended to fight the high number of deaths and overdoses. Classifying drugs into various legal categories is one way in which policy enforcement is attempting to help contain this drug epidemic. By classifying drugs into higher categories, the punishment for misuse of these drugs is much more severe, which, arguably, serves as a deterrent.

Public policy is also concerned with supporting and promoting a positive change in lethal drug use by offering needle exchanges in various states and cities. Needle exchange programs promote public safety in various ways, including providing clean needles to drug users that are either at high risk for HIV or already HIV positive.

Jason Bertrand

See also: Alcohol; Tobacco.

Further Reading

Austin, C. L. *D.A.A.P.E Drug and Alcohol Addiction Prevention Education.* Bloomington, IN: Author Solutions, 2012.

Mahato, R. *Pharmaceutical Dosage Forms and Drug Delivery.* Florence, KY: CRC Press, 2011.

Perrine, D. *The Chemistry of Mind-Altering Drugs: History, Pharmacology, and Cultural Context.* Washington, DC: American Chemical Society, 1996.

DYING TRAJECTORY

The concept of a dying trajectory refers to the perceived course(s) of dying that health care providers come to expect based on their experience of working with dying patients. The concept was first deployed by Glaser and Strauss (1968), who identified three trajectories of dying commonly recognized by hospital staff: (1) sudden swift death, (2) sudden unexpected death, and (3) lingering death. Since then, the notion of a trajectory of dying has been used more generally to describe the pattern and process by which dying unfolds, especially in regard to how this "journey" affects not only the experiences of those who are dying, but also the family, friends, and those charged with caring for them.

In some instances, the duration of a dying trajectory may be short, unexpected, and almost instantaneous, as in the case of a heart attack. In others, it may be long and drawn out, unfolding over weeks, months or years, as in the case of Alzheimer's disease (see **Alzheimer's Disease**). While dying trajectories vary from person to person, they are characterized by two overarching properties: (1) duration, that is, the length of time between the onset of illness and eventual death; and (2) shape, that is, the course in which dying unfolds. In the latter, the progression of illness is sometimes uneven and difficult to predict, involving periods of remission and relapse in ways that can complicate and confuse the experiences of dying. Most *communicable diseases*, perhaps with the exception of HIV/AIDS, are characterized by a relatively brief dying trajectory; while *degenerative diseases*, such as motor neuron or Parkinson's disease, are likely to be more protracted, more difficult to predict, and will likely involve some degree of pain, suffering, and the loss of physical and/or mental functioning.

Finally, we can distinguish two different stages in the dying trajectory: (1) a period when the person knows he is terminally ill and is living with a condition that will eventually culminate in his death; and (2) a short-term period when death is imminent and the person is said to be "actively dying" (see **Active Dying**).

Michael Brennan

Further Reading

Glaser, Barney and Anselm Strauss. *Time for Dying*. Chicago: Aldine, 1968.
Pattison, E. M. *The Experience of Dying*. Englewood Cliffs, NJ: Prentice Hall, 1977.

E

EATING DISORDERS

Eating satisfies one of the most basic of human needs, but is also subject to individual, social, and cultural intervention. The food a person eats, how they eat it, as well as the frequency and quantity of food intake are influenced not just by individual appetite and the availability of food, but also by factors that include family, peers, and cultural norms about food and body size. All of these variables affect how a person views and modifies food intake. An eating disorder involves disturbances in eating behaviors that negatively affect physical and mental health such as extreme dieting, binge eating, and severe anxiety due to negative body image. The three most commonly known eating disorders are anorexia nervosa, bulimia nervosa, and binge eating disorder (also known as compulsive overeating).

Risk factors and correlates of eating disorders include gender, race/ethnicity, childhood eating and gastrointestinal problems, elevated shape and concerns about weight, negative self-evaluation, sexual abuse, and a range of biological, psychological, emotional, interpersonal, and social factors. In spite of the risk factors involved, the practice of restricting food intake so as to control weight and/or body shape is one that is today engaged in by a significant number of young women and men.

An eating disorder may begin with a preoccupation with food and weight, but it is most often about much more than food. People with eating disorders often use food and the control of food in an attempt to compensate for feelings and emotions that may otherwise seem overwhelming. Dieting, bingeing, and purging may begin as a way to cope with painful emotions and to feel in control of one's life, but these behaviors will ultimately harm a person's physical and emotional health, self-esteem, and sense of competence and control.

Types of Eating Disorders

Anorexia nervosa: The American Psychiatric Association defines anorexia nervosa as an abnormally low body weight (15 percent below normal body weight for age and height), coupled with an intense fear of gaining weight or becoming "fat," disturbance and preoccupation with body weight and shape, and, in females, amenorrhea (the absence of three consecutive menstrual cycles). Despite the fact that many anorexic patients engage in compulsive exercising, restrictor-type anorexic patients are distinguished by their resolute refusal to eat above a bare minimum, whereas bulimic-type anorexic patients regularly engage in binge eating and purging.

Bulimia nervosa: Commonly known as bulimia, bulimia nervosa is an eating disorder in which the person engages in recurrent binge eating followed by feelings of guilt,

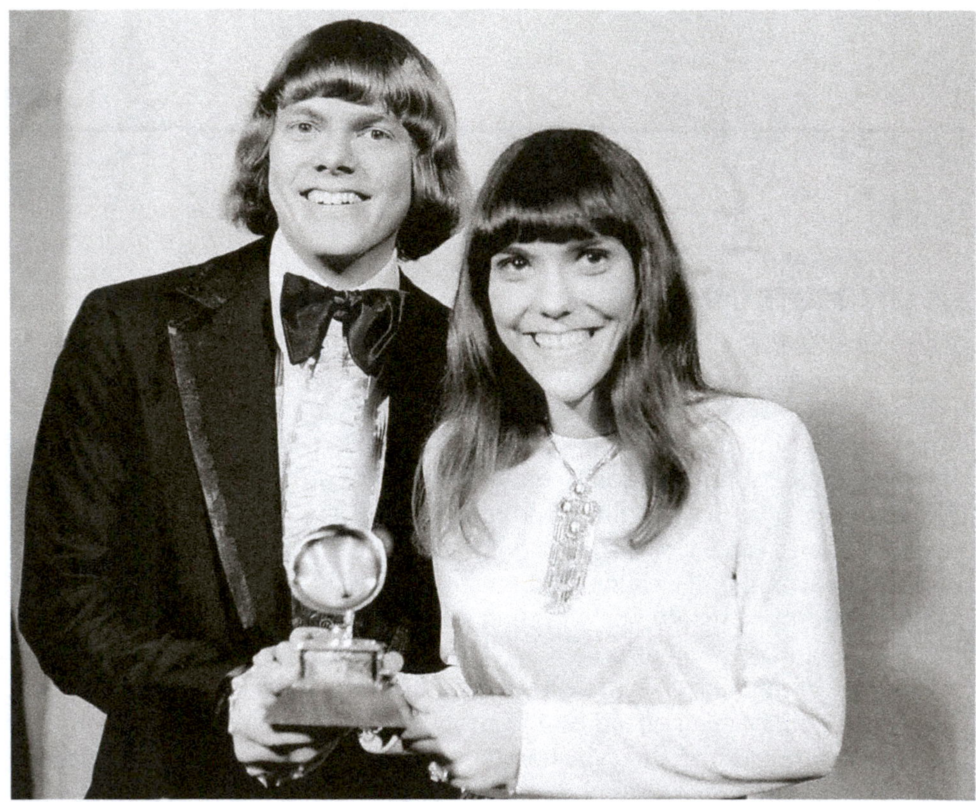

Karen Carpenter achieved fame and success, together with her brother Richard, as part of the musical duo The Carpenters. Karen died in 1983 from complications related to her long battle with anorexia nervosa. (AP Photo)

depression, and self-condemnation. The person will then typically engage in compensatory behaviors, referred to as "purging," to counter the excessive eating. Purging may take the form of vomiting, fasting, the use of laxatives, enemas, diuretics or other medications, or overexercising.

Binge eating disorder: Binge eating disorder (BED) is a type of eating disorder not otherwise specified and is characterized by recurrent binge eating without the regular use of compensatory measures to counter binge eating.

Eating disorders not otherwise specified (EDNOS): Eating disorders not otherwise specified (EDNOS) can include a combination of signs and symptoms of anorexia, bulimia, and/or binge eating disorder, but not meet the full criteria. While these behaviors may not clinically constitute a full-syndrome eating disorder, they can nevertheless still be physically dangerous and emotionally draining.

Incidence and Prevalence of Eating Disorders

There are great variations in estimates of the incidence and prevalence of eating disorders, doubtless because sufferers from these disorders are often hesitant to reveal their condition. In spite of the lack of solid data, the majority of those who have researched or treated eating disorders are in consensus that the incidence and prevalence of both anorexia and bulimia have increased noticeably in the past 50 years. A proportion of this increase may be attributed to greater public awareness, and thus to greater identification, of disordered eating. Statistically, eating disorders are most common in young, middle to upper-middle class white women living in food-abundant countries. These data are the basis for linking eating disorders with culturally defined gender role expectations. Only an estimated 5–15 percent of those with anorexia or bulimia and an estimated 35 percent of individuals with binge eating disorders are male. Studies on the epidemiology (the distribution and patterns of health events) of anorexia in Western industrialized countries suggest an incidence of between 8 and 13 cases per 100,000 persons per year using strict criteria for diagnosis. There are at least twice as many bulimic patients than there are anorexic patients. The prevalence of partial eating disorders (e.g., restrictive dieting) is at least twice that of full-syndrome eating disorders. Longitudinal studies indicate a progression from less to more severe eating disturbances, with normal dieters occasionally becoming pathological dieters, who in turn occasionally progress to partial or full-syndrome eating disorders. Even though eating disorders are most common among young, middle-class white females, anorexia is becoming increasingly common among young black, Hispanic, Asian and Asian American, Native American, and lesbian women and girls.

Mortality and Eating Disorders

Those with eating disorders have significantly elevated mortality rates, with the highest rates occurring in those with anorexia nervosa. The mortality rate for anorexia nervosa is some 12 times higher than the death rate associated with all causes of death for females aged 15–24, and between 5 and 10 percent of people diagnosed with anorexia will die as a result of eating-disorder-related causes within 10 years of diagnosis. Among anorexics, suicide is the second leading cause of death, while for those with bulimia nervosa, care accidents and suicide are the most frequently reported causes of death. Even though self-starvation is a fundamental aspect of anorexia, the exact cause of death for people with severe anorexia is less likely to be malnutrition than it is a starvation-related medical complication, such as heart disease and electrolyte imbalance.

Theoretical Models of Eating Disorders

Eating disorders are complex conditions that stem from a mixture of long-standing behavioral, biological, emotional, psychological, interpersonal, and social factors. Theoretical models used to explain the epidemiology, etiology (causation or origination), and treatment of eating problems include biomedical, psychological, and sociocultural models. Researchers are continuing to acquire knowledge about the underlying causes of these conditions, having already identified some general issues that can contribute to the development of eating disorders.

Biomedical/biological models: Scientists are still researching possible biochemical or biological causes of eating disorders. Early theories of eating disorders, such as biomedical (i.e., of or relating to biology and medicine), emphasized "individualistic factors" that affect both eating and body size. Biomedical models of eating disorders posit that they result from physiological rather than psychological disturbances. From this perspective, eating disorders are involuntary illnesses rather than (un)conscious choices. For example, biomedical models trace the origins of eating disorders to physiological factors, such as chemical and hormonal imbalances, that may lead to metabolic changes in the body, including depression and anxiety, or imbalances of chemicals in the brain that control hunger, appetite, and digestion. Furthermore, as eating disorders often run in families, current biomedical research indicates that there may be a significant genetic component to eating disorders. A combination of psychotropic drugs, hormone replacement, nutritional therapy, and exercise are typically prescribed and monitored as the preferred forms of treatment from the biomedical perspective.

Psychological factors: Psychological models identify eating problems as "multidimensional disorders" that are influenced by biological, psychological, and cultural factors. Theories of etiology have generally fallen into three categories: *psychoanalytic* (involving pathological responses to developmental conflicts), *family systems* (implicating enmeshed, rigid families that impede an individual's growth and development), and the *endocrinological* (involving a precipitating hormonal defect). Psychological studies explore the possibility that problems of identity and control are central to eating disorders, with the individual attempting to resolve these problems by investing emotionally and behaviorally in the pursuit of slimness.

The underlying psychological causes of eating problems may also include a woman's ambivalent relationship with her mother or father, as well as familial attitudes toward dieting and history of obesity. Other factors include an individual's perception of the self, issues of control, a predilection toward addiction, issues of perfectionism, and a response to physical and/or sexual trauma. As with the biomedical model, treatments may include medication, exercise, and nutritional interventions, as well as individual therapy, group therapy, and family counseling. In severe and/or chronic cases, interventions may involve hospitalization or alternative residential treatment centers designed for prolonged treatment and recovery through a combination of intensive therapies.

Sociocultural models: The sociocultural model is useful for understanding the social, cultural, and social group dynamics of eating disorders. Sociocultural models locate the source of eating disorders in influences within the wider social environment, including the media and advertising, which create social, cultural, and economic pressures on women to lose weight in order to conform to highly unrealistic standards of beauty and body size. These wider social and cultural influences are thought to be at the root of most, if not all, eating disorders; helping to shape the behaviors of young girls and women precisely because females are rewarded for thinness, both socially and economically. For example, dieting to a body weight leaner than needed for health is highly promoted by current fashion trends, sales campaigns for special foods, the exercise and fitness industry, and many other elements of an appearance-conscious culture.

What is more, there are well-documented biases against "fat women" in the job market. In linking women's successes, their perceived value, and even their economic survival, to culturally constructed and unrealistic standards of beauty, women are diminished and controlled in society. From a sociocultural perspective, women and girls with anorexia, bulimia, and binge eating disorders thus become victims of a merciless consumer culture that teaches them that their only value lies in their ability to maintain a weight below normal standards of health.

Treatment Options

There are a number of treatment options available for people with eating disorders. However, there is little research to document the success of these treatments because of the difficulty of recruiting sufficient numbers of participants for treatment trials, inducing compliance with treatment, and retaining patients for the duration of the trials. Psychological and medicinal treatment plans for eating disorders may include medical care and monitoring, medications, nutritional counseling, and individual, group, and/or family psychotherapy. Some patients may also need to be hospitalized or may find treatment in specialized recovery centers designed to treat malnutrition, weight loss, and self-esteem issues. Without intervention from significant others, individuals with eating disorders rarely seek treatment; they are often in denial and refuse to accept the seriousness of their eating problems.

Melissa Sandefur

Further Reading

Claude-Pierre, Peggy. *The Secret Language of Eating Disorders: How You Can Understand and Work to Cure Anorexia and Bulimia.* New York: Random House, 1999.

Costin, Carolyn. *The Eating Disorder Sourcebook,* 3rd edition. New York: McGraw-Hill, 2007.

Hesse-Biber, S. *Am I Thin Enough Yet? The Cult of Thinness and the Commercialization of Identity.* New York: Oxford University Press, 1996.

http://www.nationaleatingdisorders.org

http://www.nimh.nih.gov/health/publications/eating-disorders/what-are-eating-disorders.shtml

http://www.nlm.nih.gov/medlineplus/eatingdisorders.html

Menzie, Morgan. *Diary of an Anorexic Girl: Based on a True Story.* Nashville: W Publishing Group, a Thomas Nelson Company, 2003.

ELEGY

A poem or song to memorialize the dead, the elegy is usually pensive, reflective, or plaintive; an expression of suffering or woe. Elegies typically describe feelings of sorrow, sadness, mournfulness, melancholy, nostalgia, lamentation, or some blending of these qualities. The origins of the word elegy are found in the Greek *elegeia,* meaning a poem or song of lament, or mourning, for the dead. Synonyms include dirge (a hymn of grief) and threnody (a song of lamentation for the dead). The requiem, a musical composition played at a mass for the dead, is related to the elegy. Although somewhat similar in function, elegy is not to be confused with eulogy (oratory or praise in honor of the deceased) or epitaph (a brief statement commemorating the deceased, often inscribed as a memorialization on a tomb) (see **Epitaphs; Eulogy**).

As a poetic form, the elegy began as an ancient Greek metrical form that was written or spoken in response to the death of a person or group. A traditional elegy embodies three stages: First is the lament, in which the speaker or writer expresses grief and sorrow. The middle stage is given to praise and admiration of the idealized dead. Finally, the elegy offers solace and consolation to the mourners. Elegies have been represented in various artistic media, including literature, music, and painting, as well as in film, television, and theater.

In traditional Hawaiian culture, chants known as *mele kanikau* were used as laments. Some *kanikau* were carefully composed; others were chanted spontaneously during the funeral. Imagery of the natural world is called upon to portray the experience of loss. Memories of shared experiences amid natural surroundings are mentioned: "My companion in the chill of Manoa" or "My companion in the forest of Makiki." Such chants fondly recall the things that bind together the deceased and his or her survivors.

Early examples of the genre of elegy in English literature include John Milton's "Lycidas" (1637) and Thomas Gray's "Elegy Written in a Country Churchyard" (1750). Examples from American literature include "O Captain, My Captain" (1865), Walt Whitman's elegy on the death of President Abraham Lincoln, and "For the Union Dead" (1965), Robert Lowell's elegy based on the story of Colonel Robert Shaw who led the first all-black brigade during the American Civil War.

Elegies have been written not out of a personal sense of grief, but rather a generalized feeling of loss and metaphysical sadness. Examples include the series of 10 poems in *Duino Elegies* by the German poet Rainer Maria Rilke and poems by Czeslaw Milosz, which lament the cruelties of totalitarian government. Other examples are Wilfred Owen's poems of moral objection to the pain wrought by the industrialized warfare of World War I; Allen Ginsberg's *Kaddish* after the death of his mother; Seamus Heaney's memorials to the suffering caused by political violence in Ireland; and the "parental elegies" in the poetry of Sylvia Plath, Anne Sexton, and Adrienne Rich. In the modern period, the poetry of mourning assumes an exceptional diversity and range, with more anger and skepticism, more conflict and anxiety.

When Pan Am Flight 103 was brought down by a terrorist bomb over Lockerbie, Scotland, in 1988, Suse Lowenstein's son was among those killed. As a sculptor, she expressed her grief and the grief of other women bereft by the crash by making a series of female nude figures that compose an exhibit titled *Dark Elegy*. The larger-than-life figures are shown in the throes of grief. Some look mute. Others are obviously screaming. Some look as though they were eviscerated. The artist expressed the hope that this visual elegy would serve as "a reminder that life is fragile and that we can lose that which is most precious to us so easily and have to live with that loss for the remainder of our lives."

Elegies offer a way for people to give voice to their stories of loss. They convey the notion that we can be deepened by heartbreaks, not so much diminished as enlarged by grief and by our refusal to let others vanish without leaving some kind of record. Thus, the elegy is an important "cultural space" for mourning the dead. It gives artists and writers a medium for creating credible responses to loss.

Albert Lee Strickland

Further Reading

Kay, Dennis. *Melodious Tears: The English Funeral Elegy from Spenser to Milton.* New York: Oxford University Press, 1990.

Kennedy, David. *Elegy.* New York: Routledge, 2007.

Ramazani, Jahan. *Poetry of Mourning: The Modern Elegy from Hardy to Heaney.* Chicago: University of Chicago Press, 1994.

Weisman, Karen (ed.). *The Oxford Handbook of the Elegy.* New York: Oxford University Press, 2010.

EMBALMING

Embalming is a chemical process that preserves and sanitizes the dead human body for the purpose of anatomical study in medical schools, or for viewing the body during a public or private funeral. According to the American Board of Funeral Service Education, embalming is defined as "the process of chemically treating the dead human body to reduce the presence and growth of microorganisms, to retard organic decomposition, and to restore an acceptable physical appearance." Embalming for the purpose of funerals is temporary; the goal is not to create mummy-like results, but rather to help recreate the natural form and color that have been lost in death. This preservation process also provides valuable time in which family and friends can gather together to pay their respects and say their farewells. Embalming is thus one of the ways in which the living can take care of the dead, while at the same time attending to the needs of the living.

Methods

There are two key methods by which a body can be preserved. One is achieved in nature when a body is subjected to the harsh conditions of extreme heat and dry environments (such as those found in the desert), or extremely cold environments (such as those found in areas where the temperature is consistently below 32°F). The second method of preservation is performed artificially with the use of chemicals such as formaldehyde, glutaraldehyde, alcohols, and phenol.

Restoration

In the United States, embalming is performed not solely for reasons of preservation, but also for restoration, helping to create a "memory picture" that allows family and friends to remember the deceased as they were in life rather than in death. The dead human body inevitably undergoes chemical and physical changes, including changes in appearance, regardless of whether death was due to illness, trauma, or natural causes. Special materials are used, such as cotton and eye caps for recreating the proper shape to the eyes; modeling wax and wire for recreating the natural form to the mouth and lips; and a variety of cosmetics for the recreation of natural skin color and facial features. Embalming thus helps reduce, and in many instances remove, the appearance of pain and suffering that a person may have endured, instead, leaving the deceased with a peaceful and restful appearance.

Chemical Process

The chemical process of embalming is achieved by injecting chemicals into the vascular system, which work on the proteins present in the body. Proteins are attracted to water and once death occurs, these proteins take on more water, which then creates an environment that allows microorganisms and bacteria to thrive and multiply. The end result is decomposition of the human body. Decomposition causes adverse effects, such as foul odor, bloating, and changes in texture and complexion of the skin. Embalming stops the growth of microorganisms, which in turn stops the process of decomposition. It does so chiefly because embalming chemicals are attracted to proteins, which then cling to the chemicals and in so doing lose their ability to retain water. Without the ability to hold water, protein can no longer be a food source for bacteria and microorganisms.

The length of time that preservation lasts depends upon factors such as bacterial growth and moisture content inside the body, as well as how effective the embalming chemicals have worked throughout the body. Other factors include the strength of the embalming chemicals used and the surrounding environment in which the embalmed body (contained in casket or vault) is placed, such as moisture content, temperature, and the presence of insects and air.

A History of Embalming

Whether accomplished through the use of chemicals or by nature, embalming has been practiced for more than 6,000 years. This span of time can be divided into three historical periods: the ancient, anatomist, and the modern.

Ancient period: This occurred between 6000 BC and AD 650. It was the Egyptians, and their belief that the soul would revisit the body as long as the body stayed intact, who gave us the first examples of embalming. Unlike today, embalming was not simply a choice given to an individual but was essential in order for the body to be resurrected. Embalming techniques varied depending upon the wealth of the deceased. The most elaborate and expensive consisted of several distinct stages, which included (1) the removal of organs followed by their washing in wine and spices; (2) laying the body in a salt solution for several days; (3) bathing and drying the body in the desert sun; and finally (4) wrapping the body in several yards of bandages and placing it in an wooden or stone sarcophagus. The Egyptians' main goal was to create mummies that preserved the human body and allowed it to be reunited with the soul some 3,000 years later. Embalming came to a halt with the advent of Christianity and fall of the Roman and Egyptian empires, whereupon the practice was viewed as pagan and subsequently ended.

Anatomist period: This took place in Europe between 650 and 1861. The chief motive for embalming—in a period that saw tremendous growth in the pursuit of scientific discovery and knowledge in areas such as medicine, religion, and law—was anatomical study. Anatomy became a popular subject of study and anatomical dissection was performed in open amphitheaters, available to anyone who wanted to observe. This took place mostly during the winter months when the rate of decomposition was slowed due to cold temperatures. As the interest in anatomy and physiology grew, so did the demand to increase the number of months during which anatomical studies were performed. This brought about experiments of injecting the body with materials such as water, dye, mercury, and wax in order to preserve the body and be able to view blood vessels and organs. These ideas and techniques evolved over several hundred years and were later brought to the United States.

Modern period: This began in the United States in 1861 and involved similar techniques to those that are practiced today. The chief reason for embalming during this period was to allow the bodies of Union soldiers killed in the Civil War (1861–1865) to be preserved long enough so as to be buried in their Northern homes, where family and friends could pay their last respects. The first prominent military figure to be embalmed during the Civil War was Colonel Elmer Ellsworth, who was embalmed by Dr. Thomas Holmes, a Civil War surgeon widely considered to be the modern father of embalming. Thousands of people came to New York City to view Colonel Ellsworth's body, following its railroad journey from the White House in Washington, D.C., where it had been kept at the order of President Abraham Lincoln. When Lincoln too was killed following an assassination on April 14, 1865, his body was embalmed and taken by train from New York City to his hometown of Springfield, Illinois. This three-week journey included several stops along the way, allowing grieving people to see President Lincoln and pay their respects to him. Lincoln's appearance was described as looking as though he was sleeping. It was this event in U.S. history, together with the early techniques of embalming practiced during the Civil War, which helped change the funerary landscape by making embalming a mainstay of American cultural life.

Today: Embalming is still a core part of the funeral ceremony across the United States, but the number of people choosing it for their loved ones has slowly diminished over the last 30 years. Some of the reasons can be attributed to financial concerns, a change in beliefs and traditions, and the potential for emotional distress caused by seeing the body of a loved one lying in a casket. Embalming and viewing the body, however, will likely continue to be a part of the funeral ceremony because the idea of being able to say a final goodbye to a loved one continues to play an important role in the grieving process.

Jody LaCourt

Further Reading

Klicker, Ralph L. *Restorative Art and Science*. Buffalo, NY: Thanos Institute, 2002.

Mayer, Robert G. *Embalming: History, Theory, and Practice*, 5th edition. Boston: McGraw-Hill Medical Publishing Division, 2012.

Strub, Clarence G. and Lawrence G. Frederick. *The Principles and Practice of Embalming*, 5th edition. Dallas, TX: Professional Training Schools, Inc. and Robertine Frederick, 1989.
Williams, Melissa Johnson. "A Social History of Embalming." In *Handbook of Death and Dying, Volume. 2: The Response to Death*, edited by Clifton D. Bryant (pp. 534–43). Thousand Oaks, CA: Sage, 2003.

EPIDEMICS AND PLAGUES

An epidemic can be defined as the temporary upsurge in the number of cases of a communicable disease caused by pathogens (disease-producing agents such as viruses, bacteria, or fungi), within a particular geographical area, which exceeds the number of cases that might usually be expected. Perhaps the best known example of an epidemic is the bubonic plague (or Black Death) that ravaged the population of medieval Europe and parts of North Africa between 1347 and 1351, killing an estimated 100 million people in Asia, Europe, and Africa. The disease, which was highly contagious, is produced by the bacillus *Yersinia pestis* (originally named *Pasteurella pestis*), and is widely believed to have been introduced to Europe from Asia by mercantile traders via a Black Sea port. The main symptoms of the plague included swelling in the large lymph nodes (of the neck or armpit); convulsive fits; the vomiting of blood; and a blackening of the limbs, thus leading to the moniker, the Black Death. The economic impact of the plague was such that it caused a deep depression in Europe lasting several decades; while its cultural influence can still be found in artistic and architectural representations of the *danse macabre* (see **Dance of Death**).

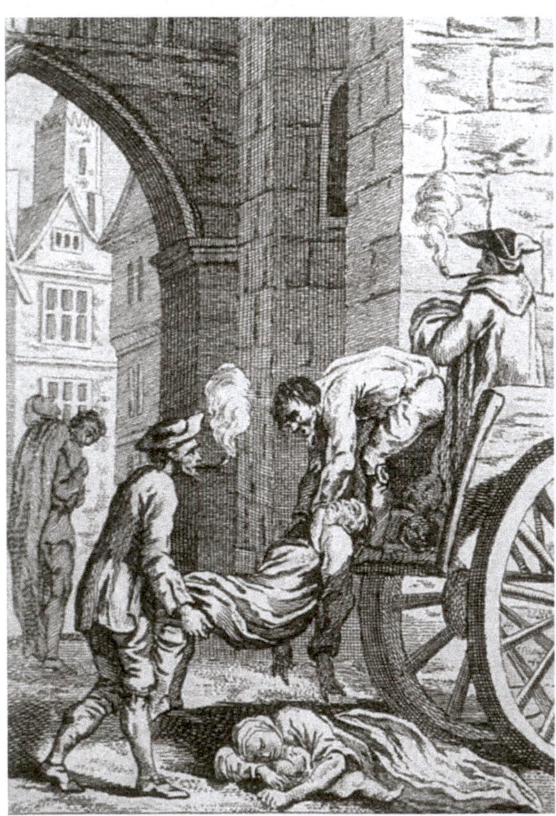

Seventeenth-century illustration of plague victims being collected and loaded on a cart. (Courtesy of the National Library of Medicine)

More recent examples of epidemics include the cholera epidemics that swept across Victorian England and were caused by a lack of public sanitation and contaminated water supplies. In the developed world, improvements in public health and the development of antibiotics and vaccines have served greatly to reduce the incidence and spread of epidemics like cholera, influenza, and scarlet fever. However, in large parts of the developing world, potentially epidemic-causing diseases such as cholera and influenza continue to pose a major threat to health; while the emergence of newer communicable diseases and infections, such as avian flu (H5N1) and dengue fever, have reached epidemic proportions in some less developed nations, the latter being a major cause of serious illness and death among children in parts of Asia and Latin America.

The study of epidemics falls largely to epidemiologists (see **Epidemiology**), who are responsible for identifying and tracking the outbreak and spread of infectious disease, alerting agencies of public health so that they can implement measures in order to prevent them, where possible, from becoming epidemics. In the United States, chief responsibility for controlling the spread of communicable diseases lies with the Centers for Disease Control and Prevention (CDC), a federal agency housed within the Department of Health and Human Services. Researchers working for the CDC and at the Pasteur Institute in France were among the first to identify the first known cases of what later became known as HIV/AIDS (human immunodeficiency virus/acquired immune deficiency syndrome) (see **HIV/AIDS**). This modern epidemic, which was first identified in young homosexual and bisexual men, was, in the early 1980s, wrongly labeled by certain sections of the media as the "gay plague." The disease, which quickly became global in its manifestation, affecting whole sections of the population and not limited to a particular region or continent, is, strictly speaking, and because it is global in nature, best described as a pandemic rather than an epidemic.

That epidemics and plagues continue to exert a powerful grip over the public imagination can be seen from the general anxiety and panic generated by the H1N1 virus. Such fears provide the basis for popular cultural representations of epidemics in movies like *Outbreak* (1995), about a fictional but deadly Ebola-like virus. In the 21st century, the threat of bioterrorism is sufficient to raise concerns among counterterrorism experts about the potential risk of an attack by terrorists using biological agents in order to spread pneumonic plague (though biodefense experts acknowledge that such an attack would require specialist knowledge and technology). Further fears have been raised most recently by the British government's chief medical officer for England, Professor Dame Sally Davies, who in March 2013 warned that a growing resistance to antibiotics, and the failure of pharmaceutical companies to develop new ones, posed as big a risk to public health as terrorism.

Michael Brennan

Further Reading

Cantor, Norman, F. *In the Wake of the Plague: The Black Death and the World It Made.* New York: Free Press, 2002.

Hays, J. N. *Epidemics and Pandemics: Their Impacts of History.* Santa Barbara, CA: ABC-CLIO, 2006.

Walsh, Fergus. "Antibiotics Resistance 'As Big a Risk as Terrorism'—Medical Chief." *BBC News,* March 11, 2013. http://www.bbc.co.uk/news/health-21737844

Wolfe, Nathan, D. *The Viral Storm: The Dawn of a New Pandemic Age.* Harmondsworth: Penguin, 2012.

Zeigler, Philip. *The Black Death.* Stroud: Sutton Publishing, 2003.

EPIDEMIOLOGY

Epidemiology is a multidisciplinary science concerned with identifying, tracking, and treating patterns of disease in populations. Epidemiologists have been influential in identifying (and helping to prevent the spread of) communicable diseases such as cholera, influenza, and smallpox, which, in previous generations, decimated whole swathes of the population. In some cases, these diseases are well known whereas in other situations the disease was not previously recognized or has occurred in new populations or manifested in new ways. Infectious disease epidemiology is concerned with patterns of disease related to infectious organisms and the manifestations in human populations and/or the transfer from nonhuman populations to humans. For infectious disease epidemiology, the public health triad of person, organism, and environment is central to any investigation

Epidemiologists investigate who is being infected and the characteristics of those infected and, in particular, what makes the infected distinctive with regard to exposure to the specific illness. Characterizing the symptoms of the illness is helpful in determining the route of infection. For example, if the symptoms are largely gastrointestinal, epidemiologists may try to identify exposure to a common venue where those affected dined or purchased food. Once a common venue is identified, further investigation is required, including the question of exposure to a pathogen in a common food that was ingested. Food may have been contaminated at many points in the trajectory including: prior to delivery at the restaurant, improper storage of food, inadequate sanitization of cooking implements, plates and cutlery, or contamination by someone doing the food preparation. The latter is exemplified by the case of Typhoid Mary, a healthy carrier of typhoid fever, who was known to spread the typhoid bacillus in the process of food preparation. Careful investigation of commonalities in those infected led to the identification of the source of the exposure. Epidemiologists are essentially detectives tracking a chain of evidence in order to identify the cause of illness. Laboratory personnel are essential to the identification of the details of the pathogen and its confirmation as the source of disease.

Historically, the examination of illness in populations is related to potential causes and one of these is the water supply. John Snow (1813–1858), an English physician and anesthesiologist, investigated an outbreak of cholera in Victorian England by distinguishing the source of the water supply and the location of the domiciles of those who became ill with cholera from those who remained well. The pattern indicated that those who were unwell lived in homes that all shared the same water source. This hypothesis was verified by shutting off the Broad Street pump in Soho, London, thereby reducing the incidence of new infections as people were no longer able to draw water contaminated with raw sewage.

Epidemiological investigations have followed this pattern of careful observation, development of a hypothesis, testing the hypothesis, and then taking appropriate action.

The approach to hypothesis testing includes case counts that are expressed as absolute numbers, incidence and prevalence, cohort studies, and case-control studies. The cohort study is useful in determining whether a stated exposure is related to the development of a particular disease. The efficacy of a given flu vaccine can be determined by tracking the development of flu in those who did and did not receive the flu vaccine. If there is no difference in the occurrence of disease in the two groups, there may be several explanations. The first is that the vaccine was not effective. A different strain may have become prevalent and the vaccine may not have contained the materials effective for the strain that was dominant in that year. Another explanation is that there simply was not a lot of flu in a given population for whatever reason. One of these reasons is that something called "herd immunity" reduced the transmission of the flu (see **Health Promotion**). Herd immunity occurs when a sufficient percentage of the population has been immunized so that transmission from one person to the next is interrupted. Which of these explanations is correct as to why there were no differences in the two groups requires further investigation, but the initial approach is a cohort analysis.

By way of contrast, in a case of food-borne illness where the commonality was having an illness, a case-control study would be appropriate. In such an approach, those having the illness would be compared with those without this illness. The epidemiologist would seek commonalities in those with the disease. Once a likely commonality has been identified, a comparison group with the same commonality but without the illness would be sought. For example, the hypothesis that dining at a given restaurant was the common factor would be inadequate to explain the occurrence of illness if those without the disease also ate there during the same time period, or there were cases of the illness that had not frequented the specified venue. Further inquiry, however, may indicate that although some individuals in both groups had eaten at a common venue, the individuals who became ill had all ingested the same food. Laboratory analysis of the food might confirm the presence of a pathogen in the cohort who were sick but not in the control group.

The meticulous methodology utilized by epidemiologists is a model of the scientific rigor required for the successful identification of the proximate causes of disease. The use of this scientific rigor is emulated by television programs such as *CSI: Crime Scene Investigation* in the identification of the culprits in a crime.

Epidemiologists are concerned not only with tracking outbreaks of disease or investigating problems after they occur. As indicated by the example of the flu vaccine, they are also concerned with prevention of disease and identifying a previously unacknowledged problem. The former, namely the prevention of disease, is illustrated by the careful monitoring of rates of infection. Where there are high rates of a given sexually transmitted infection (STI), it is likely that other STIs will appear in the same population. Thus, where there were high rates of gonorrhea and syphilis, infection with the human immunodeficiency virus (HIV) was also likely to occur given the same route of transmission. Monitoring the rates of one of these infections provides the basis for health education in order to prevent the transmission of other diseases by the same route.

A previously unidentified problem is illustrated by the occurrence of clusters of cancer in a particular geographic area that are identified, much as John Snow did with cholera. Pinpointing the cases and looking for a commonality, such as an environmental exposure to a toxic chemical, can lead to further research that identifies the precise nature of the exposure-disease relationship. This identification provides the basis for further action, often regulatory and/or political, to eliminate or mitigate the source of the illness. As is evident, epidemiology is a science with well-defined methods that provide the foundation for identifying sources of potential harm to the public, as well as the most effective approaches to maintaining or restoring health.

Inge B. Corless

Further Reading

Frerichs, R.R. "Cholera in Haiti and the Modern 'John Snow.'" http://www.ph.ucla.edu/epi/snow/cholera_haiti.html

McKeown, T. *The Rise of Modern Population.* London: Edward Arnold, 1976.

Merrill, R.M. *Introduction to Epidemiology,* 5th edition. Sudbury, MA: Jones and Bartlett Publishers, 2010.

Rothman, K.J. *Epidemiology: An Introduction,* 2nd edition. Oxford and New York: Oxford University Press, 2012.

EPITAPHS

An epitaph is a statement about the deceased placed on their memorial. Most memorial inscriptions give basic information on the name and age of the deceased, together with family relationships and sometimes their profession. Where present, the epitaph then follows as a distinct part of the text. Modern epitaphs are usually brief, but up to the early 19th century they could be quite lengthy and detailed. Early modern epitaphs were designed to record the virtues of the person commemorated, often emphasizing the religious and charitable nature of the person, and achievements in work and with family. Other epitaphs emphasized human mortality, warning that the reader would follow to the grave only too soon. The purpose of all these epitaphs was to encourage the living to behave well through warnings and by good examples, as judgment would inevitably follow. Epitaphs were frequent for both men and women, but until the 19th century were only ever affordable by the most wealthy in society. Thereafter, they may occur on headstones and other monuments in Britain and North America, but are less common in most of Europe.

Epitaphs reveal what the bereaved felt was most important about the lives of the deceased that they wished to be read by others; only a few are critical. For women, what was important to describe was often their family ancestry and connections, their loving nature, charitable giving, modesty, and the children they bore. Men were often celebrated not only for their character but also for their actions in society, and many record long and distinguished military or political careers. Those who died in unusual or tragic circumstances may have these recorded in considerable detail, sometimes eclipsing what they achieved in life. Those who had long illnesses frequently have these mentioned, with the suggestion that the suffering was borne without complaint. Quotations from the Bible, or verses from hymns, are frequently used as epitaphs. Communal memorials, such as war memorials or monuments to those lost in shipwrecks or industrial accidents, usually have a short, inclusive epitaph. Most epitaphs of all kinds are not unique, but occur many times over; indeed undertakers and memorial masons have, since the 19th century, had selections of appropriate epitaphs available for mourners to choose from.

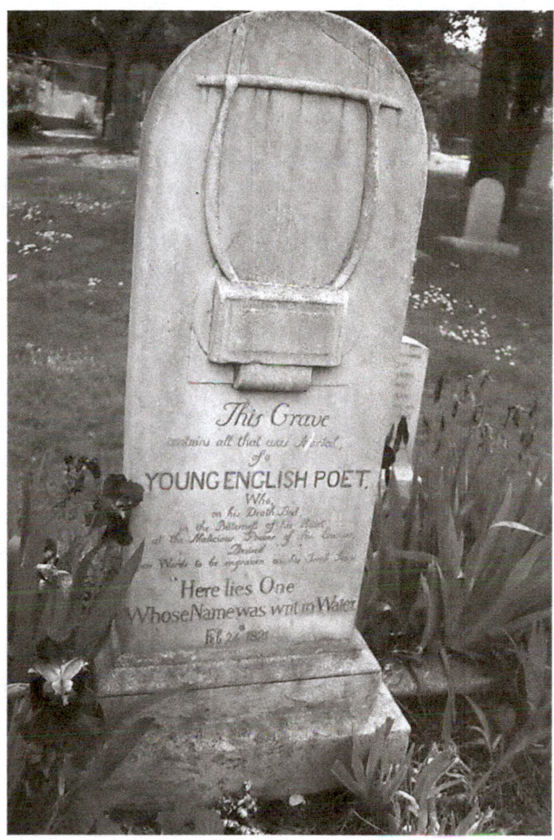

The tombstone of John Keats in Protestant Cemetery, Rome. The inscription reads: "This grave contains all that was Mortal, of a YOUNG ENGLISH POET, Who on his Death Bed, in the Bitterness of his Heart, at the Malicious Power of his Enemies, Desired these Words to be engraved on his Tomb Stone 'Here lies One Whose Name was writ in Water' Feb 24th 1821." (Giovanni Dall'Orto)

There has been a long history of recording and publishing epitaphs since the 17th century. The earlier collections were designed to improve the character and behavior of their readers, following the original purpose of the inscriptions, but more recently many collections have been compiled merely to entertain. Many of the most amusing epitaphs that have been published cannot now be located and may have been invented, and some are read as amusing now because the meanings of words and phrases have changed over time. With increasing informality during the 20th century, more epitaphs are deliberately witty or take an irreverent attitude to life or death. Epitaphs may give some insight into the lives and deaths of the commemorated, but are generally very partial and selective in what they emphasize and conform to the pattern of many others erected at the same time.

Harold Mytum

See also: Eulogy.

Further Reading

Enright, D.J. *The Oxford Book of Death.* New York: Oxford University Press, 1983.
Greene, J. *Epitaphs to Remember: Remarkable Inscriptions from New England Gravestones.* Chambersburg, PA: Alan C Hood, 2005.
Grigson, G. *The Faber Book of Epigrams and Epitaphs.* London: Faber & Faber, 1977.
Lindley, K. *Of Graves and Epitaphs.* London: Hutchinson, 1965.
Weever, J. *Ancient Funerall Monuments.* London, 1961/1631. Available on Google books http://books.google.co.uk/books?id=Um0DAAAAYAAJ&pg=PR9&lpg=PR9&dq=weever+epitaphs&source=bl&ots=h_rffgk5BX&sig=4TOy9309fHuLPqE_jQCjdszuVjk&hl=en&sa=X&ei=UDSIT_HRGqqo0QXmmoi3CQ&sqi=2&ved=0CCUQ6AEwAg#v=onepage&q=weever%20epitaphs&f=false

ESTATES

Probate or testamentary estate includes the total assets and debts of an individual at death, subject to distribution according to the terms of a will, or in the absence of a valid will, by the laws of inheritance of the state or nation of primary domicile. The individual(s) designated by the will to conduct the settlement is the *executor* or *personal agent* (or an *administrator* if appointed by the court). This individual(s) is empowered to fulfill the descendant's stated wishes. Determining what is included and excluded in the estate is crucial. Life insurance policies, for example, that name a beneficiary and funds designated P.O.D. (payable on death) are excluded.

The major goals for probate—the process of settling the estate—is determining the validity of a will, protecting the interests of any minor offspring, and insuring that taxes and creditors have been paid. A valid will must have been signed by the testator, dated, and witnessed by two people. Some states recognize a holographic will written in the decedent's handwriting and dated without witnesses. A will may be challenged by family members or individuals with interest in the settlement alleging that the decedent was mentally incompetent at the time of drafting or signing the will, or was coerced in formulating the will.

Individuals dying without a will are *intestate.* Under the laws of intestacy, heirs share equally by class; that is, children, then grandchildren, then lineal descendants (parents), and, if necessary, collateral descendants (brothers and sisters, nieces and nephews, cousins, etc.). Generally, the closest biological kin have the highest right to inherit. Each state establishes the ranking for the "right to inherit." Given the reality that the decedent may have offspring from one or more marriages or relationships, probate may be delayed until conflicting claims are evaluated.

The marital status at death and the marital history of the deceased influence probate. Some states have a "homestead law" insuring that the surviving spouse gets a "life estate" or right to own the primary residence until death; heirs then share the property. Some states restrict who can be disowned or excluded as heirs.

Many states have adopted the Uniform Probate Code standardizing probate. Estates with assets totaling over $5.25 million are subject to federal inheritance tax. Despite the protest of the "death tax," less than 1 percent of estates pay federal inheritance tax. If both parents of a minor child die simultaneously, a probate court appoints a guardian for the minor child and a conservator to manage the child's inheritance until the child reaches adulthood. If the decedent(s) died in circumstances "giving rise" to a wrongful death claim, settlement of the estate may be delayed until civil litigation is completed.

Harold Ivan Smith

See also: Advance Directives.

Further Reading

Clifford, Dennis. *Plan Your Estate*, 11th edition. Berkeley, CA: Nolo Press, 2012.
Wheatley-Liss, Deirdre, R. *Plan Your Own Estate: Passing On Your Assets and Your Values Legally and Efficiently.* New York: Apress, 2012.

EULOGY

A eulogy is the written form of a public address that is usually delivered aloud to an audience, and which marks the life, and its passing, of an honored or loved member of the community. Eulogies are usually presented soon after a death within a funeral or memorial service. Once considered the province of religious clergy who may have known the deceased personally as a member of their congregation, today relatives and friends frequently offer eulogies to deliver more personal insights about a person's character and their accomplishments. Knowledge about the function, form, and content of eulogies enables more effective composition, comprehension, and criticism of particular instances of the genre.

The functions provided by a eulogy are various and include not only honoring the life of the deceased (by bestowing upon it special significance and meaning), but also, significantly, raising the spirits of those left behind by bereavement. In this way, the eulogizer performs a vital service to the deceased as well as to the grieving audience of mourners. Since the earliest occasions when human beings spoke for their fallen peers, it has been expected that praise and memorialization of the dead would be a primary concern. Thus, after the ancient Athenians withstood a year of the Peloponnesian War with Sparta, the politician, Pericles, eulogized those lost in battle by extolling their virtues to an audience of survivors.

The deceased, then, receives honor in the exemplary eulogy, while the bereaved audience member receives some measure of comfort and consolation from the speech. Research indicates that eulogizers may draw from a variety of devices to foster a temporary relief from the grief and sadness occasioned by death. One such tactic is to promote actions that audience members may use to help them remember, or further the cherished causes of the lost loved one. A famous pair of examples can be found in the eulogies given by presidents Ronald Reagan and George W. Bush in 1986 and 2003 for the crews of the doomed space shuttles, *Challenger* and *Columbia*, respectively. Both presidents endorsed a continuation of support for the space programs that the astronauts lived and died for. Similarly, when a bomber killed four young black girls in a Birmingham, Alabama church, in September 1963, the Reverend Dr. Martin

Luther King Jr. used his eulogy as an opportunity to urge a continuation of the struggle against racism.

Another common strategy for providing solace in the eulogy is to promote the adoption of alternative, more positive mind-sets, in order to offset the morose feelings of loss. Mourners are encouraged to "look on the bright side of life," and to take solace from having been fortunate to have enjoyed and learned from the deceased. An extension of this strategy is to make meaning from the deceased's death through explicit recognition and appreciation of their life or through consoling the audience with knowledge of the deceased's existence in a better place, such as an afterlife. John Cleese eulogized Graham Chapman, a fellow member of the British *Monty Python* comedy troupe, by interpreting Chapman's penchant for offending public sensibilities as a lesson about the "momentary joy of liberation, as we realized in that instant that the social rules that constrict our lives so terribly are not actually very important."

Besides attending to the deceased and the audience, eulogizers may also address their own distress by giving voice to the intense emotion that they experience following the loss and because of the responsibilities they have assumed.

Examples in the genre of the eulogy are as varied as the number of people they have honored, yet most are characterized as bringing at least short-term respite from the devastation of loss that mourners and eulogizers share.

Michael Robert Dennis

See also: Epitaphs.

Further Reading

Copeland, Cyrus M. (ed.). *Farewell, Godspeed: The Greatest Eulogies of Our Time.* New York: Harmony Books, 2003.

Gilbert, Sandra M. *Death's Door: Modern Dying and the Ways We Grieve.* New York: W. W. Norton, 2006.

Kunkel, Adrianne Dennis and Michael Robert Dennis. "Grief Consolation in Eulogy Rhetoric: An Integrative Framework." *Death Studies,* 27(1) (2003): 1–38.

Theroux, Phyllis (ed.). *The Book of Eulogies: A Collection of Memorial Tributes, Poetry, Essays, and Letters of Condolence.* New York: Scribner, 1997.

EUPHEMISMS

A euphemism is a word or phrase that is deployed as a substitute for one that is more direct or explicit and whose use would be perceived as distasteful or causing unnecessary upset and harm. In the context of death and dying, euphemisms are routinely employed as a linguistic device for holding the emotional distress elicited by bereavement at arm's length. For some, the deployment of euphemisms reflects a careful attempt to use language sensitively so as to avoid upset and provide comfort to those in need of support. Euphemisms expressed in the language of condolence, either in verbal utterances or in the text found on sympathy cards, do this by reassuring the bereaved that the dead are not lost but are "gone before" or are merely "sleeping."

In addition to drawing upon metaphors such as sleep, much euphemistic language relies upon religious frameworks that serve to assure us of the existence of an eternal afterlife, where not only spiritual but also physical reunion with the dead is possible. Such language was popularized by the Romantic Movement in literature and art during the Victorian era, helping to fuel an anthropocentric view of the afterlife with human beings at its core. For others, however, the deployment of euphemisms in the context of death, dying, and bereavement is unhelpful, storing up problems (especially issues of psychosocial adjustment) by denying the reality of loss while at the same time adding to the social taboos and interdictions governing discourse on death and dying.

A most fierce critic of euphemisms in this context was the British aristocrat and author, Nancy Mitford, who in her book about the U.S. funeral industry, *The American Way of Death,* was searing in her criticism of the way in which language was being increasingly used to mask the reality of death. In this way, and allied to the growing professionalization of the funeral industry itself, we can see how cremated remains were transformed into "cremains," how hearses became "coaches," and how undertakers rebranded themselves as "funeral directors" or "morticians." Indeed, the term "undertaker" itself can be seen as a euphemism that was evolved to describe the business of disposing of the dead by those who, at first, agreed to "undertake" responsibility for providing various goods and materials to the bereaved (coffins, candles, carriages, etc.), and who later extended their remit by providing services including laying out, embalming, and disposing of the dead.

The potential harm caused by the use of euphemisms can also be seen in everyday informal conversation about the recently deceased, which, if overheard by the bereaved, can be deeply upsetting. To describe someone insensitively as having "kicked the bucket" or as being "six feet under" or "pushing up daises" can but add to the distress of the bereaved. The deployment of euphemisms, even with the best of intentions, to shield children from the upset caused by death can also be problematic, not least in delaying or even distorting the development of a mature understanding of death as something that is both finite and irreversible. Using the metaphor of sleep to refer to death can also induce fear in children about the nightly activity of sleep itself (lest they do not awake the following morning and suffer the same fate as a recently deceased relative).

In keeping with the deployment of euphemisms as a linguistic defense for shielding us against the terror of death, their usage can also be found in humor, which in itself is a tool for making light of a burdensome topic. Here, we find euphemisms employed by emergency care workers (such as paramedics and nurses) whose work brings them into contact with death and dying on a daily basis, often as a coping mechanism and distancing device. Health care professionals, often without necessarily realizing it, find themselves substituting explicit terms such as died or dying with phrases such as "passed away," "expired," or "terminally ill" in their outfacing encounters with bereaved relatives and the media.

Laurel Hilliker and Michael Brennan

See also: Humor; Taboo.

Further Reading

Holder, R. W. *Oxford Dictionary of Euphemisms.* Oxford and New York: Oxford University Press, 2003.

Keyes, R. *Euphemania: Our Love Affair with Euphemisms.* New York: Little, Brown & Co., 2010.

Mitford. N. *The American Way of Death.* New York: Simon and Schuster, 1963.

EUTHANASIA

The term "euthanasia" (from the Greek, meaning good death) refers to a variety of practices that involve someone other than the patient taking the final steps to end the patient's life; for example, a physician giving a patient a lethal dose of morphine. Euthanasia is distinguished from physician-assisted suicide in that the latter involves the patient taking the final steps to end his or her own life (see **Physician-Assisted Suicide**).

Euthanasia can be both voluntary and involuntary. It can be an affirmative act to end one's life (usually with a large dose of morphine or some other medicine administered by a physician), and is referred to as "active euthanasia"; or the discontinuation of means to extend life, which is described as "passive euthanasia." Hence, euthanasia is often divided into four distinct practices: voluntary active euthanasia, voluntary passive euthanasia, involuntary active euthanasia, and involuntary passive euthanasia.

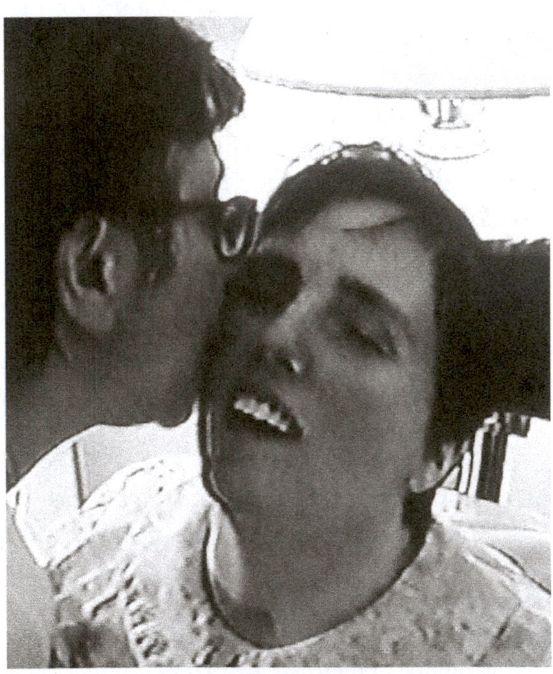

Video still of Terri Schiavo and her mother taken in Terri's hospice room in Pinellas Park, Florida, August 11, 2001. Schiavo, who suffered severe brain damage following a heart attack in 1990, was at the center of a national debate about the rights of incapacitated adults. (AP Photo/Schindler Family Video)

Most Americans approve of voluntary passive euthanasia and disapprove of any sort of involuntary euthanasia. The disagreement over the morality of euthanasia concerns the issue of whether voluntary active euthanasia is morally permissible.

The history of euthanasia, until recently, remained relatively static. The Hippocratic Oath, written about 2,500 years ago, counseled against the practice of active euthanasia: "I will give no deadly medicine to any one if asked, nor suggest any such counsel." Subsequently, active euthanasia, like suicide, was prohibited or discouraged throughout the Western world. English Common Law outlawed suicide, and in an 1877 Massachusetts decision (*Commonwealth v. Mink*), the court stated: "Now if the murder of one's self is felony, the accessory is equally guilty as if he had aided and abetted in the murder." In 1828, New York became the first in the United States to pass a statute outlawing euthanasia.

Voluntary *passive* euthanasia is legal throughout the United States. Adult patients have a right to bodily autonomy—the right to decide what happens in and to one's body—and this right includes the right to refuse or discontinue medical treatment, even if doing so will lead to the one's own death. *Active* euthanasia (voluntary and involuntary), on the other hand, is still prohibited in all of the 50 states of the United States. (Although active euthanasia is prohibited throughout the United States, a number of states have recognized or are considering recognizing the right to engage in physician-assisted suicide. For example, both Oregon and the state of Washington have passed Death with Dignity acts, i.e., legislation legalizing physician-assisted suicide.)

There are arguments both in support of, and in opposition to, voluntary active euthanasia. One of the most common arguments in opposition to voluntary active euthanasia is that as the practice becomes more prevalent, terminally ill patients may opt for active euthanasia, even if they oppose the practice or do not truly want to end their own lives. Patients may feel guilty if they do not consent to being euthanized and may come to believe that their loved ones expect them to consent; that their loved ones want to be spared the costs associated with a long, slow death (even if a patient's loved ones have never expressed such concerns).

A second argument against voluntary active euthanasia is based on the supposition that if voluntary active euthanasia becomes more widespread, health care professionals may come to resent (or treat less well than they otherwise would have treated) patients who do not opt for active euthanasia. Health care professionals are usually busy and space in hospitals is limited. Hence, health care professionals may (unconsciously) become hostile or resentful toward those who reject active euthanasia and insist on using/wasting valuable, limited resources.

A related argument is that active euthanasia is inconsistent with a physician's duty to preserve a patient's life and is therefore morally and professionally wrong.

A fourth argument against voluntary active euthanasia is that killing an innocent human is wrong because life is intrinsically valuable (e.g., life is a gift from God or every human is unique/special).

Finally, some claim that euthanasia is morally wrong because the Hippocratic Oath explicitly prohibits this practice. This is not a very strong argument, because the Hippocratic Oath contains other prohibitions that most of us do not embrace. One cannot "pick and choose" which prohibitions one wants to take seriously and which prohibitions one wants to reject. For example, the Hippocratic Oath prohibits physicians from practicing surgery. We do not outlaw or morally condemn surgery merely because the Hippocratic Oath prohibits it. Consistency dictates that we ought not, therefore, to oppose active euthanasia merely because active euthanasia violates the Hippocratic Oath.

One of the most common arguments in support of voluntary active euthanasia is based on a person's right to bodily autonomy. This argument is an extension of the standard justification of voluntary passive euthanasia. According to this argument, a person has a right to decide what happens in, and to, his or her own body. This right includes the right to decide whether she or he wants to continue living and the right to decide whether to introduce into his or her own body medications that will lead to their death. In addition, this includes the right to consent to others introducing into one's body medications that will lead to their death.

Another argument in support of voluntary active euthanasia begins with an examination of why most people believe voluntary passive euthanasia (i.e., disconnecting a person from life support or terminating other life-prolonging treatments) is morally permissible. Presumably, voluntary passive euthanasia is permissible because physicians are permitted to limit or decrease a patient's pain/suffering (both physical and/or psychological) if the patient requests pain relief. Passive euthanasia, or disconnecting a patient from life-supporting technology, is a means of limiting or decreasing the patient's pain/suffering, and is therefore considered permissible.

Advocates use this argument to assert that voluntary active euthanasia also decreases pain/suffering. In fact, voluntary active euthanasia decreases pain/suffering to a greater extent than does voluntary passive euthanasia. Hence, if voluntary passive euthanasia is justified because it alleviates pain, it follows that voluntary active euthanasia is also justified.

One response to this argument rests on the moral distinction between killing and letting die. Many of us believe, according to those who proffer this response, that killing is morally worse than letting die. Killing is an affirmative act, while letting die is an omission. It is therefore argued that because passive euthanasia consists of letting the patient die, while active euthanasia consists of killing the patient, active euthanasia is morally worse than passive euthanasia.

In an essay discussing voluntary active and passive euthanasia, James Rachels questions whether there truly is a moral distinction between killing and letting die. He suggests that they are morally comparable. Rachels asks the reader to consider a hypothetical case in which Smith stands to inherit a lot of money when his six-year-old nephew dies. While the nephew is taking a bath, Smith enters the bathroom and pushes his nephew under the water. He holds his nephew under the water until his nephew dies.

Rachels asks us to compare the behavior of Smith to that of Jones, who also intends to kill his six-year-old nephew in order to secure a large inheritance. But just before Jones reaches out to push his nephew under the water, the nephew slips, hits his head and falls face first into the water. Jones stands over the nephew waiting to drown him if necessary; however, the nephew drowns without Jones ever touching him.

Smith's behavior is an act of killing, while Jones's behavior is an act of letting die. Yet, according to Rachels, we believe Smith's and Jones's acts are morally comparable. That is, we do not believe that killing (in this example) is worse than letting die. Hence, Rachels claims the killing/letting die distinction is indefensible. If this is correct, then it is false to claim that active euthanasia is worse than passive euthanasia merely because the former involves killing while the latter involves letting die.

Finally, Rachels claims that the Smith and Jones cases reveal that what makes an act of killing (or letting die) good/bad is the intention of the agent. If an agent kills (or lets die) and his intention is morally bad, he is acting out of hatefulness and the act is morally wrong. But if the agent's intention is morally good, and he is acting out of benevolence or love, the act is morally right. Since most cases of killing flow from morally bad intentions, we have come to see killing as wrong. But in the case of euthanasia, whether active or passive, the physician's intention is good, and both practices are, therefore, morally permissible.

Courts and legislatures do recognize that acts that may *look* like active euthanasia may not actually be active euthanasia. That is, if a patient is in so much pain that the only way the pain can be controlled is by giving the patient a dose of medicine that will likely kill the patient, the act is not necessarily active euthanasia (a concept sometimes referred to as "double effect" or "terminal sedation"). In order to defend this claim, one must distinguish between foreseeable unintended consequences and foreseeable intended consequences. Consider a dentist who says to her patient: "Extracting your tooth will be painful, but I must extract it in order to cure a dangerous infection." The patient agrees to the extraction and then claims that the dentist acted wrongly, because the dentist hurt her. Most of us would say that the patient is not describing the situation accurately. We would agree that it is wrong for someone to intentionally hurt another person, but in this case hurting the patient was not the intention of the dentist. The dentist did foresee that her behavior would hurt the patient, but she did not intend to hurt her. Rather, pain was an (unavoidable) foreseeable, *unintended* consequence of the dentist's behavior. If, however, the dentist wanted to hurt the patient, we would react differently and conclude that her behavior was morally wrong.

Similarly, many recognize that if a patient is in so much pain that (adequately) controlling the pain would require a lethal dose of morphine, it does not necessarily follow that giving the patient this dose of morphine is morally wrong or that it involves the intentional killing of the patient. After all, the physician's intent is to stop pain, even though he or she knows that stopping pain will (likely) lead to the patient's death. One might describe the death as a foreseeable, unintended consequence of providing the patient with adequate pain relief. And, like in the case of the dentist, many of us believe it is wrong to conclude that an agent is morally blameworthy when his or her behavior was unintended (yet foreseeable).

Of course, if the physician provides morphine in order to kill the patient, then the death is foreseeable and intended, and the physician may be morally blameworthy. As stated above, many state legislatures recognize this distinction, as does the U.S. federal government.

Although involuntary euthanasia (both passive and active) is considered murder, philosopher Peter Singer has suggested that involuntary euthanasia may be justifiable, at least in theory. Singer considers a case in which a person is in so much agony that her physician (or others) believe her life is not worth living, yet the person does not recognize (or agree) that her life is not worth living. In such a case, Singer suggests, involuntary euthanasia may be permissible, because it is in the best interest of the patient. However, Singer points out that we are unlikely to come across this type of case in real life. After all, if a physician believes that his or her patient's life ought to be terminated because it is a life not worth living, and the patient disagrees, it is likely the case that the patient is correct. It is the patient who is living the life and is therefore in the best position to evaluate it.

Scott Gelfand

Further Reading

Brock, D. "Voluntary Active Euthanasia." *Hastings Center Report,* 22 (March-April, 1992): 10–22.

Callahan, D. "When Self-Determination Runs Amok." *Hastings Center Report,* 22 (March–April, 1992): 52–55.

Kass, L. "Neither for Love Nor Money: Why Doctors Must Not Kill." *Public Interest,* 94 (1989): 25–46.

Rachels, J. "Active and Passive Euthanasia." *New England Journal of Medicine,* 292(2) (1975): 78–80.

Singer, P. *Practical Ethics.* Cambridge: Cambridge University Press, 1993.

Wolf, Susan. "Gender, Feminism, and Death: Physician-Assisted Suicide and Euthanasia." In *Feminism and Bioethics: Beyond Reproduction,* edited by Susan Wolf (pp. 282–317). New York: Oxford University Press, 1996.

EXHUMATION

Exhumation (also known as disinterment) involves the removal of a casketed or noncasketed body from a grave, tomb, or mausoleum. In most societies throughout recorded history, the removal of bodily remains from their final resting place has been considered highly taboo and even sacrilegious; though there are some notable exceptions, such as in medieval Europe, where, due to a lack of available burial space, corpses were sometimes exhumed and placed in charnel houses (repositories for the storage of bones) (see **Charnel Houses**). In the United States, exhumation is rare and is only undertaken for legal reasons or, in exceptional circumstances, at the request of the deceased's family.

Reasons for exhumation are wide ranging and may include the need to transfer remains to a grave in another part of the cemetery from where the original burial took place. This is usually performed at the request of the family or if the body has been buried in the wrong grave. In many states, this is a straightforward procedure that does not usually require a court order but may require the written permission of the family. In parts of England (including London), because of a severe shortage of burial space, the possibility of reusing graves through a method known as "lift and deepen" has been discussed by local authorities as a serious option for resolving this shortage. Using this method, graves are excavated to their lowest possible depth. The bodily remains and any coffin furniture are then removed and reinterred in a casket at the bottom of the grave, thereby providing stacking space for up to three extra coffins. This practice is common in Germany, where graves are reused after 20 years, following the exhumation and cremation of existing bodily remains.

Another reason for exhumation would also include the need to transfer bodily remains to a grave in a different cemetery. This is usually undertaken at the request of the deceased's family, where it requires their written permission and may involve a court order and/or the issuing of a disinterment and reinterment document. It usually involves an amendment to the death certificate so as to reflect a different burial location. A document to disinter does not, however, include the opening of a casket or coffin. In Minnesota, opening a casket or coffin without a court order is a felony. In the United States, since cremation is considered final disposition, legal requirements for the exhumation of cremated remains is usually done at the request of the family and does not require a court order or extensive documentation.

A further reason for exhumation would be the need to re-examine a body in order to determine identity and to affirm or amend the cause of death (see also **Cause of Death**). This usually requires a court order and does not require family permission, unless the family is asking for the exhumation. In the United States, laws governing exhumation remain vague and vary from state to state. Most state regulations derive from English common law. One notable and high-profile example of exhumation of this sort was that of Yasser Arafat (1929–2004), former chairman of the Palestine Liberation Organization (PLO) and president of the Palestinian National Authority (PNA), whose remains were exhumed in November 2012 so that an autopsy (especially toxicology tests) could be performed to determine whether or not his death in 2004 was the result of poisoning.

Exhumation may also result from the relocation of a cemetery because of construction involving the erection or enlargement of a building or church; or some larger construction project such as the construction of a new road or the damming of a river.

Exhumation, however, is not typically granted in cases in which: the consent of the next of kin has not been given; the burial plot cannot be identified; the remains lie unidentified in a common plot (e.g., in the burial plot of a religious order); or in cases where due respect to the deceased cannot be guaranteed; the remains to be exhumed are located below a body that is not to be exhumed; public health and decency cannot be protected; graveyard ground conditions are not conducive to an exhumation; or conditions attached to the exhumation license cannot be complied with.

In the United States, when someone buys a grave site, that person is also buying the right to be buried perpetually; however, in some countries or societies, use of the grave is limited by time, such as 25 or 50 years. In Hong Kong, the body must be removed after as little as six years. Exhumation in these societies, as a preparation for double or secondary burial, is common. In many non-Western societies, secondary burial is performed as a rite for ensuring that the soul of the deceased passes to the spiritual afterlife (see **Anthropology**).

Within particular religions and faith communities, exhumation is strictly forbidden. Jewish law, for example, forbids exhumation except in the following circumstances: if the dead person is to be reinterred alongside his or her parents or close relatives; if disinterment is for the purpose of reburial in Israel; if the body of a Jew is buried in a Gentile cemetery and is exhumed for reburial in a Jewish one; if a grave is in danger of water seepage; or if the exhumation is ordered by a civil authority. In Islam, exhumation is forbidden, except in certain circumstances. In Christianity, both Catholic and Protestant churches forbid the disturbance of human remains, where possible. However, upon canonization, saints have frequently been disinterred so their remains can be dismembered and turned into relics.

In the United States and Australia, the exhumation of indigenous remains of American Indians and Aboriginal peoples by archaeologists has led to considerable controversy. Such controversy at the apparent violation of cultural sensibilities of ethnic groups, and the removal of their remains for display in museums as artifacts, helped prompt the passing by U.S. Congress in 1990 of the Native American Graves Repatriation Act. This ensured that human remains and other artifacts of American Indians were reunited with the living ancestors of their communities. In a similar move, the University of Nebraska agreed to return the remains of 1,700 American Indians to the living communities to which they belonged.

Michael Matthews and Michael Brennan

Further Reading

Kammen, Michael. *Digging up the Dead: A History of Notable American Reburials.* Chicago: University of Chicago Press, 2010.

Metcalf, Peter and Richard Huntington. *Celebrations of Death: The Anthropology of Mortuary Ritual.* New York: Cambridge University Press, 1991.

EXISTENTIALISM

Existentialism is a school of thought with its roots in the writings of two 19th-century philosophers, Søren Kierkegaard (1813–1855) from Denmark and Friedrich Nietzsche (1844–1900) from Germany. Kierkegaard believed that the duty of Christians is not to follow blindly what other people have defined as "God's will," but to serve God by finding their own way in life, making their own decisions and therefore being judged not by how loyal they were to other people's prescriptions, but by how true they were to their own authentically chosen path. His ideas have proven to be very influential, not least in his commitment to the importance of individuals being true to themselves and not just mindlessly following the crowd as a result of social, cultural, or religious expectations.

Superficially, Nietzsche's approach seems very different from Kierkegaard's, as he is famous for having declared the "death of God." That is, he believed that we should stop looking to a nonexistent (in his view) God for direction in our lives but instead find our own way. So, while their respective beliefs about God were poles apart, they shared a view that life is not simply a matter of following a preordained pattern. Nietzsche distinguished between ordinary people who largely just follow others uncritically without forming a view or a path of their own, and those people who were capable of making something of their lives for themselves. Making something of their lives was not simply a matter of achieving conventional success and wealth, as that could be seen as just mindlessly following other people's expectations. Rather, he saw it as a matter of developing our own path, something he referred to as "self-overcoming."

In the 20th century, two other European philosophers became famous for developing the ideas of their 19th-century predecessors. Martin Heidegger (1889–1976), from Germany, developed a very complex philosophy that came to be known as existentialism. This in turn influenced a wide range of thinkers who adopted what is now seen as an existentialist perspective. He emphasized the importance of "becoming," recognizing that human beings are not fixed entities, with set "personalities" (or "essences") but, rather, beings on a journey, constantly making choices and creating a sense of who they are and how they fit into the world.

One of the key writers Heidegger influenced was Jean-Paul Sartre (1905–1980), the French philosopher, novelist, and playwright. Heidegger's concept of "being-with-others" had shown that he understood human existence to have a social basis, but Sartre took this further. He argued that we are "what we make of what is made of us." That is, we have to make choices (there is no way of escaping that, as to refuse to make a choice is in itself a choice) and those choices serve to define who we are; they shape our identity to a large extent. However, those choices are not made in a vacuum, but are instead influenced by wider social factors, such as class, race, gender, and other such patterns of power and inequality.

One of the implications of this is that our identity will be forged in part by how we respond to what are known as existential challenges: the demanding situations we encounter from time to time where we have to make important decisions with significant, possibly life-changing consequences. Chief among these existential challenges are death and issues of loss more generally. This is significant in two key ways:

1. Facing up to our own mortality, recognizing that we will all die some day
2. Coping with the disruption and disorientation we encounter when we grieve a major loss

Existentialism, therefore, offers a way of understanding why death and loss are such challenging experiences: they disrupt our sense of who we are. Because existentialism presents a view of human beings as constantly changing as we move through our lives, major losses are significant because they prevent us from simply carrying on as before. They force us to rethink our understanding of ourselves and how we fit into the world. A major loss can therefore be understood as a form of existential or spiritual crisis. This is especially the case with bereavement (see **Bereavement**) as it reminds us that we are all mortal.

Neil Thompson

Further Reading

Flynn, Thomas. *Existentialism: A Very Short Introduction.* Oxford: Oxford University Press, 2006.

F

FACEBOOK

Facebook is a social networking site (SNS) with close to 1 billion members. Social networking sites, such as Facebook and Twitter, are part of social media that, in the first decade of the 21st century, have increased the interactivity of web- and mobile-based technologies by facilitating new and unprecedented opportunities for user-generated content. Not surprisingly, and because death, dying, and bereavement are social experiences, these technologies have also influenced the way people grieve as well as the way people die.

In the first instance, Facebook routinely provides a communal space—albeit a virtual one—in which people can come together to offer their condolences and provide social support to friends, family, and acquaintances following the loss of a loved one. This virtual congregational space, where people can grieve together online, is especially important in an age where our lives are increasingly geographically fragmented, separated in space and time. In the second, Facebook and other social media have the potential to reduce the sense of social isolation (see **Social Death**) often felt by those who are dying, allowing them—through Facebook updates, weblogs, and participation in Internet forums—to document their experiences and remain part of the social networks of the living. This development can in some ways be seen to reverse the modern process by which death and dying were "sequestered" or concealed from public view, marking instead a return to a time when death and dying were social events involving the whole community (see **Ariès, Philippe; Public Dying**).

A major way in which Facebook has, and continues to be, used is to memorialize the lives of people who have died. Launched in February 2004, Facebook did not have a policy on what to do with a person's account when they died—other than shut it down—until 2005, when a friend and colleague of Facebook employee Max Kelly was killed in a bicycle accident. As questions arose among colleagues as to do with his Facebook profile, the company decided to allow a person's page to remain active following death, memorializing their account by removing sensitive information—such as status updates and contact details—and adjusting privacy settings so that only confirmed "friends" can post messages of remembrance or locate that person during a search of the site. Facebook's current policy is to memorialize all deceased users' accounts unless family members request that an account be removed from their site. However, potential problems can arise if family members cannot agree on whether a loved one's Facebook account should be removed from the site. Such difficulties can be overcome by a digital will that provides instructions—including passwords to secure sites such as those for online banking—on what to do with online accounts following a person's death.

There are good reasons for believing that new technologies are modifying and expanding, if not changing, the ways we grieve by providing new opportunities for novel and innovative mourning practices. Adding "RIP" and the name of the person who has died to a Facebook status update, or changing a profile picture to one of (or with) the deceased person, are simple ways of indicating to others one's status as a mourner. Posting a message of condolence on a deceased friend's wall or on a specifically created Facebook memorial page are also increasingly common ways in which people are choosing to mark the death of a loved one. More personalized and inventive ways of Facebook grieving include the example of a teenage girl who created a memorial page for her murdered best friend: Facebook friends were invited to pen the lyrics of the murdered girl's favorite song—"Keep Breathing"—on their wrists, take a photograph, and post it.

One striking characteristic of Facebook grieving noted by observers is the tendency to address messages to the deceased directly and as if they were alive. While this is not entirely uncommon in off-line and face-to-face grieving (such as in paper-based public books of condolence or the habit of talking to the dead at the graveside when no one else is present), it can perhaps be explained as a consequence of a particular type of SNS communication that, unlike the telephone or face-to-face conversation, does not demand a response. Leaving a message to a dead person on Facebook is in this respect no different to posting a message to a living addressee. What is different, however, between off-line and online forms of communication on SNSs is that in the latter the dead appear to be listening; almost as if cyberspace functions as a metaphysical space—which is neither "here" nor "there"—where the dead reside.

This tendency toward communing directly with the dead, unselfconsciously and without embarrassment or shame, is also reflective of a desire to express a continuing bond with the deceased (see **Continuing Bonds**). This desire is reflected in Facebook policy on memorialization, which states that: "When someone leaves us, they don't leave our memories or our social network." It also, in some ways, reflects a return to a time when the living and the dead were copresent in society; when the dead, especially in premodern European societies, were buried at the heart of a living community in ways that, according to French social historian Philippe Ariès, suggested a "promiscuity between the living and the dead."

These transformations in how we communicate our experiences of death and dying reflect the technological changes that facilitate them. Early indications suggest that online grieving on SNSs provides comfort but also confusion, especially given the uncertainty surrounding what constitutes socially acceptable etiquette, such as how long after a person's death should one wait before removing the picture of the deceased from one's profile picture. Preliminary research on microblogging sites such as Twitter—which allow users to post messages of up to 140 characters to their social network—also suggest that these are less likely to be used to post messages of remembrance and condolence, than they are to share news and information, sometimes malicious, about celebrity deaths such as Michael Jackson's in 2009.

Michael Brennan

See also: Condolence (and Condolence Books); Cyberspace; Public Dying; Public Mourning; Social Death.

Further Reading

Goh, D. H. and C. H. Lee. "An Analysis of Tweets in Response to the Death of Michael Jackson." *Aslib Proceedings,* 63(5) (2011): 432–44.

Miller, Lisa. "R.I.P. on Facebook: The Uses and Abuses of Virtual Grief." *Newsweek,* March 1, 2010, 24.

Stone, Elizabeth. "Grief in the Age of Facebook." *Chronicle Review,* February 28, 2010.

Walter, Tony, Rachid Hourizi, Wendy Moncur, and Stacey Pitsillides. "Does the Internet Change How We Die and Mourn? An Overview." *Omega: Journal of Death and Dying,* 64(4) (2011): 275–302.

FAMILICIDE

Familicide is the murder of family members by another family member. In other words, familicide is a multiple-victim homicide in which the killer's spouse or partner and one or more children are killed. Although familicide is relatively rare, it is nevertheless the most common form of mass killing. It is differentiated from other types of mass murder in that victims are family members rather than being anonymous or unknown to the murderer. Despite the rarity of familicide, parents are more likely to kill their children than strangers are to abduct or kill them.

Most familicides are perpetrated by men, who, after their murders, kill themselves as well. Regardless of gender, familicide is often followed by the suicide of the murderer.

Among the reasons cited for familicide are custody disputes following marital separation, a parent's wish to stop children's suffering (perhaps due to domestic violence or sexual abuse), feelings of shame resulting from a job loss or perceived inability to provide for family members, other financial reversals, and a history of mental illness, including severe depression or psychosis. When money is the issue, the killer may see himself or herself as the breadwinner and feel that he or she must take the whole family with them when completing suicide.

Some experts find that women are more likely to kill their children than men are, whereas men are more likely to kill both their children and their spouse. Women may have different motives or reasons for familicide than do men. Women tend to kill their children because of a delusional sense of altruism or selflessness, as opposed to feeling that they have failed at adequately providing for them.

For someone who is psychotically depressed, the whole world is dull gray, and one's children are seen through their suffering and emotional pain, causing the

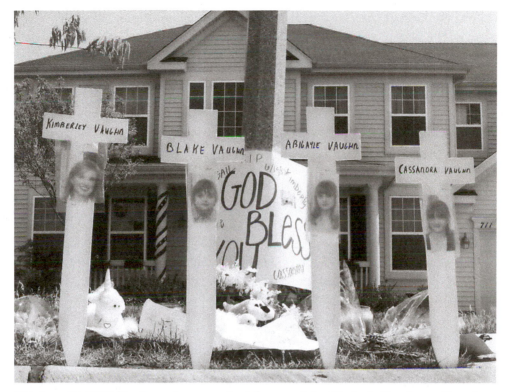

This June 15, 2007 file photo shows a makeshift memorial to Kimberly Vaughn, and her three children. In November 2012, Christopher Vaughn was sentenced by a court in Joliet, Illinois, to four consecutive life sentences for shooting dead his wife and children. (AP Photo/Charles Rex Arbogast, File)

killer to believe that the children, too, are suffering. Thus, the killer may believe that they would be better off in heaven or some other paradise. Killing is thus perceived as a selfless decision, one carried out with the hope of relieving suffering but with horrific results.

Psychosis may also lead a perpetrator to believe that the killing of a child is done with the goal of ending the child's suffering or because the child is demonically possessed. In the second case, the killer may see the child not as suffering but as unredeemingly evil. For the protection of others, he or she must be killed.

Familicide also encompasses murders in which a parent or parents and other relatives such as siblings, in-laws, or grandparents are killed. If only parents are killed, the situation can be referred to as a parricide. Parricide is most often committed by a son against the father and is commonly associated with delusional or faulty mental processes.

Terms related to familicide include filicide (the killing of one's child or children), uxoricide (the killing of one's wife), fratricide or sororicide (the killing of one's brother or sister), avunculicide (the killing of one's uncle), and nepoticide (the killing of one's nephew).

Albert Lee Strickland

See also: Homicide; Infanticide.

Further Reading

Ewing, Charles Patrick. *Fatal Families: The Dynamics of Intrafamilial Homicide.* Thousand Oaks, CA: Sage, 1997.

Websdale, Neil. *Familicidal Hearts: The Emotional Styles of 211 Killers.* New York: Oxford University Press, 2010.

FAMINE

A famine is defined as a widespread scarcity of food caused by a number of factors, such as the failure of crops to grow, the infestation of insects (locusts), the impact of disease on crops and on poultry and livestock, overpopulation, government policy (e.g., not controlling the sale of food resources to other countries), corruption in handling the production and distribution of food, and the side effects of either manmade (e.g., war) or natural (e.g., a flood or extended heat/drought) disasters. Famines commonly lead to widespread malnutrition, starvation, epidemic, increased mortality, and a period of psychosocial instability associated with the scarcity of food, such as riots, theft of food, and fall of governments caused by political instability borne of an inability to deal with the crisis created by famine. Famines are more likely to occur where poverty is widespread, where the infrastructure is not equipped to deal with food shortages, and where people are ruled tyrannically and their rights suppressed. Similarly, where a country's road system is underdeveloped, distributing food to those who need it may be nearly impossible. War or economic instability can also impede efforts to recover from the effects of famine. For countries that depend on a harvest to survive, three consecutive bad harvests create conditions ripe for famine.

Famines affect hundreds of millions of people worldwide, and are often most common and severe in sub-Saharan counties in the African continent. Famines are also quite common in some areas of Asia, such as India and China. During the 20th century, 70 million people died worldwide from famine, with 30 million dying during the 1958–1961 famine in China. The earliest recorded famine was that in Egypt in approximately 3500 BC. Historically speaking, widespread famines have occurred at one time or another in Russia, Ireland, and Bengal.

Famines are best understood at multiple levels. Most clearly, at the micro level it is individuals who suffer tremendously when starvation produces extreme malnutrition in the form of marasmus or kwashiorkor. These forms of childhood malnutrition caused by inadequate intake of calories and protein, lead to inactivity, malaise, growth retardation, weight loss, abdominal edema, and diarrhea. A most obviously recognizable symptom of kwashiorkor is a distended abdomen.

Though relatively little is known about the other effects of famine, relationships with others who people perceive as competitors for scarce food supplies, or persons whose needs they place above their own, are likely to be affected. If such people die, survivors grieve their deaths. Over and above dealing with the loss of a loved one, survivors may also feel hopeless and angry about their lives, especially their governments' inability to prevent or control the effects of famine and because of the loss of relationships with others. As more people die, disposing of their bodies in a publically healthy way, minimizing the spread of disease, and dealing with food riots and corruption, are challenges that overwhelm many countries, perpetuating both the short-term and long-term effects of famine on individuals and their families, friends, neighbors, and coworkers.

While famine cannot always be prevented, its effects can be minimized by providing the people affected with vitamins and minerals to supplement their diets, providing foodstuffs to afflicted countries, targeting malnourished children, providing cash or vouchers for people to purchase food or providing subsidies to farmers for fertilizer, seed, and water so they can grow food. Ultimately, people can avoid famine by becoming as self sufficient as possible, so as to minimize their dependency on others in the event of a mass shortage of food. Educating farmers about how to fertilize and irrigate their land effectively can be a way of dealing with the effects of famine by preventing them from reoccurring or, at the very least, from being as devastating in their impact. Treating diseases (e.g., diarrhea, cholera, dysentery, and infection) that are consequences of famine can also be an effective way of minimizing its multiplicative effects. The effects of famine are most severe for children and older adults, and males generally are more likely to die than females (who may be more resilient and better placed biologically to withstand the effects of famine, with less body mass on average than men, meaning they need less food to survive, and with more body fat on average than men). Those who survive the effects of malnutrition often never recover fully, experiencing brain damage and an inability to fight disease and infection. Famine also undermines fertility, with birthrates increasing after the famine has ended, the result of which is termed a "rebound effect." The effects on populations are usually overcome in several years after the end of a famine. This was the case for China (1958–1961) and Ethiopia (1983–1985); after a few years, the previous effects of mortality were virtually eliminated, and population growth was restored.

The effects of famine are commonly evaluated in terms of degrees of "food insecurity," which vary from near scarcity, to scarcity, to famine. Currently, an intensity scale is used by such agencies as the U.S. Agency for International development, with intensity being graded as "food secure, food insecure, food crisis, famine, severe famine, and extreme famine." Here, mortality is assessed in terms by which less than 1,000 deaths are defined as a minor famine, and over 1 million deaths are defined as a catastrophic famine. Evaluating famines in these ways allow governments to anticipate the occurrence of famine, permitting the monitoring of, and attention to, the distribution of available food supplies as well as enabling them to enact measures that may prevent famine from occurring in the first place. For example, making sure that adequate water is available to allow for the growing of crops, and ensuring that adequate grain (i.e., wheat, soybean, maize)—the price of which is impacted by oil prices—is available to feed poultry and dairy cows, are ways in which the (re)occurrence of famines can be minimized. The use of fertilizers to stimulate crop production, however, may have long-term negative effects on soil quality, which actually increases the odds of famine (re)occurring.

Bert Hayslip Jr.

Further Reading

Bloy, Marjie. "Famine." In *Encyclopedia of Death and the Human Experience,* edited by Clifton D. Bryant and Dennis L. Peck (pp. 445–49). Thousand Oaks, CA: Sage, 2009.

Kastenbaum, Robert J. *Death, Society, and Human Experience,* 10th edition. Boston: Allyn & Bacon, 2009.

FORENSIC SCIENCE

Forensic science is the term given to a somewhat amorphous array of academic specialisms whose techniques and expertise are brought to bear in helping to establish the likely cause, time, and location of a person's death. It is especially pertinent in circumstances in which a death is unexplained, out of the ordinary, or suspicious. In such instances, the cause of death must be determined by a death investigator, usually a coroner or medical examiner, the latter being a physician equipped with specialist knowledge and advanced training in the fields of anatomy and forensic pathology. In cases of suspicious death, the role of the forensic pathologist—which includes performing an autopsy to determine the cause of death—involves providing evidentiary knowledge that can be used in a court of law. Such knowledge is pivotal in ensuring justice and providing answers to questions of grieving relatives who would want to know more about the circumstances in which a loved one died.

The origins of forensic science can be traced to series of developments which occurred toward the end of the 19th and beginning of the 20th century. Among the most significant of these events was the development of fingerprinting technology based on the ideas of Frances Galton, who, in 1892, had discovered that no two persons had the same curved lines on the tips of their fingers; that they were instead unique to the individual and were thus an invaluable tool in helping identify those responsible for a variety of crimes, including murder. These ideas were taken up and developed by Edward Henry, and by the early 1900s, had been widely adopted by criminal investigators the world over.

Further breakthroughs during this period included the pioneering development by Alexandre Lacassagne of forensic ballistics. Lacassagne established that bullet casings fired from guns left their own indelible "fingerprints" in the marks made by gun barrels as bullets passed through them. Forensic ballistics was further developed in the 1920s and 1930s by Calvin Goddard, who is today widely regarded as its founder. Attempts to recover and identify spent gun casings from the scenes of crime are nowadays a taken-for-granted aspect of criminal investigations and a crucial element in the panoply of forensic science.

In similar vein, and based on the shared assumption that every criminal leaves some trace of himself behind at the scene of a crime, Karl Landsteiner contributed at the very beginning of the 20th century to the burgeoning field of forensic science through the discovery of serology (the scientific study of blood and bodily fluids such as semen and saliva). Like fingerprints, Landsteiner discovered that blood types were unique to the individual and were routinely left behind at the scenes of murder (as drops, stains, or splatters) in ways that could be traced to both victims and perpetrators, providing forensic evidence that could be used to secure a criminal conviction. Drawing upon developments in these separate fields (especially the assumption that every criminal not only leaves behind but also takes something away with them from the scene of a crime), Edmund Locard established in 1910 the first laboratory for analyzing trace material (hair, clothing fibers, dirt, leaves, etc.) recovered from crime scenes.

More recently, the discovery in 1984 of "genetic fingerprints" in the form of DNA (deoxyribonucleic acid) by Alec Jeffreys at the University of Leicester in England, has added another, albeit even more sophisticated, layer to the armory of weapons available to forensic scientists. These forensic technologies have been tremendously influential, helping to secure criminal convictions as well as to exonerate the wrongly accused and redress miscarriages of justice.

Even more recently, sophisticated DNA techniques have been employed by forensic scientists for identifying human remains in instances where all that is left is a badly decomposed corpse, skull, skeletal remains, or bone fragments. Together with the work of forensic anthropologists (who have been able to determine the sex, age, and time of death from the analysis of bone fragments), such techniques have been used to identify the victims of plane crashes, serial killers, genocide, terrorism, war, and state-sanctioned killing in places where political opponents were the subject of human rights abuses and violations. Forensic science of this sort, especially under the auspices of Clyde C. Snow, has been used since the 1980s to identify murder victims and convict perpetrators in places such as Argentina, Croatia, and Rwanda, among others. In Argentina, for example, following the end of the military junta and election of a civilian government, Snow led a forensic team charged with identifying the remains of the *desparecidos,* "the disappeared," who had been murdered by death squads during seven years of military rule.

A major discovery within the broadly constituted field of forensic science (encompassing archaeology, osteology, history, forensic pathology, and genealogy) came in February 2013, when scientists at the University of Leicester in England were able to confirm the identity of remains discovered in a city center parking lot were those of the last Plantagenet King of England, Richard III, who had died in battle some 500 years earlier. Using DNA analysis, skeletal examination, and radiocarbon dating, researchers were able not only to confirm the identity of Richard III but also, remarkably, to determine the likely cause of death and when he was killed. Beyond this, researchers were also able to determine his diet (as high in protein and consistent with that of a person of high status), to reconstruct how Richard might have looked, and to disprove the myth of his "withered arm" promulgated in Shakespeare's portrayal of him.

All of this, especially in light of popular cultural fascination with forensic science (e.g., the popularity of television shows such as *Bones*, *Silent Witness*, and *CSI*, whose principal characters are forensic pathologists and anthropologists), might lead one to assume that the results of analysis are always precise and are arrived at quickly (usually within a matter of hours). The reality, however, is somewhat more complex, and the results of forensic testing are often not known for a matter of weeks, even months, and may in some instances remain inconclusive. What is clear is that forensic science, as is often portrayed in fictional and real-life accounts of forensic scientists (such as the PBS documentary series *Secrets of the Dead*), does give voice to the dead, who can no longer speak for themselves nor communicate the circumstances surrounding their death; as well giving some comfort and "closure" to the relatives and loved ones of the deceased, who, in some instances, can reclaim the dead for ritual disposal and begin a process of grieving that had hitherto been inhibited or delayed.

Michael Brennan

See also: Archaeology; Autopsy; Coroner/Medical Examiner.

Further Reading

Buckley, R., M. Morris, J. Appleby, T. King, D. O'Sullivan, and Lin Foxhall. "The King in the Car Park: New Light on the Death and Burial of Richard III in the Grey Friars Church, Leicester, in 1485." *Antiquity*, 87(336) (2013): 519–38.

Manhein, Mary H. *The Bone Lady: Life as a Forensic Anthropologist.* New York: Penguin Books, 2000.

Snow, Clyde C., Lowell J. Levine, Leslie Lukash, Luke G. Tedeschi, Cristian Orrego, and Eric Stover. "The Investigation of the Human Remains of the 'Disappeared' in Argentina." *American Journal of Forensic Medicine and Pathology*, 5(4) (1984): 297–99.

Tilstone, William J., Kathleen A. Savage, and Leigh A. Clark. *Forensic Science: An Encyclopedia of History, Methods, and Techniques.* Santa Barbara, CA: ABC-CLIO, 2006.

Yount, Lisa. *Forensic Science: From Fibers to Fingerprints.* New York: Chelsea House, 2007.

FREUD, SIGMUND

Sigmund Freud was the founder and father of psychoanalysis, a subspecialism within the broader disciplinary field of psychology. Born in 1856 in Freiberg Moravia (then part of the Austrian Empire, now the Czech Republic), Freud's family moved to Vienna when he was a child, and he attended school and university there (studying medicine). The rise of the Nazi party and the persecution of Jews made life in Vienna increasingly dangerous, Freud's books were burnt in Berlin in 1933, and he followed his family to London in 1938. He died of cancer on September 23, 1939, three weeks after the beginning of the Second World War.

From his consulting room in Vienna, and via his extensive writing and the energies of those who built on his ideas, he promoted a new way of understanding what it means to be human and what underpins society. His ideas of the importance of early experience—the impact of the irrational and the unknown on our actions, the importance of sexuality across all aspects of our life, and how dreams illuminate our wishes and fears—have become part of our intellectual terrain. The terminology of psychoanalysis—the unconscious, neuroses, repression, taboos, "the Oedipus complex," and "Freudian slips"—have become part of everyday discourse. Psychoanalysis, a method of illuminating the complexities of different parts of the psyche, characteristically via encouraging a person to "free associate" and to recount dreams, is widely used. While psychoanalysis constitutes a specific method with a rigorous training, it has exerted a wider influence on a range of "talking cures" for emotional distress.

Freud's twin focus on both the individual and society is evident in those aspects of his work that directly engage with death. In considering the individual's experience of loss, he compared normal and pathological mourning; in looking at society, he explored the reasons for there being social taboos about the dead. He also examined destructiveness in individuals and society. But, his approach involves assumptions and terminology that are complex. To appreciate his contribution to death and dying, we must locate these aspects of his work within his overall approach to the mind.

Freud's Theory of Mind

Freud worked with patients throughout his professional life. His insights were developed from reflecting on things they told him, including their dreams. The adult personality, Freud argued, is the outcome of experiences and conflicts beginning in early childhood. Conscious thought is a surface activity and underneath it the unconscious operates according to its own rules. Freud's early works, such as *The Interpretation of Dreams* (1899), described how our lives are structured by a pleasure principle and a reality principle, with the latter constraining the former. Dangerous or socially unacceptable desires are repressed and resurface in other guises. Many of these desires are sexual in nature. They can only be fulfilled in dreams (although often in a disguised form) because they cannot be allowed to dominate waking life.

Freud's clinical work and his experience of the world around him, most significantly the death and destruction of World War I, prompted a reworking of his theory of mind. He now described the psyche as comprising the id, ego, and superego. The instinctual realm (id) is divided between life instincts (*Eros*) and a death drive (later described by other psychoanalysts as *Thanatos*).

Individual Responses to Death

Freud's patients told him about their dreams of the death of close relatives. He interpreted these dreams as a manifestation of unconscious hostility. For example, a reported sense of guilt and a feeling of responsibility for a death may disguise an inadmissible and unconscious sense of satisfaction that this person has died. Such feelings exemplify a phenomenon central to Freud's approach, ambivalence. We can unconsciously feel hostility, even wish for someone's death, and at the same time exhibit affection toward them.

In his 1917 paper, "Mourning and Melancholia," Freud compared normal responses to irreparable loss that are found in grief to pathological responses found in clinical depression. In the normal process of mourning, the person works through attachments to the person who has died and, since reality confirms that they are absent, the instincts of self-preservation characteristic of the ego, lead to severance of those attachments and thus, eventually, to detachment. In pathological forms of mourning, ambivalence distorts this process. Rather than ensuring a self-preserving detachment, there is an unconscious identification with the dead person. The hostile feelings that were the unconscious source of the ambivalence toward the person who has died are directed against the ego. The result is a state of depression or melancholia. In an extreme form, this hostility toward the ego, toward oneself, can result in suicide.

For Freud, grief is a normal response. It requires time and hard work, not therapy. It is a human misfortune, not a pathological condition. Pathological forms of mourning justify the use of therapy, as a means of exerting some control over unacknowledged influences of the past by bringing them to light. But the aim of both the normal response and the therapeutic response is the same: to preserve the ego via the elimination of the tensions that can beset it. That is achieved by the severance of emotional ties with the person who has died.

Death and Society

Just as Freud saw life instincts and a death drive as coexisting elements of the id in each individual, he also saw an ongoing struggle in society between competing impulses for activity and survival on one hand, and withdrawal and death on the other. There is an ambivalence manifest in society as well as in individuals.

In *Totem and Taboo* (1913), Freud described a different way in which unconscious hostility to the dead can be resolved. Here, rather than ambivalence being expressed via hostility toward oneself, it is projected onto the dead—now constructed as a category, not a specific person. Avoidance, fear, and demonization of the dead are all manifestations of ambivalence at a social level. One way this occurs is via the establishment of ritualized taboos about the dead. Taboos are both expressions of mourning and forms of self-defense, ways of disguising unconscious hostility.

Shortly after the end of World War I, Freud, in *Beyond the Pleasure Principle* (1920), explored an opposition between a sexual life instinct (Eros), which moves us to reproduce and so to guarantee survival, and a death drive that moves us to return to an earlier condition of tension-free stability. Aggression is the death instinct directed outward toward others as obstacles, while self-destructive behavior is the death instinct directed inward toward the self as an obstacle to the right kind of death. The right kind of death is one that achieves a tension-free stability. This internal process of linked aggression and self-destructiveness are manifest also in nations. For example, war can be a way of avoiding self-destructive internal feuds by redirecting energy elsewhere.

Holding Instincts in Check

For Freud, the individual seeks to preserve the ego by negotiating a route between different tensions. One is a tension between our instinctive desires and our fears of social sanctions. The other is a tension between *life instincts*, a tendency toward survival that is manifest in sex, in having children, and in other creative activities; and a *death drive* that is manifest when we keep returning to things that traumatize us or when we are self-destructive or aggressive to others. We will feel grief when those we are close to die, but with time and effort we can reassemble the ego without them and carry on. But if we do not escape our ambivalence we will battle with ourselves, a battle manifest in depression. More generally, we will deal with the psychic disruption caused by death by projecting our ambivalence, and our fears, onto socially shared symbols (totems) that are taboo. Or we might succumb to self-destruction or aggression when, as a society, we can neither acknowledge nor overcome our ambivalence. In these ways, a concern with death is at the heart of Freud's project because it is at the heart of the preservation of both the self and society.

Neil Small

See also: Mourning.

Further Reading

Freud, Sigmund. "Beyond the Pleasure Principle." In *The Standard Edition of the Complete Psychological Works of Sigmund Freud*, edited by James Strachey, Vol. 18 (pp. 1–64). London: Hogarth Press, 1955/1920.

Freud, Sigmund. "Civilization and Its Discontents." In *The Standard Edition of the Complete Psychological Works of Sigmund Freud.* edited by James Strachey, Vol. 21 (pp. 64–145). London, Hogarth Press, 1963/1930.

Freud, Sigmund. *The Interpretation of Dreams.* Harmondsworth: Penguin, 1976/1900.

Freud, Sigmund. "Mourning and Melancholia." In *The Standard Edition of the Complete Psychological Works of Sigmund Freud*, edited by James Strachey, Vol. 14 (pp. 152–70). London: Hogarth Press, 1957/1917.

Jones, Ernest. *Sigmund Freud: Life and Work.* London: Hogarth Press, 1955.

Storr, Anthony. *Freud: A Very Short Introduction.* Oxford: Oxford University Press, 2001.

FUNERAL DIRECTOR

The terms funeral director, mortician, and undertaker are all used interchangeably to describe the after-death care provider in modern Western societies. In the past, care of the deceased—including disposal of the body—fell largely upon family, friends, and the wider community, who were responsible for "looking after their own." As societies developed, each characterized by an increasingly complex division of labor (in which employment became segmented into particular fields of expertise), specialists gradually assumed responsibility for tasks that people had once carried out themselves. Initially, it was coffin makers who began to "undertake" more and more responsibilities associated with after-death care, such as providing ornaments with which to conduct mourning rituals and a carriage in which to transport the body to a place of burial. As societies continued to develop, so this list of services provided by undertakers was extended to include a place of storage for the deceased's body in the period between death and burial. Traditionally, the dead had been kept at home in the family's parlor, yet as modern societies became increasingly concerned with issues of hygiene (in which death itself was viewed as repugnant), undertakers began to offer "chapels of rest" for storage of the deceased—a precursor of the funeral parlor or mortuary chapel provided by today's modern funeral directors.

Today, the full range of services provided by funeral directors can be divided into four main parts: (1) helping to administer the legal and bureaucratic formalities triggered by death, including liaising with agencies such as the police, hospitals, and coroners; (2) taking possession of the body by providing a place of storage before burial or cremation; (3) embalming the body to enable visitation and facilitate grieving; and (4) organizing the funeral ceremony, arranging for floral tributes, disposal of the dead, and so on. Funeral directors may also provide "aftercare" services, such as helping the bereaved find counseling or a support group. In some instances, this "aftercare" has replaced the services once provided by clergy, while in others it may include helping facilitate a link to local clergy. In other instances still, some hospices and funeral homes have joined forces to provide an integrated package of "aftercare" support to the bereaved. Unlike many other careers, the job of funeral director requires round-the-clock commitment, 24 hours a day, 365 days a year. A glimpse into this commitment, and the many services provided by a funeral director, is provided by the PBS documentary film *The Undertaking*, which focuses on the Lynch and Sons family-run funeral home in Milford, Michigan.

Despite the generally high levels of customer satisfaction reported by the consumers of funeral services, funeral directors are often perceived in a less-than-positive light by the public at large. Part of this perception stems from a belief that funeral directors profit financially from the bereaved by charging them for services and items they do not actually need or had not requested. The Federal Trade Commission's ruling, implemented in 1984 and known as The Funeral Rule, was intended specifically to protect consumers by insisting that funeral directors provide a fully itemized list of services provided. A further criticism sometimes leveled at funeral directors is that the bereaved are "decentered" from practical and ceremonial proceedings in ways that are disempowering. Some of this criticism has provided the impetus for a movement in "do-it-yourself" funerals, in which the bereaved have attempted to reclaim some of the responsibilities and rites conceded to professionals. At the same time, many funeral directors have responded to this criticism, and an apparent desire on the part of consumers, by providing greater choice, flexibility, and involvement of the bereaved in funeral arrangements.

Michael Brennan

See also: Embalming; Funeral Industry.

Further Reading

Haberstein, Robert W. and William M. Lamers. *The History of American Funeral Directors.* Milwaukee: Bulfin Printers, 1962.

Howarth, Glennys. *Last Rites: The Work of the Modern Funeral Director.* Amityville, NY: Baywood, 1996.

Lynch, Thomas. *The Undertaking: Life Studies from the Dismal Trade.* New York: W. W. Norton and Co., 1997.

FUNERAL INDUSTRY

While in most societies, funerals and their accompanying rituals are systematically organized, it is in only in Western societies that they have attained the status of an industry, with an expert funeral director at the heart of the proceedings. The roots of the modern funeral industry lie in the medieval art of heraldry that planned and controlled the funerals of royalty and the aristocracy in Europe. These funerals were extremely grand affairs that were largely designed as a highly public display of the handover of power from one monarch or high-status individual to another. It was during the 17th and 18th centuries that undertakers began to take over the role of the College of Arms (who were in charge of Heraldic funerals), in centralizing the services of a range of agencies involved in provision of the funeral.

With the growth of towns, and as societies became increasingly industrialized, the traditional social order was changing and there was less emphasis on the hierarchies that were prevalent in rural societies. This was also a period in which people became more individualistic and family oriented and, as a result, when death and grief were more private affairs and focused around the family, rather than the community. At the same time, the demands of industrial society meant that people had less time to organize what might be (for the wealthier sections of society at least) elaborate and complex funeral rituals. Handing over responsibility to an expert was a way of unburdening the family, and also of ensuring that the rituals were observed in what was considered to be the socially correct fashion.

The new funeral industry began by handling the funerals of the emerging middle classes, commonly imitating the procedures adopted by the College of Arms. The funeral thus became a means by which families could publicly display their wealth and status. Undertakers (the forerunners of funeral directors) handled the provision of all that was considered necessary for a funeral, and they controlled the work of other industries that were involved such as drapers, carpenters, wreath makers, and metal workers. During the 19th century, with the creation of large cemeteries located on the edges of towns and cities, there was a new requirement for vehicles to transport the body and mourners to the graveside, and this resulted in increasingly flamboyant funeral provision. The industry thus provided an ever-multiplying range of commodities presented as essential to the "respectable funeral" and based on a code of status that varied according to social rank and wealth. For example, *Cassells Household Guide, 1870,* described the requirements of a middle-class funeral in London as including a hearse with four horses, two mourning coaches and horses, plumes made of ostrich feathers, velvet coverings, a cushioned elm coffin with a further coffin made of lead, brass handles, mutes with gowns, 14 men as pages, men to carry elaborate feathers, coachmen, and further attendants.

As the 19th century progressed, however, the funeral industry was subject to increasing criticism from the Church, which accused it of using pagan symbolism; and from other reform movements, who, in Great Britain, depicted undertakers as greedy, heartless men enforcing an expensive range of funeral goods on their clients that resulted in millions of pounds each year being "thrown into the grave." If the industry was to survive, it needed to change its image, and this was largely achieved by a process of professionalization involving industry regulation, educational and training programs, innovation in services, and a greater focus on care for the bereaved family.

Despite reform, or possibly as a result of it, the industry has retained control over the services and rituals associated with the funeral. While demonstrating that they now offer more practical and affordable procedures for disposal, they have effectively expanded the range of services they offer. For example, it was during the 20th century that funeral homes were established to relieve the family of the problem of housing the body of the deceased, and to take account of new public health concerns that questioned the practice of keeping the corpse in the home prior to disposal. In the United States, this led to an increase in the practice of embalming, which was thought to address these health concerns while preserving the body for viewing (see also **Embalming**). Modern embalming differs dramatically from the practices of ancient Egypt, and was first employed during the American Civil War, when it was used to preserve the bodies of dead soldiers to enable them to be returned home for burial. The skills needed for embalming have led to it become a profession in and of itself, requiring training and scientific knowledge of the body (see also **Mortuary Science**).

Further, major changes that took place in the industry during the 20th century included offering clients a greater range of coffins and, in the United States, the introduction of the casket. A coffin has shaped shoulders and was traditionally made by the local carpenter (who was commonly also the local undertaker), whereas a casket is rectangular. Until the mid-20th century, caskets were usually made of wood, but the increasing popularity of the metal casket, which required more complicated manufacturing processes, meant that dedicated companies were established, thus expanding the funeral industry. By the 1990s, over 60 percent of caskets sold in the United States were made of metal.

During the 1960s, a number of large companies moved into the funeral industry, buying up small local funeral homes. While retaining the outward appearance of a small business (and often keeping the original name), these organizations benefit from the economies of scale that are gained by sharing services such as vehicles and staff.

In the United States, the funeral industry is subject to regulation on a state-by-state basis. Although regulations differ, most states require funeral homes to be licensed

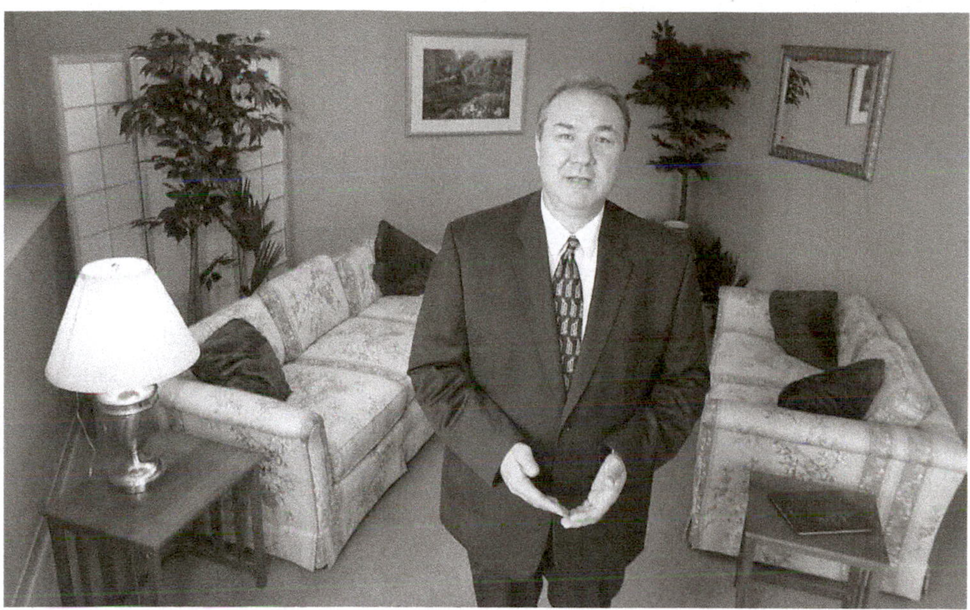

John Bucci, a licensed funeral director, talks in the reception area of his recently opened Wisconsin Chapels and Cremation Society in a strip mall in Verona, Wisconsin, on September 28, 2005. His business was threatened with a proposed bill in the Wisconsin Legislature that aimed to ban funeral parlors from strip malls. (AP Photo/Andy Manis)

and funeral operatives to be appropriately qualified. There are commonly other restrictions in place. For example, in some states, companies are prevented from owning both funeral homes and cemeteries, and the prearranged funeral package is highly regulated to avoid intrusive sales practices and to ensure that monies are paid into trusts that guarantee that service will be delivered when needed.

Glennys Howarth

See also: Funeral Director.

Further Reading

Howarth, Glennys. *Last Rites: The Work of the Modern Funeral Director*. Amityville, NY: Baywood, 1996.

FUNERALS

A funeral service, or funeral, is an event where family and friends gather before burial or cremation to honor the life of the person who has died. In addition to commemorating the person who died, a funeral service serves as a symbolic ritual for survivors in which it is traditional for family and friends to offer social, spiritual, and emotional support. A funeral visitation time, also referred to as a wake or a viewing [of the body], typically occurs a day or two before the funeral (see **Wakes/**

Visitations). A funeral service may be lawfully conducted anywhere. Nevertheless, a funeral home, operated by a funeral director, is typically the chosen place for the visitation and funeral service.

Funeral Symbolism

The funeral memorial service serves to commemorate the dead person's life and his or her passage from that life. In addition, and as a matter of practicality, the funeral service allows family members to make a public statement, akin to issuing a death notification, to the community at large that their loved one has died.

Families have many decisions to make regarding the specifics of their loved one's funeral, but there is a growing trend toward people making active choices about their own funeral service before they die. This way, people are assured that their funeral service will be representative of who they were and what they liked. For example, one person, who enjoyed working at children's birthday parties as a clown, specified that he wanted to be dressed as a clown in his casket. In another example, a biker stipulated that, from his funeral service to his burial site, bikers on Harley Davidson bikes should lead the hearse. Another new funeral custom is to use fewer hymns and more popular music, such as Frank Sinatra's "My Way" or Celine Dion's "My Heart Will Go On." Regardless of whether a person makes his or her wishes known before their death or whether the family makes the decision after the person dies, it seems clear that a new age of funerals exists that comes from a blending of a variety of traditions and styles—secular with religious, old with new, popular with classical, and Eastern with Western, and so on.

In addition to commemorating the life of the deceased, the traditional American funeral service provides a place for friends to show sympathy, as well as provide emotional and spiritual support. Support may include talking, praying with the survivors, and preparing food for the extended family. As survivors transition from a life with their loved one to a life without, the support of others is helpful, especially for those whose identity may have changed. For example, a man who lost his wife is suddenly a widower; a woman, who lost her husband, is now a widow.

Decisions for Family Members

After the death of a loved one, one of the first decisions family members must make is to select a casket or coffin (a coffin is usually made of wood and has an octagonal shape and is wider at the shoulder area, a casket is typically rectangular in shape and is made of more durable materials, such as steel or bronze, and is often expensive).

Another decision family members must make is whether to have a burial or cremation, the process of burning a dead body and its container (see **Cremation**). Overall, cremation is less expensive. Also, unlike with a burial, a casket is not required in cremation. If opting for burial, the family may choose between an earth burial or interment of the body in an above-the-ground building known as a mausoleum (see **Tombs/Mausoleums**).

Other family decisions include deciding the type of funeral service. For example, will the service be religious or nonreligious? Will there be music? Who will sing? Who will speak? Who will write the obituary (an account of the dead person's life) for the local newspaper? Another decision includes selecting pallbearers, the people who carry the casket or coffin at the funeral and burial. A decision must also be made about where the burial plot will be as well as deciding on grave markers/tombstones.

A family may also choose to remember a loved one who has died by a eulogy, the words spoken about the deceased at the funeral (see **Eulogy**), or by an epitaph, words engraved on a tombstone (see **Epitaphs**).

Religious and Cultural Traditions

Religious traditions have had a central role in ritualizing death. These traditions offer structured ways to celebrate and remember the deceased. Ritualistic examples include the Hindu practices of the people of India. Here, at death, male relatives carry the dead body to a river where it is immersed for purification. Next, cremation follows to liberate the soul for reincarnation. After cremation, family members, all of whom are dressed in white, come together for a meal and prayers. Friends visit the family for 13 days (see **Hinduism**).

When a loved one is near death, Buddhists, living chiefly in South Asian countries, whisper the name of Buddha, into the ear of the dying person in an effort to bring good to the person after death. As soon as the person dies, relatives begin wailing to express sorrow and to notify neighbors. After funeral rights are spoken, a man carries a white banner on a long pole, leading the procession to the cremation grounds. When they arrive at the cremation site, mourners toss lighted candles into the cremation coffin (see **Buddhism**).

Another example of religious customs involving funerals is that practiced by Muslims, whereby burial takes place without a coffin so that the body can decompose into the original four elements (earth, air, water, and fire). If possible, Muslims bury their dead within 24 hours. The dead body, wrapped in white, is placed with his or her head facing right toward Mecca, Islam's holiest city. The official mourning period is three days (see **Islam**).

When death occurs in a family in China, all mirrors are removed from sight to avoid the death of another family member, lest he or she catches their reflection in a mirror. As mourners arrive to visit the bereaved, they enter the house through a door draped in white cloth. In Japan, the dead person is transformed into a revered ancestor whose spirits gradually fade away (see also **Ancestor Worship**).

Orthodox Jews, about half of whom live in North America, typically prepare the dead body for burial and remain with it continually until burial. With the belief by many that cremation is a desecration of the body, most Jews are buried in a cemetery. Many mourners make a symbolic tear (*keriah*) in their clothes to represent the tearing of the deceased from life. During the seven days of mourning (*shiva*), family members do not shave, bathe, wear makeup, use perfume, wear leather shoes, or get haircuts.

Christianity, it should be noted, began as a Jewish sect, and, traditionally, most Christian mourners wear black; however, that custom is not as common as it once was. Funeral services typically include singing and readings from the Bible before the body is transported to a cemetery for burial or crematory for cremation.

In earlier times, and regardless of their religious preferences, people lived in a world of fear regarding death, for it was attributed to divine powers or spirits, which could not be seen. To make a truce with these spirits, people devised ceremonies and rituals, many of which were initiated to protect the living from the sprits that were believed to have caused the death. Some of these primitive examples include the following:

- Mourners wore mourning clothes of different colors (e.g., black, white) to disguise themselves from returning spirits.
- The dead person was covered with a sheet to prevent the person's spirit from escaping through the mouth.
- People kept watch over the dead in hope that life would return and in the belief that the deceased were merely sleeping, hence the term "wake."
- Lighted candles were used so that fire would devour spirits.
- Bells were rung in medieval times to drive away evil spirits.
- Flowers were placed around a coffin to gain favor with the spirit.
- Funeral music began as ancient chants to calm the spirits.

Today, in the United States, sheets are placed over a dead body, and, in many religious funeral services, music is played, bells are rung, flowers are placed on the coffin, candles are lit, and people, typically dressed in black, attend wakes/visitations. Many religious traditions have their beginnings in nonreligious customs.

Dixie Dennis

Further Reading

Lynch, Thomas. *The Undertaking: Life Studies from the Dismal Trade.* New York: W. W. Norton and Company, 1997.

Mitford, Jessica. *The American Way of Death.* New York: Simon and Schuster, 1963.

O'Connell, Laurence J. "Religious Dimensions of Dying and Death." *Western Journal of Medicine,* 163(3) (1995): 231.

G

GENDER

It was often assumed that men and women would exhibit distinct patterns in the way they experience, express, and adapt to grief as a result of either inherent biological differences or cultural differences in the socialization of males and females. In much popular commentary, it was further suggested that the traditional male role would inhibit grieving, since it emphasized the regulation of emotional expression and inhibited seeking support from others. Women, on the other hand, were seen as more ready to accept help and express emotions, both of which are seen as facilitating the grieving process.

Theoretical Explorations of Gender Differences in Grief

These ideas are rooted in early research on grief, which tended to focus on surviving widows. Early research tended to feminize grief; since the experience of grief became explored from the perspectives of women, their experiences were viewed as a model for both genders. This perspective, referred to as the "feminization of grief," was often expressed in the literature about grief and went largely unchallenged until the late 1980s. In many ways, this perspective corresponds with the affective bias that is, in some ways, part of the "culture of counseling," including the way in which counselors often focus more on conversations about inner feelings rather than on thoughts or behaviors.

In the late 1980s and early 1990s, the notion of "masculine grief" emerged in the literature. This approach emphasized that due to biological or cultural-socialization differences, men and women did exhibit distinct differences in the ways that they grieved. Men tended to grieve in more active and cognitive ways. However, these approaches were no less effective. The clinical implication was that, when assisting male clients, therapists should use different approaches such as cognitive-behavioral therapies; that is, therapies that place more attention on thoughts and actions rather than feelings.

These ideas further evolved in the late 1990s to *styles* of grief. This approach, evident in the work of Terry Martin and Kenneth Doka, viewed gender as only one variable affecting the ways that individuals experienced and expressed grief and adapted to loss. Thus, while gender *influences* grieving styles, it does not determine that style; other factors, including culture, personal temperament, and other variables such as formative experiences affect the style.

Doka and Martin propose that grieving styles are best perceived as a continuum. On one end of this continuum are persons whose style may be described as *intuitive*. Intuitive grievers experience, express, and adapt to grief on an affective or feeling level. They are likely to report the experience of grief as waves of affect or feeling. They are also likely to express these emotions strongly as they grieve—crying, shouting, and/or displaying emotion in a variety of other ways. Intuitive grievers are likely to be helped in ways that allow them to ventilate and to explore their emotions. Help for intuitive grievers may come in the form of self-help and support groups, counseling, and other opportunities to ventilate and to assess their feelings. This style may often be found in women and is generally validated by counselors.

On the other end of the continuum are *instrumental grievers*. Instrumental grievers are more likely to experience, express, and adapt to grief in more active and cognitive ways. Instrumental grievers tend to experience grief as thoughts, such as a flooding of memories or in physical or behavioral manifestations. They are likely to express grief in ways consistent with this—doing something related to the loss, exercising, or talking about the loss. For example, a man whose daughter died in a car crash found solace in repairing the fence his daughter had destroyed. "It was," he recollected, "the only part of the accident I could fix." Instrumental grievers are often helped by strategies such as bibliotherapy (the use of literature, including self-help manuals, to relieve intrapersonal distress) or other interventions that make use of cognitive and active approaches. This style is often used by many men.

Toward the middle of the continuum are *blended grievers*. These grievers deal with a range of responses as they experience and express grief. They may draw on numerous coping strategies—cognitive, behavioral, spiritual, or emotion-based—as they cope with the loss. It is not unusual in blended grievers to see different types of loss bring out varied responses.

Doka and Martin posit one other form of griever in their typology—the *dissonant griever*. Dissonant grievers experience grief in one pattern, but are inhibited in finding compatible ways to express or adapt to grief in ways consistent with their experiences of grief. For example, a man may intuitively experience grief, but feel inhibited from expressing his grief or adapting to it because he perceives it as inimical to his male role. Similarly, a woman may also experience grief intuitively but believe she has to curb her feelings of grief in order to protect her family.

Martin and Doka suggest that many men, at least in Western culture, are likely to be found on the instrumental end of this continuum, while women are more likely to be found on the intuitive end. They do, however, stress that while gender does influence the style of grief, that style is not determined by gender. It is crucial to bear in mind that any discussion of gender differences in grief or even of patterns of grief that are gender influenced, should take into account cultural differences. Culture impacts grief in several ways. First, each culture has norms governing the ways in which grief is expressed. In some cultures these norms may differ between genders. For example, a study that surveyed 60 societies found that 32 had no differences in the expectation of crying between men and women. In the remaining 28 societies, women were afforded greater emotional expressiveness. Second, each culture defines its relationships in different ways, in turn influencing the level of attachment. These, too, may vary by gender. For example, in some societies, the relationship of a father with a child may be more remote.

Research on Gender Differences in Grief

Research on spousal loss has emphasized that widows and widowers face distinct problems in loss and respond differently. Widows reported financial problems and greater emotional dependence on their late husband. Widowers tended to stress the need to be realistic about the loss and to show a narrower range of affect than that of widows. While women tended to seek emotional support, men found solace in exercise, religion, work, poetry, or in some more destructive patterns such as excessive alcohol consumption. Men were more reluctant to reach out to others, but they were more likely to return to work, date, and remarry. In a study of resilient widowers, these widowers used strategies that included cognitive reorganization (i.e., interpreting adversity to find benefit or make meaning of the loss), taking pride in developing new skills necessitated by the loss and in supporting and helping others, readjusting role priorities, and increasing social involvements.

Many of these same differences were found in the loss of a child. Studies have shown that mothers tended to experience a more intense level of grief or distress than fathers. Similar patterns were observed in perinatal loss, though others found that these patterns tended to converge over time. In one study, mothers expressed a greater need to talk about the loss than fathers.

Strategies for dealing with the loss also differed. Mothers were more likely to seek outside support and ventilate their feelings. Fathers were less likely to express feelings and felt a need to continue to provide for and protect their families. Women were inclined to use strategies that were more emotion focused and support seeking. Men tended to use more problem-focused strategies and controlled affective expression and intellectualized grief. Where men did show affect, it was generally in anger or aggression.

The research on grief outcomes has varied considerably. Some research has indicated that men generally fare better on measures of mortality and physical and psychological morbidity, while other research has suggested that women fare better. These results are generally reflected in research on counselors' perspectives of gender differences. In one study, for example, a random sample of counselors and educators who were certified by the major professional organization within the field agreed that there were significant differences between men and women grievers. Men were viewed as less likely to exhibit strong emotions and more likely to evoke distractions such as work, sex, play, or alcohol. Men were also seen as more likely to respond cognitively, or, when affect was experienced, to show anger. Women, on the other hand, were seen as more expressive and willing to seek out the support of others. Their grief tended to be experienced on a deep, affective level. These counselors also expressed a belief that men needed less time to grieve. Despite the recognition of differences, most counselors believed that there were no significant differences in outcome. Other research suggested that those who respond in ways conforming to their gender role are more likely to receive social support than those who do not.

Clinicians should clearly be concerned about the ways a client's gender is influencing the client's experience of grief and develop counseling approaches and interventions sensitive to the client's grieving style. However, at the same time, clinicians need to take care that neither gender stereotypes nor the affective bias in the culture of counseling color their approach to the client.

Kenneth J. Doka

Further Reading

Chethik, N. *Father Loss: How Sons of All Ages Come to Terms with the Deaths of Their Dads.* New York: Hyperion, 2001.

Doka, K.J., E.N. Heflin-Wells, T.L. Martin, L. Redmond, and S. Schacher. "The Organization of Thanatology." *Omega: Journal of Death and Dying,* 63 (2001): 113–24.

Doka, K.J. and T.L. Martin. *Grieving beyond Gender: Understanding the Ways Men and Women Mourn.* New York: Routledge, 2010.

Field, D., J. Hockey, and N. Small (eds.). *Death, Gender, and Ethnicity.* New York: Routledge, 1997.

Levition, D. "The History of the Forum." *Forum for Death Education and Counseling Newsletter,* 1(1) (1976): 1,7.

GENOCIDE

Genocide is the intentional and systematic killing of an ethnic, racial, national, or cultural group. The term was coined by Raphael Lemkin and first appeared in print in his work, *Axis Rule in Occupied Europe,* published in 1945. Lemkin created the word from the Greek and Latin roots, *genos* (Greek for family, or race) and *-cide* (Latin for killing). The term "genocide" was originally used in referring to the execution of the Jews under Nazi rule before and during World War II (see **Holocaust**). The meaning was subsequently broadened to include the deliberate killing of any group with an identifiable ethnic, racial, cultural, religious, or national membership. Examples include race (Jews killed by the Nazis); ethnicity (Rwandan Tutsis killed by the Hutu); religion (Jews killed by Christians, Bosnian Muslims killed by Serbian Christians, and Christian Armenians by Muslim Turks); and language—a genocide which is intended to destroy a culture without necessarily killing all of the group's members (linguistic genocide practiced by slave masters against African American slaves in North America to destroy the culture that gave slaves a group identity). None of these examples suggests a single cause of genocide. They are offered only to highlight what was the main focus in a particular historical event.

Because the term *genocide* is so closely linked to the Holocaust, a new term has been suggested—*democide.* Democide is defined as the murder of a person or group of people by a government. It may include events labeled as genocide or as politicide (killing by a government for political purposes) but goes beyond those terms. For example, democide includes the killing of noncombatants in time of war, while excluding the death of noncombatants killed during attacks on military targets so long as the primary target is military. It can, however, be difficult to make such a distinction.

Convention on the Prevention and Punishment of the Crime of Genocide

A basis for defining genocide is the *Convention on the Prevention and Punishment of the Crime of Genocide*, adopted by Resolution 260 (III) A of the United Nations General Assembly on December 9, 1948. The convention was to last for 10 years with automatic renewal every 5 years, unless a member state withdrew from the agreement with written notice delivered six months before the scheduled date of renewal. The convention defines genocide as any of the following acts, when such acts are committed with the *intent to destroy* a national, ethnic, racial, or religious group:

- Killing members of the group
- Causing serious bodily or mental harm to members of the group
- Deliberately inflicting on the group conditions of life calculated to bring about its physical destruction, in whole or in part
- Imposing measures intended to prevent births within the group
- Forcibly transferring children of the group to another group

This is perhaps the broadest definition of genocide, since it includes more than killing. Causing "serious bodily harm" to members of a group or transferring children from one group to another (as the Nazis did with Polish children who had "Aryan" features) would constitute genocide according to the U.N. Convention. Politics too play a pivotal role in determining whether or not a particular event constitutes genocide. "Intent" is often assumed where the actions of a "rogue" regime result in a significant loss of human life. In contrast, where the regime in question is viewed favorably, similar actions may be viewed as "unintentional," even where these actions too result in considerable loss of human life.

There are three 20th-century events that are offered as clear examples of genocide. They are the killing of Jews by the Nazis before and during World War II, the killing of Christian Armenians by the Muslim Turks during World War I, and the killing of the Tutsi (and moderate Hutu) by the predominantly Hutu government in Rwanda in 1994.

The Holocaust

The most well-known case of genocide is the deaths of six million Jews during Nazi rule in Germany before and during World War II. The term *Holocaust* comes from the Greek *holokauston*, meaning to "sacrifice by fire." The National Socialist Party in Germany came to power in January 1933. They preached the natural racial superiority of Germans and labeled other groups as inferior, making them a threat to a strong German state. The Holocaust is the attempted extermination of European Jewry (and, indeed, world Jewry had the Nazis triumphed). However, the Nazis also targeted and sought to exterminate other groups that were seen as "inferior," including gypsies, the mentally ill, and physically disabled. Others were incarcerated and killed for political and ideological reasons. Among these groups were German socialists, communists, trade unionists, and Jehovah's Witnesses. In addition, Nazi officials persecuted homosexuals and others whose behavior did not match prescribed social norms.

Many of the political and military leaders who carried out this genocide were judged for "crimes against humanity" in trials held in Nuremburg, Germany (a city chosen, among other reasons, because it had been a center for Nazism, home to the infamous Nazi Party Rallies, and would therefore be the place that, symbolically, would mark the party's demise). The first trials were held between November 20, 1945 and October 1, 1946 and others were conducted later as more of the accused were taken into custody. It was the revelations of the extent of the genocide conducted by Nazi Germany that eventually led to the adoption of the Convention on the Prevention and Punishment of the Crime of Genocide in 1949.

Armenian Genocide

To be considered genocide, the killing of a group, whether in whole or in part, has to be established as deliberate. It is precisely the difficulty in establishing the intentionality of killing that has led to decades of debate over whether or not the mass deaths of Armenians during World War I were, in fact, genocide. Most modern scholars agree that the deaths of over one million Armenian Christians under the Ottoman Empire were the result of actions that were deliberately planned, ordered, and executed. They see this as the first genocide of the 20th century. Few, if any, deny that Armenians died in large numbers in the years between 1915 and 1918. It has been claimed that the Committee of Union and Progress, formed from the Young Turks who came to power in 1908, developed a plan to eliminate all of the Armenians. In actions that would become familiar in the accounts of the Holocaust, Armenians were targeted for deportation. When they were moved, valuables were confiscated. They were mistreated and malnourished as they were relocated. Armenian members of the Turkish military were disarmed and prevented from returning to their families, leaving these civilians defenseless. As the Armenian population was being transported in convoys, it was common for these vehicles to be attacked and the civilians killed. The government had made no provisions to feed or care for the deportees and many, especially the elderly, young children, and the infirm, died from starvation, exhaustion, and disease.

To this day, Turkey officially denies that this was the result of any government action or plan. Relocation of civilians in time of war is common and is not, by itself, the cause of deaths that took place. The Turkish government says there was no "intent" in any of this and that the deaths of the Armenians occurred during a time of chaos as the Ottoman Empire was collapsing. Political pressure from the Turkish government has led political figures in the United States and other Western countries to be reluctant to label the deaths as genocide. The issue remains contentious, even to the present day. It is estimated that between 1 and 1.5 million

Armenians died in this genocide. Their deaths are remembered and commemorated by their descendants, and by all Armenians, on April 24 every year.

Rwandan Genocide

The destruction of the Tutsi people occurred in the last decade of the 20th century, but its tribal roots went back for many years. Tutsi had once ruled the Hutu and when the Hutu came to power, there were old scores to be settled. From the start, the killing was systematically organized under government direction. A 1993 peace agreement gave some hope that genocide might be avoided. But the government imported over half a million machetes for Hutu use in killing Tutsi.

There was little or no attempt to conceal what would happen. Rwandan Prime Minister Jean Kambanda testified later at an International Criminal Tribunal that the genocide was *openly* discussed in cabinet meetings. At such a meeting, one cabinet minister was quoted as saying that the deaths of all Tutsi would mean the end of Rwanda's problems. It would be, to use the Nazi phrase, a "final solution" to the ethnic division in the country. The United Nations Peacekeeping Forces, led by the French, tried to move the Tutsi to a place of safety. However, because this was not formally declared to be genocide (which would have authorized United Nations intervention), they did not receive full United Nations support and were eventually ordered to leave the country. It is estimated by the United Nations that over 800,000 Tutsi were killed in this genocide.

Robert G. Stevenson

Further Reading

Kiernan, Ben. *Blood and Soil: A World History of Genocide and Extermination from Sparta to Darfur.* New Haven: CT: Yale University Press, 2007.

Melvern, Linda. *Conspiracy to Murder: The Rwanda Genocide and the International Community.* London, UK: Verso, 2004.

Power, Samantha. *A Problem from Hell: America and the Age of Genocide.* New York, NY: Basic Books, 2002.

Rummel, Rudolf J. *Democide: Nazi Genocide and Mass Murder.* New Brunswick, NJ: Transaction Publishers, 1991.

Schabas, William A. *Genocide in International Law: The Crime of Crimes.* Cambridge, UK: University of Cambridge, 2000.

GHOSTS

Ghosts take many forms, but they are most commonly portrayed as the nonphysical souls of people who have died. This definition, however, is not without exception in legend and folklore. A ghost is the essence of a person, the part that lives on and retains the individual's characteristics when physical body is decomposing. To believe in ghosts is to believe that, in some way or other, it is possible to survive one's own death.

Ghost legends have changed through time, and so have the ways in which they are claimed to appear to their viewers. Early stories portray apparitions (i.e., ghostly figures) as monster like, with horns or other such nonhuman characteristics. Later, and more commonly, ghosts are portrayed as looking exactly like the physical body of the person who has died, except perhaps that they are more transparent and less substantial. Often they will appear just as they did when they died. If their death was bloody, they may appear bloodstained or if they died at sea, they might appear wet or covered in seaweed. Recently, ghosts have been described as orbs, or balls of light that are capable of being recorded in photographs or video.

The term "ghost," in contrast with the term "soul," is frequently used to refer to the spirit of someone who, for one reason or another, remains on earth rather than moving on to an eternal destination, whatever that may be. When a ghost remains in the same place, the place is said to be "haunted" by that ghost. Traditionally, ghosts may remain on earth for a number of reasons. If the person died suddenly or traumatically, they may be unaware that they are dead. They may have unfinished business or a message to convey to someone who is still alive, like *Hamlet*'s father or the spirits from Dickens's *A Christmas Carol*. A spirit may remain on earth because it was not given a certain kind of burial. Ghosts may also be vengeful—committing to remain on earth in order to haunt a person who did them wrong in life.

In most ghost legends, ghosts are conscious and active. They are aware of their current surroundings and can interact with its particulars in one way or another.

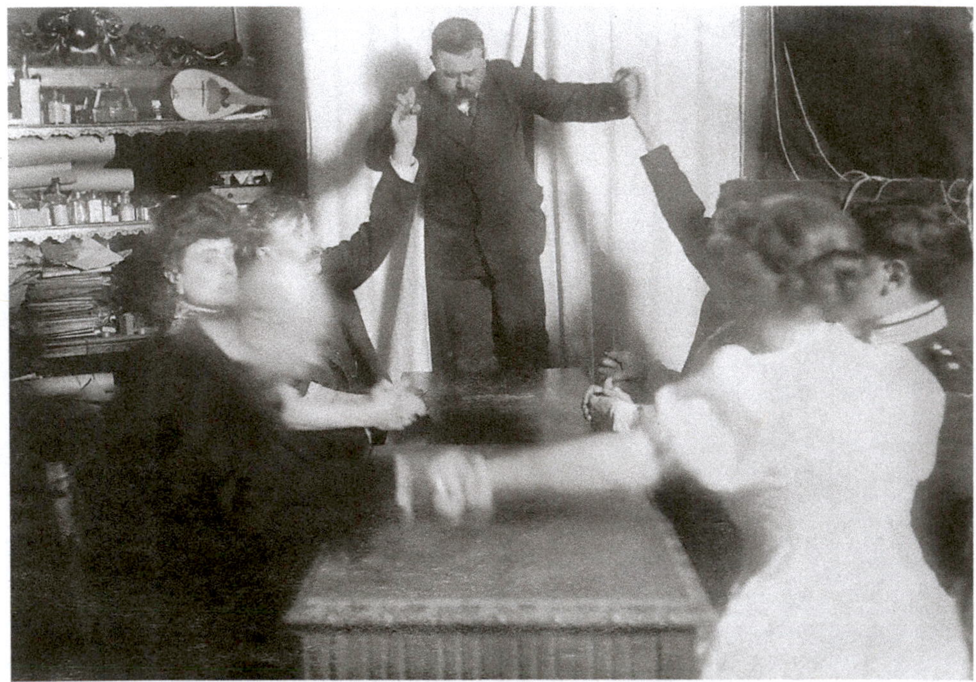

Late 19th- or early 20th-century image of a levitating medium holding a seance. Although the image was probably taken for entertainment purposes, it is indicative of the popularity of communicating with ghosts spread by the Spiritualists in the 19th century. (Library of Congress)

Some ghosts, however, are not the conscious manifestation of an active soul, but are rather the imprint of some traumatic event in history. For example, the ghost of one of the ill-fated wives of Henry VIII, Katherine Howard, is rumored to haunt Hampton Court Palace. But she haunts in a peculiar way: she is seen to break free of the guards that hold her and run down the hall to the chapel, where she knows the king is hearing mass to beg for her life. This event plays over and over again in an endless loop.

Apparitions are not always human. Every April, the train that transported Abraham Lincoln's body from New York to Illinois for burial is claimed to be seen running the same fateful course. Similarly, *The Flying Dutchman* is a ghost ship doomed to sail the seas for eternity.

Contemporary ghost hunters challenge the idea that a ghost is a wholly non-physical thing. They maintain that ghosts interact with the world in ways that can be quantified and recorded. They measure changes in temperature in locations with alleged ghost activity. They may also try to capture electronic voice phenomena (EVP) in an attempt to confirm the existence of a life after this one.

Rachel Robison-Greene

Further Reading

Cavendish, Richard (ed.). *Man, Myth and Magic: An Illustrated Encyclopedia of the Supernatural.* New York: BPC Publishing Ltd., 1970.

Izzard, Jon. *Ghosts.* London: Spruce, 2010.

GOOD DEATH

The concept of a good death has changed over time and is affected by the medical, spiritual, and cultural environment. In the United States, the idea of a good death has evolved over the past 50 years. In the 1960s and 1970s, the primary use of the term "good death" was as a synonym for euthanasia (see **Euthanasia**). In the 1980s, a broader view of the concept emerged and the first attempt at defining it was provided by Richard O'Neil. For a death to be considered "good," O'Neil claimed the following conditions needed to be met: (1) that the timing of the death is appropriate, (2) that the dying person remains in control, (3) that those involved in the death observe basic moral principles, and (4) that the "death style" of the person is logical. While it is still occasionally used to refer to euthanasia, the concept of a "good death" more often describes the elements that are necessary for a good experience surrounding a death by the patient, family, health care providers, and others.

The Nature of a Good Death

Whether a death is considered "good" or "bad" is complex and may change based on an individual's beliefs, values, and preferences; it may also depend upon where one is in relation to death, be that as a dying person, the family member of a person who is dying, a physician, or nurses caring for a dying person, or as a member of the clergy ministering to the dying. For example, some people may want to die in their sleep, while others may prefer to be alert and aware at the time of death. A person's death may be considered "good" by their spouse and "bad" by the nurse who was present.

Since individual preferences have such an important role in determining whether a death is "good" or not, it is important for people to communicate their preferences. One means of communicating these preferences is in an advance directive document or living will (see **Advance Directives**). While each individual has an idea of what a good death would be, there are some characteristics of a good death that seem to be important to everyone, although how important they are and how they are expressed may vary from one person to the next. These characteristics seem to be important across most cultures in the United States and across the world. These seemingly universal characteristics include the following:

- ***Being in control***. This can refer to a patient's sense of autonomy and of being in control of the medical choices they make, including being able to make clear decisions and to exercise some degree of control over the death, such as the location, timing, and presence or absence of other people. This is considered the most important aspect of a good death by many Americans. For some people, being in control includes being able to choose assisted suicide (see **Physician-Assisted Suicide**).
- ***Being comfortable.*** This includes pain and symptom management, as well as having a comfortable physical, social, psychological, and spiritual environment, in which one's needs are accommodated and catered for.
- ***Having a sense of closure.*** This includes having the ability to say goodbye to loved ones, to complete unfinished business, resolve any outstanding conflicts, engage in some form of life review, and make adequate preparation for death, such as estate planning and funeral arrangements.
- ***Affirmation or recognition of the value of the dying person.*** This includes acceptance of the whole person, including his or her physical, emotional, social, and spiritual attributes; it involves treating the dying person with dignity and respect, attempting to maximize the person's overall quality of life, and treating him or her as a person and not simply a "disease."
- ***Having trust in health care providers.*** This includes good communication with physicians and nurses in ways that foster a sense of trust that health care providers will honor the dying person's wishes.
- ***Having one's beliefs and values honored.*** Respecting a person's ethnic/racial, spiritual/religious, cultural, and personal beliefs is especially important when the dying person may have needs and desires that differ from those of the dominant culture.
- ***Minimizing burden to the family.*** This may include freedom from the physical burden of care giving and alleviating the family's financial concerns. It includes the idea of the dying person being independent until the end of his or her life and/or contributing to the quality of the family's life by continuing to play as active a role as possible within it.
- ***Optimizing relationships.*** This includes spending sufficient time with family and friends, and being able to communicate with them meaningfully. Forgiveness is often an important part of optimizing personal relationships.

- ***Appropriateness of the death.*** Whether a death is considered "appropriate" or timely is affected by the age of the dying person, whether the person had a terminal illness, and whether technology such as ventilators was used and/or stopped appropriately. In contemporary Western societies, the archetypal "good death" is widely considered to be at the end of a person's natural life span, rather than in the prime of life.
- ***Leaving a legacy.*** Most people want others to remember them and want to contribute to the well-being of others. A legacy can be tangible or intangible: it can be financial (such as an estate), physical (such as an heirloom), or the social and emotional impact a person has had on those with whom he or she came into contact.
- ***Family care.*** This has two aspects: care for the family of the dying person; and allowing the family to participate in care of the dying person, in the death itself, and the rituals that follow.

When a death is "good," those involved should have a sense of peace and a feeling of closure. While a good death will not prevent grief, it may leave good, positive memories for those left behind. Whether a death is considered "good" or "bad" can affect how family members and others involved in the death view death in general. Crucially, it may also have an effect on the choices they make when facing their own deaths.

Karen A. Kehl

Further Reading

Hirai, K., T. Miyashita, T. Morita, M. Sanjo, and Y. Uchitomi. "Good Death in Japanese Cancer Care: A Qualitative Study." *Journal of Pain Symptom Management,* 21(2) (2006): 140–47.

Iranmanesh, S., H. Hosseini, and M. Esmaili. "Evaluating the 'Good Death' Concept from Iranian Bereaved Family Members' Perspective." *Journal of Supportive Oncology,* 9(2) (2011): 59–63.

Kehl, K. A. "Moving toward Peace: An Analysis of the Concept of a Good Death." *American Journal of Hospice and Palliative Care,* 23(4) (2006): 277–86.

O'Neil, R. "Defining a 'Good Death.'" *International Journal of Applied Philosophy,* 1(4) (1983): 9–17.

GRAVE ROBBING

The term "grave robbing" (or "bodysnatching") has traditionally been used to describe the "theft" of freshly buried corpses that were dug up and sold to medical schools for their use in anatomical dissection. The practice of bodysnatching became most widespread during the 18th and 19th centuries, when, due to the growth of medical science and the use of autopsy, the demand for cadavers began to outstrip supply. Until this point, the only legal source of cadavers for use in medical research were the bodies of executed criminals, for whom postmortem dissection was itself viewed as a form of punishment. The social stigma surrounding dissection as a form of punishment, together with the popular belief that dissection would make physical resurrection of the body impossible, helps explain the widespread public fear of bodysnatching in the 18th and 19th centuries.

Intriguingly, and because in law a body cannot be owned, bodysnatching in most places was not classified as a criminal offense until the second half of the 19th century. In Great Britain, before the Anatomy Act of 1832 (which effectively outlawed bodysnatching), grave robbers would carefully remove any valuables from the corpse, such as jewelry, as well as the shroud in which it was buried, placing these back in the coffin so as not to be culpable of theft. Freshly buried corpses exhumed before decomposition set in were in high demand by medical schools, providing a lucrative source of income for criminals prepared to engage in this macabre activity. Those with the financial means to do so, would often go to great lengths to protect the corpses of their loved ones from theft, paying undertakers large sums of money for reinforced coffins and iron straps by which the dead were firmly secured. Some families even resorted to keeping guard over the dead from "watching huts" until such a time that the corpse had decayed and was no longer of any use to anatomists, while others paid to have their loved one's grave encircled with spiked iron railings so as to deter would-be thieves.

In Victorian England, it was, however, the poorest in society who were at greatest risk of grave robbing, where paupers' graves (large pits containing the bodies of those who could not afford proper burial) provided easy pickings for teams of what became known as "resurrectionists." In the United States too, it was social groups on the margins of society who provided a rich supply of cadavers for anatomists, such as in New York, where the corpses of African Americans were regularly snatched by medical students. Between 1785 and 1855, such activities prompted dozens of anatomy riots at medical colleges across the United States, whereby families attempted to reclaim their dead, eventually leading to legislation, first in New York, and later in many other states, that outlawed bodysnatching. The "anatomy acts" passed in Massachusetts in 1831 served to reassure the "respectable" classes that their graves were safe by allowing medical schools to legally take possession of the corpses of the "unclaimed" (the poor and destitute without money for burial who died in workhouses and hospitals). Sadly, it seems, the poor were worth more dead than they were alive.

More controversially, the term "grave robbing" has also been used to describe the removal of human remains and artifacts by archaeologists who have been accused of plundering the ancient burial grounds of indigenous peoples. In recent years, there have been growing demands from indigenous groups that artifacts and human remains displayed in museums of the West be repatriated to the living members of the cultures from which they were taken.

Michael Brennan

Further Reading

Howarth, Glennys. "Grave Robbing." In *Encyclopedia of Death and the Human Experience*, edited by Clifton D. Bryant and Dennis L. Peck (pp. 525–27). Thousand Oaks, CA: Sage, 2009.

Sappol, Michael. *A Traffic in Dead Bodies: Anatomy and Embodied Social Identity in Nineteenth-Century America.* Princeton, NJ: Princeton University Press, 2002.

GREEN BURIALS

Also referred to as "woodland," "natural," or "ecological burials," green burials eschew the use of materials known to be harmful to the environment in favor of those that minimize lasting damage to the environment. Biodegradable coffins made from cardboard rather than less sustainable hardwoods, the preference for tree planting over headstones fashioned from granite, and the rejection of embalming because of the toxic properties of substances such as formaldehyde, are all part of the practice and philosophy underpinning green burial. Even cremation, which is less environmentally damaging than traditional burial, but which is nevertheless a source of mercury and carbon emissions, is typically avoided as a source of bodily disposal in ecological funerals. (This though may soon change, with the development of "green" or "flameless cremation" in which the body is heated to 300°C in a pressurized vessel containing potassium hydroxide. Makers of the "alkaline hydrolysis" or "Resomation" machine, which reduces the body to skeletal remains that can be processed into a white powder and presented to the family of the deceased, claim it uses a seventh less energy than conventional cremation, produces a third less greenhouse gas, and allows for the complete separation of dental amalgam for safe disposal). Woodlands rather than heavily manicured suburban cemeteries routinely provide the site for green burials, thereby avoiding the environmental pollution caused to soil, water, and air by pesticides and fertilizers used to maintain traditional lawn cemeteries.

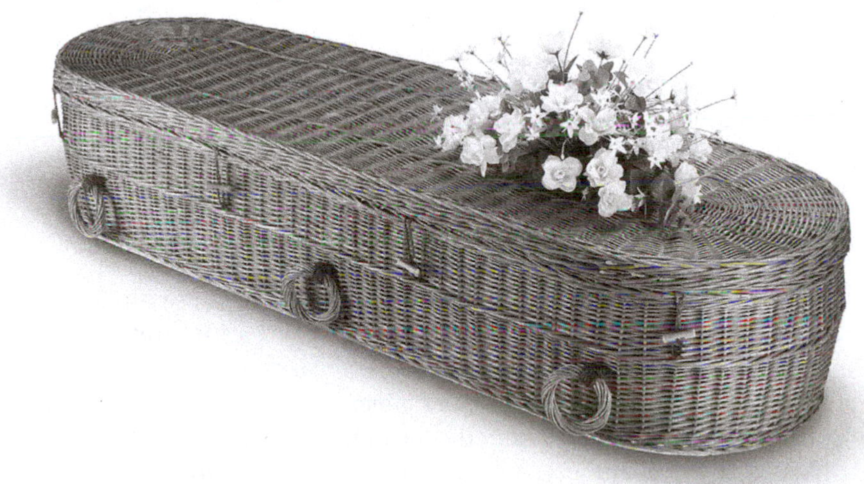

Biodegradable caskets, like this wicker coffin, are part of the new "green burial" movement. (Shutterstock)

The origins of green burials can be traced to Great Britain in the late 1980s. Taking their cue from the natural birth movement, and its attempt to resist control of childbirth by the medical profession (see **Medicalization**), the natural death movement advocated a philosophy that espoused inexpensive, ecologically friendly funerals that permitted family involvement in postmortem rituals and practices. Founded in April 1993 by Nicholas Albery, the Natural Death Centre provides advice and support to those wishing to plan and undertake a funeral without the intervention of professional funeral directors. Part of the impetus behind the emergence of the natural death movement stemmed from a desire to reclaim family control of funerals which, as they saw it, had been "sequestered" (or seized) by professionals within the funeral industry. Advocates of natural burial argue that personal involvement in funerary practice can be meaningful, enriching and empowering, providing a counter to the uniform, depersonalized and sometimes meaningless funerals offered by large funeral chains.

While green burials are growing in popularity, they nevertheless remain a less-favored option than mainstream burials, and are chosen primarily by the educated middle classes. Great Britain continues to lead the way in woodland burial with some 250 natural burial sites, compared to Germany, which has 25, and the United States, which has 13. In the United States, the independent and not-for-profit Green Burial Council was established in 2005 to promote the practice of ecological burial. In an age of the increasingly environmentally conscious consumer, it remains to be seen whether the popularity of green burials will continue and the extent, if at all, to which the choice of green burial will eventually be offered by mainstream funeral directors keen to obtain a market share of the green economy.

Michael Brennan

Further Reading

Green Burial Council: www.greenburialcouncil.org

Harris, Mark. *Grave Matters: A Journey through the Modern Funeral Industry to a Natural Way of Burial*. New York: Simon and Schuster, 2007.

The Natural Death Centre: www.naturaldeath.org

GRIEF

Grief can be defined as a distinct, personal reaction to the loss of any object to which an individual is attached. Grief reactions may occur in any situation of loss, whether the loss is physical or tangible (such as a death, significant injury, or loss of property), or symbolic and intangible (such as the loss of a dream). The intensity of grief will vary, depending upon many variables such as the nature of attachment, the relationship to the lost object, and the meaning of the attachment, prior experiences of losses, physical and psychological health, familial dynamics, informal and formal social support, and other social, spiritual, and cultural factors.

This definition of grief distinguishes it from other terms such as bereavement or mourning. Bereavement refers to an objective state of loss. If one experiences a loss, one is bereaved. Bereavement refers to the fact of loss, while grief is the subjective response to that state of loss. It should be recognized that loss does not inevitably create grief. Some individuals may be so disassociated from the lost object that they experience little or no grief.

Mourning has had two, interrelated meanings within the field. On one hand, it has been used to describe the intra-psychic process where a grieving individual gradually adapts to the loss, a process that has also been referred to as grieving or grief work. It has been used, as well, to refer to the social aspect of grief: the norms, patterned behaviors, and rituals through which an individual is recognized as bereaved and socially expresses grief. For example, in America, wearing black, sending flowers, and attending funerals are common illustrations of appropriate mourning behavior.

Manifestations of Grief

Individuals can experience grief in varied ways. Physical reactions are common. These include a range of physical responses such as headaches, other aches and pains, tightness, dizziness, exhaustion, menstrual irregularities, sexual impotency, breathlessness, tremors and shakes, and oversensitivity to noise. Bereaved individuals, particularly widows, do have a higher rate of mortality in the first year of loss. There may be many reasons for this: the stress of bereavement, the change in lifestyle that accompanies a loss, and the fact that many chronic diseases have lifestyle factors that can be shared by both partners. It is, therefore, important that a physician monitors any physical responses to loss.

There are affective manifestations of grief as well. Individuals may experience a range of emotions such as anger, guilt, helplessness, sadness, shock, numbing, pining, yearning, jealousy, and self-blame. Some bereaved individuals experience a sense of relief or even a feeling of emancipation. This, however, can be followed by a sense of guilt. As in any emotional crisis, even contradictory feelings, such as sadness and relief, can be experienced simultaneously.

There can also be cognitive manifestations of grief. Included here is a sense of depersonalization in which nothing seems real. There can be a sense of disbelief and confusion, and an inability to concentrate or focus. Bereaved individuals can be preoccupied with images or memories of the loss. These cognitive manifestations of grief can affect functioning at work, school, or home. Many people also report experiences where they dream of the deceased, have a sense of the person's presence, or even sense-based experiences of the other.

Grief has spiritual manifestations as well. Individuals may struggle to find meaning and to reestablish a sense of identity and assumptive order in their world. They may be angry at God or struggle with their faith. Others may even become religious as they seek to find solace in their spirituality.

Behavioral manifestations of grief can also vary. These behavioral manifestations can include crying, withdrawal, avoiding or seeking reminders of the loss, searching behaviors, over activity, and changes in relationships with others.

In other cases, there may be dysfunctional behaviors such as self-destructive acts or acts destructive toward others. In other situations, the grieving individual may seem unable, even after time, to function in key social roles (e.g., work, school, or home). In such situations, grieving individuals may benefit from professional help (see **Grief Counseling**).

The critical point is that reactions to grief are both multifaceted and highly individual. Moreover, grief reactions are likely to occur in waves, sometimes more intense than others. And while there is no timetable to grief, many individuals experience reactions less intensely and less often after the first year or two. However, it is not unusual to have surges of grief years after the loss, often triggered by a significant event. For example, a woman may experience the loss of her father in early adolescence. Her wedding, a decade later, may trigger a surge of grief as she realizes that her father never lived to participate in this event.

The Process of Grief

There have been a number of approaches to understanding the process or course of acute grief. Earlier approaches tended to see grief as proceeding in stages or phases. Colin Murray Parkes, for example, described four stages of grief: (1) shock, (2) angry pining, (3) depression and despair, and (4) detachment. Elisabeth Kübler-Ross described the process of coping with grief much like coping with dying. She believed individuals experienced five stages: (1) denial, (2) anger, (3) bargaining, (4) depression, and finally, (5) acceptance (see also **Kübler-Ross, Elisabeth**).

Recent approaches have emphasized that grief does not follow a predictable and linear course, stressing instead that it often proceeds in a "roller-coaster" like pattern, full of ups and downs, times when the grief reactions are more or less intense. Some of these more intense periods are predictable—holidays, anniversaries, or other significant days; others may have no recognizable trigger.

More recent approaches have emphasized that acute grief involves a series of tasks or processes. Psychologist William Worden describes four tasks of grief: (1) recognizing the reality of the loss, (2) dealing with expressed and latent feelings, (3) living in a world without the deceased, and (4) relocating the deceased in one's life. Two Dutch researchers, Margaret Stroebe and Henk Schut, described bereaved individuals as oscillating or moving back and forth between two sets of processes: *Loss-Oriented Processes* that acknowledge the reality of the loss, as well as *Restoration-Oriented Processes* that assist the bereaved person in adjusting to a life now changed by the loss. These and other similar models reaffirm the very individual nature of grief, acknowledging that these tasks or processes are not necessarily linear and that any given individual may have difficulty with one or more process or task.

Grief reactions can persist for considerable time, gradually losing intensity after the first few years. Recent research emphasizes that one does not "get over the loss." Rather, over time, the pain lessens, and grief becomes less disabling as individuals function at levels comparable to (and sometimes better than) preloss levels. However, bonds and attachments to the lost object continue. We never, in fact, forget a person who is significant, as that person remains in our memory.

Recent work has also emphasized that a loss, like any significant change, can be a catalyst for growth. Studies have indicated that many individuals struggling with a significant loss reported that, as result of the loss, they experienced greater empathy, enhanced spirituality, heightened the value of relationships, reoriented and reprioritized life, increased skills, or changed their own health practices.

The Study of Grief

Unsurprisingly, since loss is a universal experience, grief has long been the subject of a variety of writings, going back to antiquity. References to grief in loss are found in the scriptures of all faiths, in some of the oldest manuscripts such as the Egyptian *Book of the Dead* and the Babylonian *Gilgamesh Epic*. Poets, dramatists, and novelists constantly address the experience of grief.

However, the psychology of grief can be said to begin with Sigmund Freud's 1917 seminal essay "Mourning and Melancholia," where Freud begins to cover a topic still vexing today—the relationship of grief to depression. Eric Lindemann's research on survivors of the Coconut Grove fire, a night club in Boston, Massachusetts, where many young adults perished, was an early and still influential empirical study. While some research was done in the 1940s and 1950s, much significant research was done after the 1960s, as academic interest in the study of grief significantly increased (see **Death Awareness Movement**).

Getting Help in Grief

People experiencing acute grieve can help themselves in a number of ways. Since grief is a form of stress, lifestyle management, including adequate sleep and diet, as well as other techniques for stress reduction, can be helpful. Bibliotherapy or the use of self-help books can often validate or normalize grief reactions, suggest ways of adaptation, and offer hope. Self-help and support groups can offer similar assistance, as well as social support from others who have experienced loss. For example, widow-to-widow groups have helped individuals adapt to the death of a spouse, while The Compassionate Friends organization assists parents, siblings, and even grandparents in coping with the death of a child. Other groups exist on both a national and local level, offering self-help for a wide variety of losses, including deaths by homicide, suicide, military deaths, or deaths from particular diseases, such as cancer or HIV/AIDS.

It should be noted that most individuals seem to deal effectively with grief in that, over time, they can remember the loss without the intense reactions experienced earlier and function at similar or even better levels.

However, anywhere between 20 and 33 percent of bereaved individuals seem to experience more complicated grief reactions. Some people, such as those experiencing sudden or traumatic losses, the death of a child, highly ambivalent or dependent relationships, or people with prior psychiatric problems, among other factors, may be especially vulnerable. These individuals may benefit from grief counseling, particularly if their health suffers or their grief becomes highly disabling, impairing functioning at work, school, or home, or if they harbor destructive thoughts toward self or others. A number of specialized approaches have been developed to treat varied complications of grief.

Others may find counseling valuable when other support, from family or friends, is not forthcoming. Such losses may be called disenfranchised. *Disenfranchised grief* is defined as grief that a person experiences when he or she incurs a loss that is not, or cannot, be openly acknowledged, socially sanctioned, or publicly mourned. The concept of *disenfranchised grief* integrated a sociological perspective into the study of grief and loss by emphasizing that the grief process is heavily influenced by the degree to which others around, and the society at large, acknowledge and validate that loss. Grief is complicated when others do not acknowledge that the individual has a right to grieve. In such situations, people are not offered the "rights" or the "grieving role" such as a claim to social sympathy and support, or such compensations as time off from work or the diminishment of social responsibilities. Grief may be disenfranchised for a number of reasons: the relationship is not recognized (i.e., friend, coworker, etc.); the loss is not acknowledged (i.e., pet loss, loss of a job, etc.); the griever is not recognized as capable of grief (i.e., a young child, person with developmental disabilities, etc.); the circumstances inhibit support; or the way the person grieves is viewed as inappropriate by the cultural or gender norms of a society.

In recent years, there have been efforts to have categories encompassing complicated grief reactions in the *Diagnostic and Statistical Manual of Mental Disorders* (*DSM-5*) that mental health professionals use to characterize disorders. One such proposed category is *prolonged grief disorder.* At the time of writing, it is likely that a diagnostic category for some form of complicated grief will be included in the *DSM-5*, but it is premature to assess how grief complications will be recognized.

In helping individuals deal with loss, pharmacological interventions, that is the use of medications to alleviate depression, anxiety, or other manifestations of grief, can sometimes be helpful, particularly when the grief is disabling, that is, severely compromising the individual's health or ability to function. Such interventions should be focused on particular conditions such as anxiety or depression, for example, which are precipitated or exacerbated by the bereavement. Pharmacological interventions generally should be accompanied by psychotherapy.

Kenneth J. Doka

See also: Bereavement; Mourning.

Further Reading

Humphrey, K. *Counseling Strategies for Grief and Loss.* Alexandria, VA: The American Counseling Association, 2009.

Rando, T. A. *How to Go On Living When Someone You Love Dies.* New York: Bantam Books, 1991.

Sanders, C. *Grief: The Mourning After: Dealing with Adult Bereavement.* New York: John Wiley and Sons, 1989.

Worden, J. W. *Grief Counseling and Grief Therapy: A Handbook for Mental Health Professionals,* 4th edition. New York: Springer, 2009.

GRIEF COUNSELING

Grief counseling is a specialized form of counseling for people who are grieving over the death of someone close to them or adjusting to significant experiences of loss and change—such as divorce, redundancy, or migration—which may also generate a grief-like response in those who experience them. Grief counseling is usually offered by a qualified mental health professional, such as a psychologist or specialist counselor. It may also be provided by social workers, trained volunteers, spiritual care workers, and clergy. A core distinction can be made between *formal* grief counseling, which is provided by trained professionals (such as counselors, psychologists, nurses, and social workers), and *informal* grief counseling, provided by clergy, mutual support groups, and community or volunteer-based organizations.

History

Grief counseling was developed in the late 1960s when the first modern hospice and palliative care services were established in the United Kingdom and the United States. This was a time when the needs of dying and bereaved people began to be recognized, and research showed that support for the bereaved led to better health outcomes and reduced social isolation, anxiety, and depression.

Training

A grief counselor is usually trained in counseling and communication skills and will be familiar with a wide range of grief and bereavement responses in many different circumstances. Desirable qualities in the counselor include a capacity for compassion, empathy, and a nonjudgmental attitude. By listening carefully and providing information and guidance, the counselor helps the bereaved and grieving person feel less alone and more able to cope with the impact of the death or loss. Counseling is often short term and focused, in contrast to psychotherapy, which tends to be provided for a longer term.

Aims of Grief Counseling

The aim of grief counseling is to relieve the grieving person's distress through empathic listening, reassurance, and education about normal responses to loss and bereavement. By validating and authenticating the loss, the grief counselor aims to help the person feel stronger and more hopeful about the future. Loss and bereavement experiences can be painful and disruptive, but may also offer opportunities for personal growth and the strengthening of social connections and support. Grieving people may turn to a professional counselor when support from friends and family is not available or does not meet their perceived needs. The pain and intensity of grief reactions are not always recognized, nor are they are always well tolerated, and the bereaved may feel that their grief has been disenfranchised (see **Grief**).

Effectiveness of Grief Counseling

In recent years, research into grief counseling has found that counseling is most effective when provided for people experiencing complicated or prolonged grief reactions, and when family and social support systems are inadequate or non-existent. When people experience traumatic bereavements that are violent and untimely, such as homicide and suicide, they may experience rejection and stigmatization, which complicate their grief. There is some evidence to suggest that grief counseling is of more limited effectiveness for the treatment of grief triggered by less-exceptional losses. This suggests the resiliency of most people in making the psychosocial transition from life before a loss to life following it.

Grief counseling may also be effective for people who have a history of mental illness or family dysfunction that puts them at a greater risk of prolonged periods of crisis and instability. When people experience a large number of significant losses in a short period of time, their capacity for coping and adjustment may be overwhelmed, and counseling and support can help them regain their equilibrium. Grief counseling has also been found to be more effective when people are proactive in seeking help. Counseling that is imposed, or offered when people are extremely vulnerable, or immediately after a death, may actually undermine rather than strengthen the grieving person's natural coping ability and existing support systems.

Grief Support Organizations

The growth and development of self-help groups and support organizations for particular groups of bereaved people such as widows, widowers, and bereaved parents, began over 50 years ago in the United Kingdom and the United States. Their role has been to provide mutual aid and social support rather than grief counseling, although qualified helping professionals have often been involved in shaping these services and training volunteer members. One of the first "widow-to-widow" programs was established in Boston, Massachusetts, by social worker and researcher Phyllis Silverman, in the late 1960s, after widows themselves suggested that meeting with other widows, who were facing similar challenges, was more beneficial than turning to family physicians and clergy.

One of the largest of these organizations, Cruse Bereavement Care, was established in the United Kingdom in 1959 by social worker and Quaker Margaret Torrie. While initially providing care for widows and their children, Cruse opened its doors to all bereaved people in 1988. Using highly trained volunteers, many of whom are also qualified mental health professionals, Cruse has over 200 local branches throughout the United Kingdom. Its volunteers are often called upon to provide support in times of national emergency. Cruse publishes journals, helpful literature on coping with grief and loss, and provides training for counselors.

Also originating in the United Kingdom, and established by hospital chaplain Simon Stephens in 1969, The Compassionate Friends (TCF) is today a large, worldwide, self-help organization for bereaved parents and siblings. Group support, information, and education are offered in many locations and by members who have undergone training in counseling and group facilitation. Conferences are held regularly and a wide variety of publications are made available to bereaved parents, helping professionals, and the wider community. There are many other organizations that assist grieving people following deaths from cancer and HIV/AIDS, but also suicide, homicide, and other accidental and traumatic deaths.

Theoretical Foundations of Grief Counseling

While counseling and support services for grieving and bereaved people were first developed in response to the unmet needs identified by helping professionals, their quality continues to be shaped by an ever-expanding knowledge base that includes: feedback from members of support groups, evaluation of existing services, formal research into bereavement, and scholarly debate.

Early conceptualizations of grief counseling based on Freudian psychoanalytic theory (see **Freud, Sigmund**) led to a belief that grieving people recovered from bereavement by relinquishing their emotional investment in the deceased. Many grief counselors therefore believed that their task was to help the bereaved forget the person who had died and to "let go and move on." However, research into childhood bereavement at Harvard Medical School by William Worden, Phyllis Silverman, and others in the early 1990s challenged this notion and found that a "continuing bond" with the deceased was a source of strength and comfort for the bereaved (see **Continuing Bonds**). Bereaved children reported having mental conversations, dreams, and memorial activities that helped them stay connected with the deceased parent. This body of knowledge has been highly influential in encouraging counselors to help their clients establish continuing bonds with the deceased.

Bereavement research at the University of Utrecht in the Netherlands by Henk Schut and Margaret Stroebe also identified patterns of grief response that challenged previous assumptions about the importance of expressing emotion. This research found that healthy grieving and adaptive coping involve an ongoing fluctuation between, on the one hand, experiencing grief reactions by *focusing on* the loss, and, on the other, avoiding grief reactions by *moving away* from the loss. Known as the dual process paradigm or oscillation theory, this knowledge has helped practitioners to design support and counseling programs that recognize gender differences and coping styles (see **Gender**), assisting the bereaved to develop a more balanced and effective way of coping. Other theoretical approaches have been derived from philosophical perspectives on death and suffering. One of the greatest challenges for grief counselors is to help the bereaved make sense of their experiences of loss and ultimately to find meaning and purpose in life.

Research into widowhood in the 1950s by English sociologist, Peter Marris, found that widows struggled with the loss of meaning as well as with the practical aspects of life without their partner. He concluded that life had become unmanageable because it had become meaningless, and bereavement involved both a "crisis of discontinuity" and a crisis of identity for the survivor. Marris also conducted research into urban renewal and other significant experiences of loss and change and found similar patterns of adaptation and adjustment.

Colin Murray Parkes, a leading British psychiatrist and researcher who developed the first bereavement counseling services at St. Christopher's Hospice in London, refers to bereavement as a "crucial transition" or "psychosocial transition" ushering profound changes in the way that people perceive and manage the world around them. American psychologist Robert Neimeyer has described the work of forging a new way of life and new identity in bereavement as a form of meaning making and meaning reconstruction.

All of these perspectives illustrate the important link between theory and practice, especially ways in which theoretical innovations feed into, and have helped shape, clinical practice. These perspectives have also served to expose the limitations and oversimplification of the stage model of grief made popular by Elisabeth Kübler-Ross in the 1960s (see **Kübler-Ross, Elisabeth**). These perspectives address the complexity of grief and grieving, and the need for people to have access to skilled support and counseling should they feel the need for it. Criticisms of grief counseling have focused on the adherence of some grief counselors to rigid stage and phase models of grieving that ignore the individual's gender, personality, and cultural differences. For this reason, organizations such as the Association for Death Education and Counseling (see **ADEC [Association for Death Education and Counseling]**) has established education, counselor accreditation, and supervision programs for the maintenance of high-quality, culturally sensitive, and ethically minded grief counseling.

Irene Renzenbrink

See also: Bereavement; Grief; Hospice Movement; Palliative Care; Terminal Illness and Care.

Further Reading

http://www.crusebereavementcare.org.uk
http://www.compassionatefriends.org/home.aspx
Jordan, J. R. and R. A. Neimeyer. "Does Grief Counseling Work?" *Death Studies,* 27(9): 765–86.
Marris, P. *Loss and Change.* London: Routledge and Kegan Paul, 1974.
Neimeyer, R. A. "The (Half) Truth about Grief." *Illness, Crisis and Loss,* 20(4) (2012): 389–95.
Parkes, C. M. "Bereavement as a Psychosocial Transition." *Journal of Social Issues,* 44(3) (1988): 53–65.

HEALTH PROMOTION

Health promotion refers to efforts to achieve optimal well-being for the individual and population at large and to reduce premature deaths from preventable causes. It is not limited to persons of a particular age or physical condition. Health promotion efforts occur either at the individual or population level and concern infectious diseases, chronic diseases, prevention of accidents, and other threats to health and well-being. Health promotion activities aim to enable patients to improve health, often with the adoption of healthy behaviors.

At the individual level, and for prevention of infectious diseases, health promotion frequently represents the efforts of a health care provider to prevent the onset of illness by such procedures as childhood vaccination or annual flu vaccination. Thus, one aspect of health promotion is direct prevention of specific diseases. This also occurs at the population level. Annual flu vaccinations are usually initiated by government action in developing a vaccine based on the assessment of the bacterial strains likely to be prevalent at a given time. These efforts are intended to prevent the debilitating results of a massive influenza epidemic. Individual actions affect the population and efforts at the population level affect the individual. If a certain percentage of the population is immunized, "herd immunity" is developed and diseases are less likely to be spread throughout a community. The costs of morbidity, mortality, absence from work, and decreased economic and other productivity make government prevention of influenza and other such outbreaks a priority.

Health promotion also refers to the efforts of individuals or governments to institute changes to enhance health and prevent the onset of debilitating diseases. The typical "New Year's resolutions" often involve initiating or enhancing exercise programs. The point of such programs from the individual perspective may be to "lose weight." From a medical perspective, such programs may result in a decreased likelihood of the onset of cardiac and other diseases. Modifications to one's diet can lessen the intake of saturated fat and sodium, both of which have been linked to metabolic diseases.

At the population level, prevention of childhood obesity by changing the foods available in school lunch programs and educating children and their parents about the benefits of foods low in fat, sugar, and salt is also an element of health promotion. Federal regulations as to the components of processed foods, while not typically considered under the rubric of health promotion, clearly are such an effort, although some individuals may consider such endeavors as overreaching. Fluoridation of water to prevent tooth decay is another example of a population-level intervention. Fluoridation of drinking water illustrates an initiative where the population at large is affected without having to make individual behavioral changes. With other interventions, whether at the individual or population level, some degree of individual participation is required.

An example of the need for individual participation is when an individual has been diagnosed with a health-threatening condition and the effort is to achieve cure and/or prevent debilitation. Prevention of other conditions secondary to the primary illness is also a form of health promotion and more particularly so when the individual must assert some initiative in making lifestyle changes, such as diabetics engaging in careful foot care to prevent the development of foot ulcers. Indeed, much of health promotion concerns lifestyle changes at the individual level. These are typically more difficult to achieve than a government intervention such as fluoridation of water or a one-time annual occurrence, such as flu vaccination. Having mentioned fluoridation, such changes are not easy to achieve politically, but once implemented demand no further action on the part of the individual.

To the degree that health promotion requires change in individual behavior, such change may be more difficult to achieve. For example, health promotion may involve engaging in certain behaviors such as hand washing or the selection of protective suntan lotions for their ability to screen out harmful rays rather than for the achievement of a certain level of tanning. Health promotion also involves the avoidance of certain types of behaviors such as the use of "tanning beds" or drinking alcohol while driving. The former endangers one individual; the latter may endanger others.

A population-level intervention to prevent loss of life or physical injury in automobile travel is the law mandating the wearing of seat belts. This legislation is bolstered by automobile design that incorporates repeated sounds indicating seat belts have not been used. These sounds cease only when the desired behavior of using the seat belt has been achieved. Such reinforcement, while ideal from a behavioral change perspective, does not typically occur elsewhere in health promotion, unless the individual has taken proactive steps in order to pursue lifestyle changes aimed at curbing health-damaging activities. An individual may thus join a group such as Alcoholics Anonymous so as to help reinforce abstinence. Other groups attempting to achieve behavior change may also use harm reduction, substituting less-dangerous behavior for one that is potentially more lethal. An example of the latter is the use of clean needles by injecting drug users in which the harm of transmission of infectious diseases is reduced even though the dangers of drug use are still present.

Tasks that promote wellness, like fluoridation of water, require no action by the individual and the use of seat belts require a minimal amount of initiative. Behavior change that is more demanding requires a commitment to make the necessary changes and may or may not have the benefit of reinforcement. In either case, the readiness of the individual to engage in the change is a necessary consideration for those promoting the change and for the individual for whom the change is recommended. While the concept of health promotion may be positively accepted in theory, implementation may be far more challenging. This is particularly the case when the change is at a population level and may challenge what some individuals and/or groups perceive to be their fundamental rights, for example, the right to bear arms and the right to engage in health-damaging activities like cigarette smoking. Health promotion under these circumstances is far more complex. Prevention of lung cancer by restricting cigarette smoking is one example of the collision of health promotion with the perceived right of individuals to engage in certain behaviors. Health promotion at the population level may involve the development of consensus and negotiation to achieve what most people would consider desirable.

Inge B. Corless

See also: Accidental Death; Alcohol; Cardiovascular Disease; Drugs; HIV/AIDS.

Further Reading

Duaso, Maria Jose and Philip Cheung. "Health Promotion and Lifestyle Advice in a General Practice: What Do Patients Think?" *Journal of Advanced Nursing,* 39(5) (2002): 472–79.

Endelman, Carole L. and Carol L. Mandle. *Health Promotion throughout the Life Span.* St. Louis, MO: Mosby Elsevier, 2010.

Olden, Peter C. and Keith E. Hoffman. "Hospitals' Health Promotion Services in their Communities: Findings from a Literature Review." *Health Care Management Review,* 36(2) (2011): 104–13.

Pack, B. E., O. L. Deniston, S. W. Bates, and W. Beery. "A Review of Hospital-Based Health Promotion Programs in Michigan Non-Governmental Hospitals." *Patient Education and Counseling,* 7(4) (1985): 345–58.

World Health Organization (WHO). *Declaration of the 39th World Health Assembly.* Geneva: World Health Organization, 1986.

HEARSE

Hearses are funerary vehicles used to carry the body of the deceased from a church, funeral home, or some other place of worship to a cemetery or crematory, where the body is ritually disposed of. They are sometimes referred to as funeral coaches, and were at one time used by funeral directors to make the "first call" in the event of a death. The word *hearse* is derived from a Roman term for a rake or *hirpex* (the Latin name for a rake or "harrow") used by farmers for breaking up clods of ploughed land. When it was inverted and held aloft, this wooden frame fitted with iron teeth resembled the candelabra of Norman invaders' funerals. Hearses evolved from being plain and horse-drawn to being more ornate and self-propelled, with the first horseless funeral procession in the United States taking place in 1909 in Chicago. The necessity for transporting coffins became more apparent as local churchyards were replaced by larger cemeteries on the outskirts of cities as places for burial, and as undertakers evolved from people whose skills involved the preparation of the body for burial to persons who became skilled in not only building and designing coffins but also in hiring vehicles to transport the coffin to the cemetery. Hearses later became limousine-like, carrying flowers for the funeral ceremony and allowing the coffin to be mechanically lowered to the ground. In the event of cremation, the hearse would carry an urn, in lieu of a casket or coffin in the funeral procession. Symbolically, hearses are objects that reflect what Robert Kastenbaum refers to as our culture's "death system," in that the word or image of a hearse is inevitably associated with thoughts and fears about death and dying.

Bert Hayslip Jr.

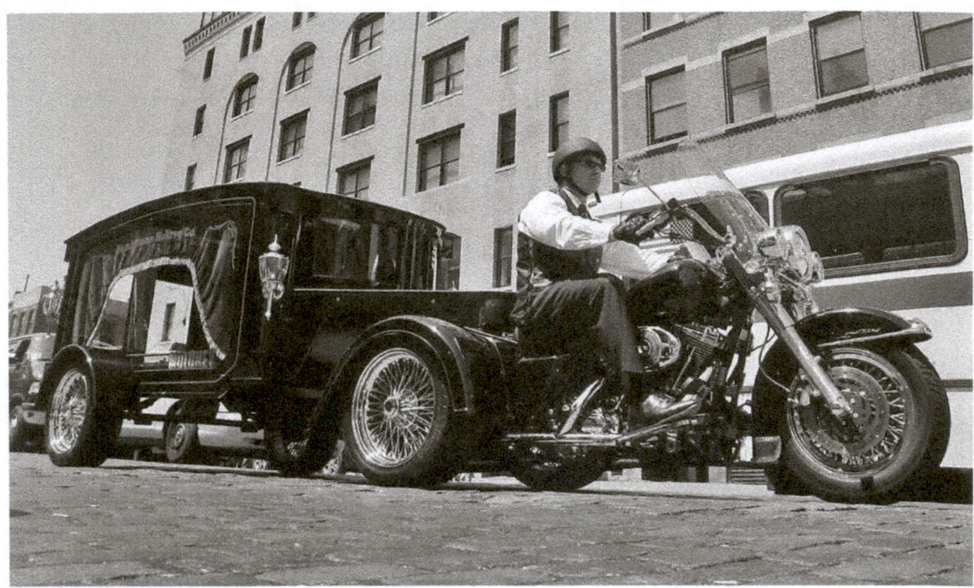

Peter Moloney, of Moloney Family Funeral Homes in Lake Ronkonkoma, New York, rides his Harley-Davidson hearse in New York, May 24, 2007. (AP Photo/Richard Drew)

See also: Funeral Director; Funeral Industry; Funerals.

Further Reading

Kastenbaum, Robert J. *Death, Society, and Human Experience,* 10th edition. Boston: Allyn & Bacon, 2009.

Merksame, Gregg D. "Funeral Conveyances." In *Encyclopedia of Death and the Human Experience*, edited by Clifton D. Bryant and Dennis L. Peck (pp. 465–69). Thousand Oaks, CA: Sage, 2009.

Schechter, Harold. *The Whole Death Catalog: A Lively Guide to the Bitter End.* New York: Ballatine Books, 2009.

HEAVEN

Heaven is the traditional Christian and Jewish designation for the abode of God. It links to "the Heavens," the sky and stars, and an entire symbolism of transcendence, sovereignty, and all-wise benevolent ordering of the worlds "below." "To ascend to the Heavens" meant to visit the place where God dwells, where God can be encountered in all God's glory, majesty, and power. Heaven in this meaning precedes any beliefs about life after death for human beings. For in the Hebrew Bible (Christian Old Testament), individuals die and "sleep with their fathers" or "descend to Sheol," but Heaven remains above, as an eternal realm belonging to God and God's messengers. Only later, during the intertestamental period (i.e., the period between the writing of the Hebrew Bible and the Christian New Testament), Heaven becomes the home of the blessed dead (at least for some Jews), and later still, among Christians, the hoped-for destination for all the faithful dead.

How did this happen? The early Christian communities proclaimed the resurrection of Jesus, and his continued existence in Heaven "at the right hand of the Father." They anticipated his return—the "second coming" or *parousia*—and the completion of God's plan for the salvation of *all* creation. They expected that they themselves would wait in a holding pattern for this consummation. Even the martyrs, clearly the privileged dead, might not be fully conscious and active in the interim state. Yet, Christians also hoped to be "with Christ," and therefore with God in Heaven. None of these ideas were very fully developed into doctrines until roughly the second Christian millennium.

When these ideas were more systematized, the vision of three eternal realms, as found in Dante's *Divine Comedy,* shows Heaven as the destination for the blessed, purified dead who no longer are burdened by the weight of the sins they committed in life, and who rejoice eternally in the beatific vision; that is, direct communion with God. That keeps them occupied, satisfied, and at peace even when they can predict dire events on earth. Those in the "lower" levels of Heaven are absolutely content, and it would offend divine order and justice were they to be elevated into the "higher" tiers.

Essentially, both Roman Catholics and Protestants accepted this "theocentric" vision of Heaven until the 18th century, at least officially. "The Celestial City" of John Bunyan's 17th-century Puritan classic *The Pilgrim's Progress* is filled with gold, light, and joyous band of triumphant arrivals, but it is not a place of domestic household contentment (this ideal only emerges as family ties take on more intense emotional meanings). By the mid-19th century, authors such as Elizabeth Phelps, writing about Heaven in *The Gates Ajar,* portrayed family reunions, growth, and personal development, and (most controversial of all) material satisfactions and consumer goods as part of what made Heaven attractive for the living to anticipate. Heaven as our "home" was a place of return to our first homes here on earth, and although God and Jesus were never displaced completely, this vision of a thoroughly "anthropocentric" heaven is what has endured in popular piety to this day.

Lucy Bregman

See also: Afterlife Beliefs; Angels; Hell; Purgatory.

Further Reading

Alighieri, Dante. *The Paradiso,* Volume 3 of *The Divine Comedy.* Translated by John Ciardi. New York: New American Library, 1961/c.1320.

McDannell, C. and B. Lang. *Heaven: A History.* New Haven, CT: Yale University Press, 1988.

HELL

For Christians, Hell is the traditional destination for the unhallowed, sinful dead. It is a place of punishment and torment, from which there is no release, ever. The equivalent in Islam is "the Fire," to which Allah sends the unrepentant on the Day of Resurrection. In Judaism, while Hell may not be eternal as a destination for the soul, it was traditionally part of the framework for the afterlife. Buddhism teaches a variety of Hells, presided over by deities who serve as judges. In all these cases, Hell is associated with burning and misery, unbearable remorse, and eternal despair.

Hell was not originally part of the cosmology of the ancient near East's religions. Everyone after death was believed to inhabit a shadowy underworld; dark and miserable but not a place of punishment or burning. In the period of Babylonian exile and after, Jews began to accept more elaborate ideas of afterlife, resurrection, and universal divine judgment. The term Hell or Gehenna came from the valley where Canaanites burned their children in sacrifice. Hence the association with fire. By the time of Jesus, the parable of the rich man and Lazarus (Luke, 16, 19–31) shows belief that at least some souls after death experienced immediate torment. "I am in agony in this fire," says the regretful rich man. The assumption is that God gives us the chance in life to follow "the law and the prophets," and beyond this life there is no opportunity to escape divine justice. There is, in Christian teachings on death and afterlife, all but universal acceptance of this view until the 17th century. Those who rejected God in life, refusing repentance, were destined for Hell. To question Hell's reality was to question divine justice.

There were some problems within this theology. What about those who never had the chance to hear the message of salvation? Virtuous pagans and unbaptized infants did not seem to belong to the same category as other inhabitants of Hell. Nevertheless, Christian thought could accommodate them, as Dante's "Inferno" in *The Divine Comedy* shows. What eventually challenged the traditional picture of Hell were modern ideas of justice and punishment. If the purpose of punishment is retribution, then an offense against God is infinite, and deserves infinite punishment. But if the purpose of punishment is rehabilitation, then the eternal agonies of Hell make no sense. No one ever emerges wiser or reformed. Moreover, the deterrent function of Hell did not seem plausible, as most persons do not consider themselves sufficiently wicked to warrant *eternal* punishment. Once these arguments were introduced, the antipathy between traditional Hell and a truly loving God seemed apparent. The debate over the reality of Hell wages on among Christians. In polls, about 25 percent of Americans say they accept Hell as a belief, but only a tiny percentage worry personally that they may end up there. Meanwhile, the traditional Hell has been the model for concentration camps in the 20th century, sometimes intentionally. Literary use of Hell has flourished too, such as in Jean-Paul Sartre's play *No Exit*. It has not been banished from Western imagination.

Lucy Bregman

See also: Afterlife Beliefs; Angels; Heaven; Purgatory.

Further Reading

Alighieri, Dante. *The Inferno,* Volume 1 of *The Divine Comedy.* Translated by John Ciardi. New York: New American Library, 1954/c.1320

Walker, D. *The Decline of Hell.* Chicago: University of Chicago Press, 1954.

HINDUISM

"Hinduism" is an umbrella term that covers a copious variety of beliefs and practices sharing certain family resemblances. Two such generic features are the belief that the immortal soul will probably be born again, and the belief in *karma*. For Hindus, death is the end of a particular embodied life, but it is not final. It is a presupposition that rebirth really happens, and this provides the essential context for their thinking about dying.

Most Hindus believe that human beings are immortal by nature: that is to say, one is essentially an indestructible soul or spirit (*jīva-ātman*) that is contingently attached to an embodied life in space and time. In other words, there is a real distinction between *what you really are* and your lives in this and other worlds of experience. This present life—in the sense of an assembly of interests and identifications striving to perpetuate itself—is not what continues after one's death. Death is the destruction of the physical organism that includes the ego (*ahaṃkāra*—the individual personality with which unenlightened beings misidentify themselves), and the psychological functions, including memory. At death, the psychologically continuous stream of phenomenal and intentional mental states that I call "mine" ceases. When Hindus say that *the soul* continues, they usually mean the permanent reflexive consciousness that accompanies all mental states. (There is no agreement on whether that consciousness is an individual substance.) This essence is indestructible and it is this that will be reborn—except in the case of those rare beings who have achieved freedom (*mokṣa*) from the round of births and deaths (*samsara*). The soul is still you at a level deeper than the everyday sense of yourself as an embodied being—it is a core identity, albeit one that is often occluded in the course of normal life. So, even though one is going to die, there is the consoling thought that, at the deepest level, there is something about me that will not become extinct.

The doctrine of *karma* says that our intentional, deliberate actions generate a sort of residue that awaits fruition in experiences occurring in the future of this life or in a subsequent life. Hindus believe that this massive accumulation of dispositions to act and experience in certain ways—it is called "the subtle body"—is attached to the soul. It is this subtle body, with which the soul is associated, that is reborn. It is reborn in an embryo produced by a couple whose circumstances provide an appropriate context for the actualization of a dominant set of potential dispositions. Inheritance is karmic, not genetic. One's karma is believed to fix the initial conditions of one's life and also its length. A soul associated with a stock of dispositions where virtue predominates will be reincarnated in a Brahmin womb (Brahmin being the highest or priestly caste in the Indian caste system). There is no recollection of previous lives. The process continues until one achieves *mokṣa* release from the cycle of death and rebirth, and for the majority that is but a remote prospect.

Rites of Passage (*saṃskaras*): Funerals and Subsequent Ceremonies

The corpse is ritually impure and treated with appropriate care. It is bathed and dressed in new clothes. Close relatives carry the deceased, usually covered by flowers, on a stretcher to the cremation ground (*śmaśāna*). The funeral rite (*antyeṣṭi*) is primarily understood as the disposal of the body. Dead bodies are usually incinerated on an open-air pyre in a specially consecrated fire. The skull is perforated to mark the departure of the soul, but this is symbolic. The soul has already departed—which is why the body is dead. Still, the ceremony is understood as fortifying the soul of the deceased for its journey to whatever new world awaits it. Death confers a status of temporary impurity on the immediate family. This means that they are excluded from normal social relations. In other words, they are secluded for a period of mourning (10 days for Brahmins—longer for others—up to 30 days for low castes.) After a day or two, one of the family members will return to the cremation ground and collect the ashes which will be scattered in a river.

Funerals are one factor marking the transition between lives. Rebirth is not immediate; it is dependent upon the occurrence of appropriate initial conditions. There is an intermediate stage when the soul plus subtle body is called a *preta*—"one who has departed" or simply "the deceased." If not properly cared for, these disembodied but *karma*-laden spirits may become dangerous ghostly presences (called *bhūtas*) that cause trouble if their relatives are neglectful of them. So, during the period of mourning it behoves the family to perform rituals (called *śrāddha*) that "feed" the departed spirit who rests content in the world of the ancestors (*pitṛ-loka*). The merit accruing from the ritual performances is transferred to the deceased. It may be a while before he or she finds an appropriate womb, so these rituals are performed for a year after death.

Other sorts of post-mortuary rites (called *Nārāyaṇa-bali* or *Sūrya-bali*) are performed for those who have suffered inauspicious or impure deaths, such as suicide or murder. These occur on the first anniversary of the death. The aim is twofold: to rescue the deceased from the hellish realms to which they have been consigned by the manner of their deaths, and to enable them to become recipients of the benefits of the usual postmortem rituals. Initially, an artificial figure representing the corpse is burnt and the procedures culminate in a ritual that confers the status of an ancestor on the deceased.

It is unsurprising that the global diaspora of Hindu people has on occasion led to conflict, and mortuary practices have been no exception. The public and visible immolation of corpses has been forbidden in British law since 1902. Subsequent to protracted legal wrangling, the Court of Appeal ruled in 2010 that a cremation within a walled but roofless structure fell within the terms of the act. This decision appears to have been acceptable to Hindus.

Christopher Bartley

See also: Reincarnation.

Further Reading

Lipner, Julius. *Hindus*. London: Routledge, 2010.
Parry, Jonathan. *Death in Banaras*. Cambridge, UK: Cambridge University Press, 1994.

HIV/AIDS

Human immunodeficiency virus/acquired immune deficiency syndrome (HIV/AIDS) is a disease that begins as a retrovirus (HIV) and, if left untreated, weakens the immune system and leads to the progression of AIDS. This weakening of the immune system leaves the body open to the risk of acute infections (such as pneumonia, tuberculosis, and meningitis), which, without medical intervention and care, are life threatening and lead to death in the vast majority of cases where people do not have access to treatment. The symptoms of AIDS are quite devastating on sufferers and those caring for them, and include extreme weight loss; a decline in stamina, memory, and physical appearance; lack of coordination; loss of energy; and, eventually, confusion, incontinence, and AIDS dementia, as well as a host of other physical conditions that result in total dependence. By the end of 2011, there were 34 million people living with HIV/AIDS worldwide and 1.7 million deaths from AIDS-related illnesses.

Emergence of HIV/AIDS

HIV/AIDS was first identified in the United States in 1981 in two separate reports by physicians in Los Angeles, and subsequently in New York City, although at the time the cause of the illness was not known. In Los Angeles, pneumocystis carinni pneumonia was identified in young men, which was considered remarkable, as this condition typically affects much older men. In New York, a number of young men were diagnosed with Kaposi's sarcoma (KS), a rare malignancy. The publication of these reports in the *Morbidity and Mortality Weekly Report* (*MMWR*) engendered considerable interest and scattered reports of similar findings emerged. Careful sociological analysis of the network of relationships of those infected in Los Angeles by Dr. William Darrow and the Centers for Disease Control (CDC) led to the hypothesis that this was a blood-borne disease similar in transmission to Hepatitis B. And while popular books such as *And the Band Played On* attributed the spread of the disease to one flight steward, scientists made no such assertion. There is some agreement that the initial infection occurred in sub-Saharan Africa and there was a likely transmission from animals to humans through the consumption of uncooked meat.

Although evidence accumulated to suggest that blood-borne transmission was the likely mode of transmission (with the report of infected hemophiliacs followed by an account of a baby infected after receiving a blood transfusion), efforts to regulate blood donation were hampered by blood banks' concerns about the availability of adequate blood supply. This concern conflicted with those of physicians and others who wanted to impede one mode of likely transmission. Ultimately, changes were made restricting men who had sex with men from donating blood. This continues to be a cause of irritation for some gay men who are in long-standing relationships and wish to be able to donate blood to the community as they had done previously.

AIDS Enters the Mainstream

One of the persons early in the epidemic who never acknowledged his infection was actor Rock Hudson, who, like Rudolf Nureyev and other talented individuals, died of the disease. Magic Johnson acknowledged his infection and in doing so, showed that this was not a disease solely of white men. This was significant because, contrary to the assumption that HIV/AIDS was a disease exclusively confined to white gay men, the highest rate of infection and contraction of HIV/AIDS is among African Americans, who are disproportionately affected by the disease. With the infection of popular figures, together with well-known individuals eliciting funds to support research of the disease, such as actress Elizabeth Taylor, HIV/AIDS discussion entered the mainstream for the first time. In the United Kingdom, Princess Diana helped raise the profile of HIV/AIDS, and to dispel some of the myths and stigma surrounding it, by being one of the first celebrities to physically embrace sufferers; this was especially important because, as a disease acquired through contagion, HIV/AIDS sufferers encountered widespread prejudice and were often regarded as modern-day lepers. But, it was activist and coalition groups such as "Act Up" that were most vocal in their advocacy for those with HIV/AIDS and were critical in helping initiate change, and spur government action needed to pursue the cause and treatment of this disease.

Treatment

Treatment of HIV/AIDS has evolved from one drug (azidothymidine, referred to as AZT and sold as Retrovir), to what is considered a cocktail of drugs, consisting of various classes of drugs. The important point about these medications is that they are directed at different points in the virus replication cycle, from blocking entry into the cell to blocking the emergence of new virions (i.e., entire virus particles). Use of these medications has resulted in a reduction of viral load in the blood. And while the goal of antiretroviral medications is to block replication, cure has not been achieved with currently available medications. Reducing replication is not tantamount to the elimination of virus. Although antiretroviral medications block replication, sanctuary sites harbor virus capable of replication, although at a reduced rate.

One of the benefits of the reduction in viral load in the blood is the decrease in viral transmission to uninfected partners. This has the profound potential to result in a decline in new HIV infections. Such a decline, however, is predicated on the infected person adhering to their medication regimen. And while not easy to take medication routinely and unfailingly either once or twice a day, this routine is far easier than the every-four-hour medication regimen required when AZT first became available in 1986.

Current and Future Research

Current research is attempting to find a cure for viral infection and a vaccine to prevent infection from occurring. Other research has investigated the efficacy of microbicides (compounds that can be placed inside the rectum or vagina to protect against HIV and other sexually transmitted diseases) to prevent the transmission of HIV. One of the important breakthroughs has been the reduction in mother to child transmission. Initially, the concern appeared to focus merely on the child and preserving the health of the next generation. More recently, with the availability of lower cost antiretroviral medications, the focus has expanded to pregnant women and providing HIV-infected pregnant women with access to most of the medications they would receive were they not pregnant. While this approach is state of the art in resource-adequate societies, women in low-resource countries are far less likely to have access to antiretroviral medications, in part because some major pharmaceutical companies in the United States have refused to reduce the cost of antiretroviral medications to less developed countries.

The issue of antiretroviral medication resistance is of concern as it involves switching to another medication regimen in order to maintain a low viral load to prevent further destruction of the immune system architecture and progression to AIDS. This progression is an indication that the disease is worsening and that the infected person is vulnerable to a number of other conditions.

The inventory of current antiretroviral medications in resource-adequate countries and the effectiveness of those treatments have made HIV infection manageable for most people where access to health care and medications are not limited. Nonetheless, given metabolic conditions such as cardiac disease and diabetes that appear to be occurring at an earlier age in HIV-infected individuals, infection with HIV is not to be taken lightly. Furthermore, HIV infection requires lifelong adherence to a medication regimen with no interruptions in routine daily medication ingestion so as to maintain the suppression of virus in the blood.

Death and HIV/AIDS

In the United States, as globally, the distribution and prevalence of HIV/AIDS reflect wider patterns of poverty, inequality, and oppression. Since the epidemic began, more than half a million Americans (636,000) with an AIDS diagnosis have died of the disease. African Americans are disproportionately affected by the disease, so that in 2010, while African Americans constituted only 12 percent of the population, they made up 44 percent of all new infections. In terms of gender, it is African American women who, of women of all other races/ethnicities, have the highest rate of contraction; while among men who have sex with men (MSM), young African American MSM are at highest risk of HIV and accounted for the largest number of new HIV infections in 2010.

On a global scale, HIV/AIDS has greatest prevalence among less developed nations, especially in the countries of sub-Saharan Africa, where it has had a devastating impact, both socially and economically. As a disease that disproportionately impacts the young (especially the 15–49 age group), it has left many children orphaned, while at the same time affecting the social fabric of society by killing those members of society who are economically active and most likely to contribute to the workforce. It is estimated that by 2010, 17 million children had been orphaned by AIDS, the vast majority of whom (almost 90 percent) were in sub-Saharan Africa, placing a tremendous burden of caring responsibilities on grandparents and siblings; at the same time challenging taken-for-granted assumptions about death as something that typically affects the elderly.

A measure of the impact of AIDS upon the countries of sub-Saharan Africa can be seen from the fact that almost 1 in 20 adults (4.9 percent) are HIV positive, accounting for 69 percent of people who are HIV positive worldwide. While AIDS remains the leading cause of death in sub-Saharan Africa, data from the United Nations has indicated some progress, with an estimated 1.8 million deaths in 2011 compared to 2.4 million in 2001, a decline of 25 percent.

Future efforts in HIV prevention and treatment are concerned with the development of preventive vaccines, reduction of risk behaviors, including unsafe sex practices (sex without condoms and reduction in the number of sexual partners), use of clean needles and syringes if injecting drug use occurs, and identification of protective methods for women. Strong antiretroviral medications, combined with an emphasis on active prevention, provide a means to treat those who are infected, while preventing further transmission of infection. An AIDS-free generation, as former secretary of state Hillary Clinton noted, is the goal; a goal to be achieved worldwide.

Inge B. Corless and Michael Brennan

See also: Grief; Health Promotion.

Further Reading

Centers for Disease Control and Prevention (CDC). "HIV/AIDS." www.cdc.gov/hiv/

Centers for Disease Control and Prevention (CDC). "Kaposi's Sarcoma and Pneumocystis Pneumonia among Homosexual Men: New York City and California." *Morbidity and Mortality Weekly Report,* (31) (1981): 305–8.

Centers for Disease Control and Prevention (CDC). "Pneumocystis Pneumonia: Los Angeles." *Morbidity and Mortality Weekly Report,* (30) (1981): 250–52.

Corless, I. B., C. P. Stowell, R. Fulton, and D. Weeks. "Perspectives in Conflict: The Response to Transfusion-Associated AIDS." *AIDS and Public Policy Journal,* 14(2) (1999): 47–67.

Shilts, R. *And the Band Played On: Politics, People, and the AIDS Epidemic.* New York: St. Martin's Press, 1987.

Smith, K., K. A. Powers, A. Kashuba, and M. S. Cohen. "HIV-1 Treatment as Prevention: The Good, the Bad and the Challenges." *Current Opinion in HIV and AIDS,* 6(3) (2011): 315–25.

Turkoski, B. B. "Unraveling the Mystery of HIV Medications." *Orthopaedic Nursing,* 25(1) (2006): 51–56.

UNAIDS. Global Report: UNAIDS Report on the Global AIDS Epidemic, 2010. http://www.unaids.org/globalreport/Global_report.htm

World Health Organization (WHO). "HIV/AIDS." http://www.who.int/hiv/en/

HOLOCAUST

The Holocaust was the deliberate and systematic killing of an estimated 6 million European Jews by Nazi Germany between 1939 and 1945. Underlined by a racial ideology in which anti-Semitism was key, Jews were singled out as subhuman (*Untermensch*) by the Nazis, who attempted their destruction through a program of industrial killing that, from 1942 onward, became known as the "Final Solution." In this, the worst example of genocide in recorded history, the Nazis used shootings, gassings, forced labor, and starvation for achieving their perverted goal—a world free of Jews (*judenfrei*) as a means of solving the "Jewish problem."

Although many Jews, especially before 1942, were rounded up and killed in mass shootings by mobile killing units (*Einsatzgruppen* or "emergency squads") as the Nazis swept across large swathes of territory in Poland and parts of the USSR, the vast majority of Jews were murdered in specially designated centers located in occupied Poland whose main purpose was death. These concentration camps were of two kinds: labor camps (such as Chelmno), in which inmates were enlisted in brutal and dangerous forced labor, many of whom were literally worked to death, while others were eventually gassed; and death camps (like Sobibor, Treblinka, and Auschwitz-Birkenau) where victims were gassed immediately upon arrival. Herded into the hideously overcrowded ghettos in cities like Lodz, Warsaw, and Minsk, many other Jews died of starvation, disease, or back-breaking labor while awaiting deportation to the camps.

A great deal of debate between historians has revolved around whether the extermination of Jews was part of Adolf Hitler's deliberate plans from the very outset, or whether, following discussions involving high-ranking Nazi officials during the

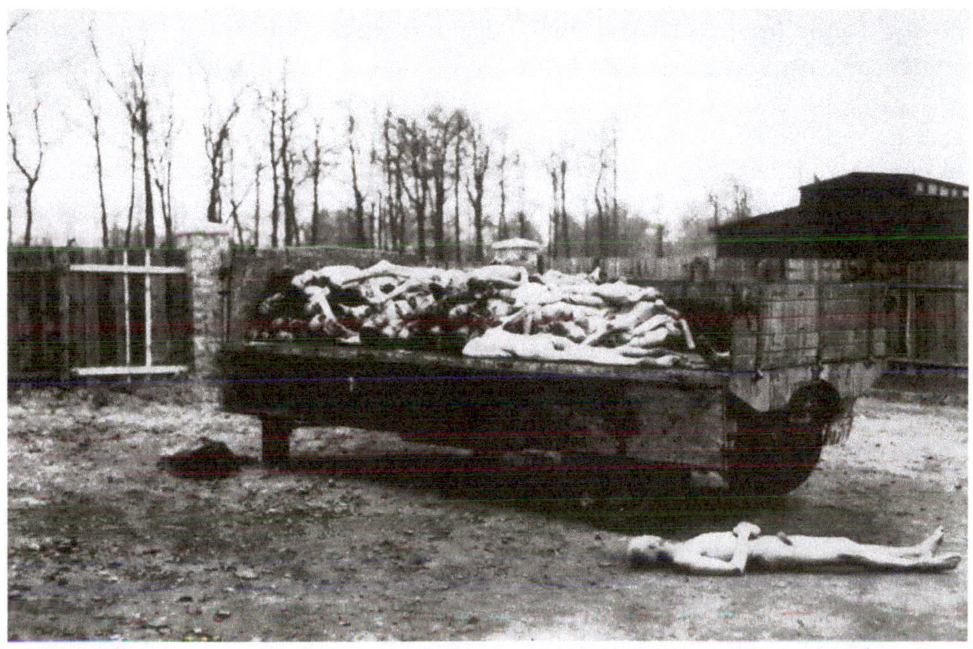

Bodies of prisoners overflow from a truck in the Buchenwald concentration camp at Weimar, Germany, in April 1945. The bodies were about to be disposed of by burning when the camp was captured by troops of the Third U.S. Army. (National Archives)

early years of World War II, it was their intended aim to deport Jews to Madagascar once victory was secured. For some, known as the "intentionalist" camp, Hitler's biographical record of anti-Semitism and seemingly congenital hatred for the Jews (witness, for example, his writing in *Mein Kampf*) is sufficient to suggest that outright annihilation of the Jews had been the Nazis' intention all along. For others, known as the "functionalist" camp, the Nazis' extermination of the Jews was born less of deliberate planning and design than it was of "practical" and prevailing circumstances, as the Nazis acquired every larger numbers of Jews under their control through the growing territorial conquest of counties in Europe with large Jewish populations and thus no longer knew how to effectively resolve the "Jewish problem."

Scholars have also been divided as to how to properly describe events that, since the 1950s, have become known as "the Holocaust." Derived from a Greek word (*holokaustos*), the term "Holocaust" translates literally as "whole burnt offering," and implies to some the suggestion that the genocide was somehow divinely sanctioned or was itself a sacrifice offered up to God. To avoid this, and reflect the unique role that events have played in Jewish history, some scholars have adopted the Hebrew term "Shoah," which translates as "catastrophe" or "disaster" and is without the sacrificial implications.

Further debate has centered around scholars who have argued that the Holocaust was a unique and incommensurable event, and those who have argued that the Holocaust can be understood and assimilated within a broader category of genocidal events, including the Turkish massacre of Armenians in 1915 during World War I, which was said to be an inspiration behind Hitler's eventual design for the Jews. One intriguing and novel explanation of the Holocaust has come from sociologist Zygmunt Bauman, who has argued that the Holocaust was as much a product of modern industrial and bureaucratic conditions as it was of centuries-old anti-Semitism. In particular, Bauman has suggested that the absence of ethical considerations in scientific thinking, namely, the optimization of industrial methods of killing, and a bureaucratic chain of command in which those who give orders for killing are physically removed from their execution, provide fertile conditions in which Holocaust-like phenomena can flourish.

The Holocaust has also provided a powerful point of controversy in terms of its representation, commemoration, and role in Jewish memory and identity. For some, the unique conditions and brutality of the Holocaust make it unrepresentable in art, literature, or film and television. A particular argument used to advance this position is that those who truly experienced the inhumanity of life in the camps did not survive to tell their stories, while those that did can never truly find the words or figurative forms to adequately describe the hellish conditions of their experience. Some, on the other hand, point to the personal testimonies and eyewitness accounts of survivors, of Primo Levi and Elie Wiesel for example, as providing the most powerful insight and best defense against a repeat of genocide.

Recent attempts at commemorating and memorializing the Holocaust have also generated significant controversy and disagreement, especially in the abstract and muted designs of memorials in Berlin and Vienna, by Peter Eisenman and Rachel

Whiteread, respectively. For some, the inverted library in Judenplatz, Vienna, is a deeply resonant and thought-provoking reminder of the attempted destruction of Jews as "people of the Book," while for others it is an ugly piece of brutalist design that sits incongruently with the beautiful baroque architecture by which it is surrounded. In defense of its design, Simon Wiesenthal exclaimed at its unveiling in October 2000 that the monument "shouldn't be beautiful" and instead that "it must hurt."

Surveys of American Jews, meanwhile, suggest that the Holocaust has surpassed religious observance and the State of Israel as a significant source of contemporary Jewish identity. Indeed, the enduring significance and legacy of the Holocaust is revealed by its generational and transnational transference in "prosthetic" and "post memory," especially its capacity to elicit trauma in those who did not experience it or are able to remember it firsthand.

A recent tendency in some strands of Holocaust research has been toward de-emphasizing its specificity as an event within Jewish history toward a focus on its "mosaic of victims," including gypsies, Jehovah's Witnesses, homosexuals, and the mentally and physically disabled. By this reckoning, the estimated 6 million victims of the Nazis extend to an estimated 11 million victims, illustrating the enormity and incomprehensibility of the Holocaust as an absolute event of history (Blanchot, 1995).

Michael Brennan

See also: Genocide; Judaism; Megadeath.

Further Reading

Bauman, Zygmunt. *Modernity and the Holocaust.* Ithaca, NY: Cornell University Press, 1989.

Blanchot, Maurice. *The Writing of the Disaster.* Lincoln, NE: University of Nebraska Press, 1995.

Gerson, Judith M. and Diane L. Wolf (eds.). *Sociology Confronts the Holocaust: Memories and Identities in Jewish Diasporas.* Durham and London: Duke University Press, 2007.

Landsberg, Alison. *Prosthetic Memory: The Transformation in the Age of Mass Culture.* New York: Columbia University Press, 2004.

Niewyk, Donald L. *The Holocaust: Problems and Perspectives of Interpretation.* Boston: Houghton Mifflin Company, 1997.

HOMICIDE

Homicide, from the Latin "*homo*" (human being) and "*cadere*" (to kill), refers literally to the killing of one person by another. It is considered justifiable or excusable—and thereby *noncriminal*—when a person is deemed to have acted in self-defense or in order to prevent harm to another (without criminal intent). Noncriminal homicide includes the use of force or violence to protect one's own person or property; or when killing is the result of an accident that occurs during a lawful act (i.e., not the result of gross negligence).

In the United States, the law has traditionally divided the category of criminal homicide into *murder* and *manslaughter.* For criminal homicide to be considered murder, the act of killing is judged to have been the result of deliberate intention (*malice aforethought*). First-degree murder is judged to have occurred as the result of careful planning, premeditation, and deliberation, and to have been committed together with some other type of serious felony, such as robbery or rape. Second-degree murder is criminal homicide committed with deliberate intention (*malice aforethought*) but without premeditation or deliberation and is often described as a "crime of passion" that takes place in the heat of the moment. In jurisdictions that permit it, capital crimes are those that are considered so heinous and abhorrent (such as the killing of a child or police officer) that the recommended punishment is none other than state-sanctioned homicide (i.e., capital punishment).

Manslaughter is criminal homicide in which the killing is unplanned and done without intention or malice but is, nevertheless, not justifiable or excusable. Manslaughter is often divided into two types: *voluntary* and *involuntary*. Voluntary manslaughter is when an assailant chose to perform an act but did not intend to kill or cause serious harm, such as an unplanned homicide that occurs when carrying out another crime, such as a robbery, or when a fight between two individuals results in the death of one of them. Involuntary manslaughter would be when a death occurs due to gross negligence or as the result of some illegal act, such as drunk driving, but is nevertheless unintentional.

Some jurisdictions have other categories of homicide, including negligent homicide, which is the least serious of criminal homicides and involves the disregard for a known and justifiable risk such that the criminal action could result in death or serious injury. Many jurisdictions also have a felony-murder doctrine, which suggests that any death that occurs during the commission, or attempted commission, of a felony that results in a death is considered to be murder. In this instance, the law assumes that the hand of one is the hand of all. Accordingly, this does not require the doctrines of malice aforethought, deliberation, or premeditation, and the person involved in the felony does not have to be the one who does the killing. Instead, simply being an accomplice in a felony that results in a death makes one liable for felony murder.

As part of the criminal justice system, and following initial determinations by medicolegal investigators (i.e., coroners or medical examiners) as to the manner of death, ultimate responsibility for the determination of homicide (following cases made by prosecution and defense teams, and under direction of the judge) falls upon the jury in a criminal trial.

While religion today has no bearing on what legally constitutes homicide, all major religions have strict prohibitions on it, including suicide, which is sometimes understood as self-homicide. The three monotheistic Abrahamic religions (after Abraham, whom they share as a common ancestor)—Judaism, Christianity, and Islam—derive part of their moral code and understanding of homicide from the Bible, including the murder of Abel by his brother Cain as told in the Old Testament. The earliest known legal document prohibiting murder was the Babylonian Code of Hammurabi, which, dating back some 3,000 years and later promulgated by Moses, is widely considered to have influenced and helped shape the legal codes of Greece, Rome, England, and the United States. It contains the principle of "an eye for an eye," which some people still cite as justification for the use of capital punishment.

Among modern industrialized nations, the United States has the highest rate of criminal homicide, but a lower rate of homicide than many Central and South American countries. Countries of the European Union, New Zealand, and Australia have much lower rates of homicide than the United States (the lowest rates are in England and Wales), though Jamaica has around 10 times more, South Africa about 25 times more, and Colombia (which has the highest rate in the world) has more than 50 times more homicides than the United States. Although rates of criminal homicide fell back in the 1990s in the United States (following a sharp increase in the 1960s and early 1970s), homicide has remained one of the top four leading causes of death between 1991 and 2007 for persons aged between 1 and 40 years according to data from the Centers for Disease Control and Prevention (CDC). According to data compiled by the United Nations, the rate of homicide in the United States in 2010 was 4.8 per 100,000 people, though rates of homicide vary considerably according to sex, race, and age, with homicide rates for men estimated to be 3 to 4 times higher than they are for women, and homicide rates among young blacks aged 10–19 estimated to be 10 times higher than among young whites of the same age.

As with other forms of bereavement that are sudden, violent, and unexpected, deaths resulting from homicide often impact survivors in ways that have the potential to complicate the grieving process. Survivors may come to face to face with the accused during their dealings with the criminal justice system, which may or may not deliver justice (thereby aggravating and intensifying the sense of unfairness and feelings of hurt caused by the loss), and these encounters may serve as "triggers" that in turn elicit painful and traumatic memories about the events that resulted in the death of a loved one. Indeed, violent death as a result of homicide may serve to shatter the assumptions and basic sense of ontological security that an individual has in the world, casting doubt upon their taken-for-granted worldview, their trust in other people, as well as in agencies of law enforcement and their ability to protect the citizens they serve.

Gerry R. Cox and Michael Brennan

See also: Capital Punishment; Coroner/Medical Examiner; Infanticide.

Further Reading

Logan, J. E., S. G. Smith, and M. R. Stevens. Homicide—United States, 1999–2007. *Mortality and Morbidity Weekly Report,* 60(Suppl.) (2011): 67–70. Centers for Disease Control and Prevention. http://www.cdc.gov/mmwr/preview/mmwrhtml/su6001a14.htm

Morrall, Paul. *Murder and Society.* Chichester, UK: John Wiley and Sons., 2006.

Rynearson, E. K., Schut, H., and M. Stroebe. "Complicated Grief after Violent Death: Identification and Intervention." In *Complicated Grief: Scientific Foundations for Health Care Professionals*, edited by Margaret Stroebe, Henk Schut, and Jan Van Den Bout (pp. 278–92). London and New York: Routledge, 2013.

United Nations Office on Drugs and Crime: http://www.unodc.org/unodc/en/data-and-analysis/homicide.html

HONOR KILLINGS

Honor killings involve the murder of female family members, usually by brothers or fathers, often in retaliation for purported premarital or extramarital sex, for refusing an arranged marriage, having been raped, for flirting, or for attempting to get a divorce. In effect, the woman is being punished for either her perceived failure to honor her societally determined commitments, or because her actions are considered to have brought shame and embarrassment upon the family. The practice of honor killings is generally found in male-dominated societies, where males feel their honor or status has been threatened or undermined by the actions of a female family member. The woman's actions are perceived to detract from her honor, which is an attribute "owned" by males in the family. Having failed in her duty to preserve and uphold the family's honor, the woman is deemed guilty and is felt to deserve the maximum punishment of death.

The practice of honor killing is centuries old, and continues today. Several thousand women a year are killed because they are thought to have sullied a family's honor. Honor killings are often concealed and are described instead as unexplained murders or suicides, if acknowledged at all. The obvious signs of a murder are ignored and such women (even infants who are predicted to bring shame upon the family) are often buried in unmarked graves. Such murders are often not prosecuted; where they are persecuted, the younger the perpetrator, the less severe the punishment.

Women in the family may be involved in the killing, whether willingly (and if only by affirming the values by which the action in question is perceived to be a "crime" that brings shame upon a family) or unwillingly, perhaps fearing a threat to their own lives.

The killers of these women feel a great sense of pressure from others (especially other men) in the community, village, or clan to engage in an honor killing. In fact, to not do so is to bring dishonor up oneself and one's family and it is the man's presumed responsibility to restore the family's honor by punishing the offending woman. Some women, in reaction to an intolerable situation (e.g., a forced marriage or history of abuse) choose to complete suicide rather than suffer interminably. Some honor killings involve questions of the woman's inability to provide an adequate dowry (the money, goods, or estate that a woman brings to a marriage); they are often referred to as "bride burning" when such women are doused with gasoline and set on fire. In some cases, such violence against women is used for political or military purposes. Short of killing them, women are often beaten, set on fire, or have their genitals mutilated. Honor killings therefore are often preceded by an extended period of abuse against women.

Despite the obvious immorality of such killings, they continue to occur. Fortunately, while cultural traditions change slowly, efforts to pursue such killings are being carried out by the United Nations Commission on Human Rights and by the United Nations International Children's Emergency Fund (UNICEF).

Bert Hayslip Jr.

Further Reading

Raouda, Najwa. 2009. "Honor Killings." In *Encyclopedia of Death and the Human Experience*, edited by Clifton D. Bryant and Dennis L. Peck (pp. 578–81). Thousand Oaks, CA: Sage.

HOSPICE MOVEMENT

The term "hospice" (from the same linguistic root as "hospitality") can be traced back to medieval times when hospice was a place, a way station, a hostel, affording shelter and rest for weary or ill travelers needing to stop for respite on a long, arduous journey. Today, hospice is a philosophy, not a place. Unlike a hospital or specific building where medical services are provided, it is a concept of care focusing on quality and value of life, not on its length. Though there are designated facilities in the United States, most services to patients and families are provided in their own private residence or long-term care institutions, including assisted-living, nursing, or medical homes.

This model for quality compassionate care for people (and their families) facing a life-limiting illness was, initially, a program for cancer patients considered terminal and expected to die within six months or less. In fact, many patients with a variety of diagnoses, including stroke, heart, liver, Parkinson's, and Alzheimer's diseases, outlive this time frame and the *possibility* rather than the *certainty* of death is now the criterion. Recognizing that the dying process is a part of the normal process of living, the principle is one of maximizing the quality of life through appropriate care and the promotion of a caring community. Affirming life, hospice neither hastens nor postpones death. Today, patients may come on and off hospice care, and re-enroll in hospice care, as needed. The Medicare benefit, and most private insurance, pays for hospice care as long as the patient continues to meet the criteria necessary.

The inspiration for the modern hospice movement came from Cicely Saunders, a British nurse who pioneered specialized care for the dying in the 1950s. Saunders, who also obtained medical-doctor and social worker degrees, emphasized focusing on the patient as a person, rather than on the disease. She introduced the notion of total pain, which includes attention to psychological, emotional, social, and spiritual aspects of suffering, as well attention to physical pain—and aggressive attention, at that, to symptom management. The hospice mission can be summarized eloquently in her own words: "You matter to the last moment of your life, and we will do all we can not only to help you die peacefully, but to live until you die." The hospice Saunders founded in 1967, St. Christopher's, exists to this day in a suburb of London.

Typically, the hospice team comprises doctors, nurses, home health aides, social workers, chaplains, counselors, and trained volunteers. This interdisciplinary team develops a comprehensive care plan which includes medications, medical supplies, and equipment needed for pain and symptom management; coaching loved ones on how to care for the person; delivering special services like speech and physical therapy when needed; providing respite care including short-term inpatient care when pain or symptoms become too difficult to manage at home, or the primary caregiver needs respite time; and providing ongoing emotional and grief support. The concept of holistic, or whole-person care, often allows for complementary therapies such as the following: massage therapy to relieve pain, reduce anxiety, and manage stress; relaxation therapy to promote a sense of calm; music therapy to manage physical symptoms, enhance mood, and stimulate memory recall; art therapy to provide a nonthreatening way to explore emotional, psychosocial, and mental states; and pet therapy to provide a warm and comforting presence for patients and families. After the person's death, bereavement support is available to families for at least one year. These services include telephone calls, visits, written materials about grieving, and support groups.

"The family," however defined, and not only the dying person, is considered to be the unit of care. It is sometimes said that it is hard to imagine anything worse than death; but there is something worse, a *bad* death, in which pain and suffering are prolonged (see also **Good Death**). Answering "yes" to any of the following questions may indicate the need for considering hospice: Are you or your loved one (1) Talking about making comfort and quality of life the most important focus of care? (2) In need of more frequent medical care? (3) Experiencing complications like pneumonia, urinary infections, anemia, and shortness of breath? (4) Experiencing any unpleasant symptoms like pain, nausea/vomiting, fear, anxiety, or loneliness? (5) Spending more time in bed or a chair? and (6) Needing more help in bathing, getting in and out of bed, dressing, eating, and with the control of bowel/bladder?

The National Hospice and Palliative Care Organization (NHPCO) defines palliative care as treatment that enhances comfort and improves the quality of an individual's life during the last phase of life. But palliative care (from the Latin *palliare*, to cloak) is any form of medical care or treatment that concentrates on reducing the severity of disease symptoms and may begin at the diagnosis of life-threatening illness and end with either cure or death (see also **Palliative Care**). The difference between palliative and hospice care is that while palliative care typically occurs simultaneous to curative treatment, hospice care is not usually administered alongside curative treatment, and the patient is required to sign a consent form giving his or her permission to end any further curative treatment. In a three-year study of lung cancer patients, those who received palliative care from the start, reported less depression and happier lives as measured on scales for pain, nausea, mobility, worry, and other problems. These patients typically lived almost three months longer than the group getting standard care, who lived a median of nine months.

A great need still exists for further education about hospice and palliative care. Only 4 out of 126 medical schools require a separate course in the care of the dying. Hospice care is also underutilized: only 40 percent of dying cancer patients are referred to hospice and the reality is that most are late hospice referrals, just days before death.

Sir William Osler, one of the most admired and honored physicians in the history of medicine, taught that: "It is much more important to know what sort of patient has the disease than what sort of disease a patient has." The palliative care approach asks: Who is this person? What does she understand about her illness trajectory? What are her hopes, values, and goals of care? Given that understanding, what are the most likely outcomes of appropriate options of care and which options are most likely to achieve those goals? Hoping for the best but preparing for the worst is a guiding principle of both hospice and palliative care. The ultimate goal, again summed up by Osler, is "to cure occasionally, relieve often, comfort always."

Sandra L. Bertman

Further Reading

Connor, S. R. *Hospice: Practice, Pitfalls, and Promise.* Washington, DC: Taylor & Francis, 1997.

Gwande, A. "Letting Go." *New Yorker,* August 1, 2010. http://www.newyorker.com/reporting/2010/08/02/100802fa_fact_gawande

McNeil, D. G. "Palliative Care Extends Life, Study Finds." *New York Times,* August 18, 2010. http://www.nytimes.com/2010/08/19/health/19care.html?_r=0

National Hospice and Palliative Care Association (NHPCO): *www.caringinfo.org;* http://hospiceofcincinnati.org

HUMOR

Death and humor do not at first sight appear to sit as easy bedfellows, each conveying a set of seemingly contradictory and irreconcilable emotions. Yet it is precisely this paradox and incongruity—between the sadness and solemnity of death, and the pleasure of laughter elicited by humor—that, in the face of death, gives humor its particular purchase and comedic value. In situations foreshadowed by death or which occur in its aftermath, humor can function effectively as a salve, helping relieve the tension and anxiety that routinely accompany death. We find examples of this in the "gallows humor" of those who make light of their impending fate, perhaps as a way of coping and coming to terms with it (in the prisoner awaiting execution who pokes fun at his imminent demise, or in the sardonic humor of the British soldiers of World War I who marched merrily toward death with songs that included lines such as "The Bells of Hell go ting-a-ling-a-ling for you but not for me" and "He's hanging on the old barbed wired").

We also find examples of humor in the context of disasters and traumatic incidents among first responders and emergency medical teams (including police, fire, and ambulance personnel) who may use humor as a defense that distances them from the horrors of death and allows them to function in what otherwise might be an unbearable and debilitating situation, as well as providing as sense of group cohesion and social support in the wake of major critical events. We find examples too in the context of hospice and hospital care of the long-term sick and dying, where humor may operate to ease discomfort in delicate and stressful situations, providing a "tool of reassurance" between patients and health care providers.

In each of these different circumstances, however, there are certain qualifications that underline the limitations of humor. In the first, while dark humor may provide a sense of bonding among emergency personnel, and be used as an informal mechanism of initiation and induction among new recruits, it may also serve to alienate those who find its use inappropriate or distasteful. In the second, there is an important distinction to be drawn in sensitive health care settings between the healthy use of humor that works by undermining the fear and anxiety surrounding death, and humor that merely masks or displaces feelings that may later resurface to cause distress.

What triggers laughter in each of us is, of course, often deeply personal and culturally specific. In some cultures, such as the Mexican celebration of the Day of the Dead (*Día de los Meurtos*), laughter and satire may be used not only to mock death but also as an anti-authoritarian device for poking fun at the political elite, by reminding them of death as a leveler that is no respecter of status and rank; while in others, such as the traditional Irish wake, laughter and joke telling are part of the social fabric by which the deceased are fondly remembered. Indeed, this kind of reminiscence, and the sometimes humorous anecdotes told during funeral eulogies (see **Eulogy**), can provide a useful source of social support, defusing the tension and silence surrounding death, while at the same time providing the bereaved with an enduring image of the deceased that can be retained and carried forward in memory.

In other circumstances, and increasingly in recent years, the death of celebrities, public figures, and people killed in tragedies and disasters has provided the basis for a subterranean culture of joke telling made possible by mass media reporting and the proliferation of the Internet technologies. This was especially true following the death of Princess Diana in 1997, and of Michael Jackson in 2009, where the Internet and social media like Twitter provided a forum by which jokes were spread rapidly around the globe. While for some these jokes are considered "sick," offending public sensibilities by violating basic standards of taste and decency, for others they provide an acceptable outlet for challenging the insincere "hegemony of feeling" and sentiment generated (and imposed) by the media for distant individuals with whom many have no affective connection.

In extreme conditions of totalitarian oppression (such as in the former USSR and Eastern bloc countries under communism), humor following the death of party leaders provided a form of clandestine resistance that could not, when expressed by word of mouth and in private, be repressed by officials. The sensitivity surrounding attempts to make light of death has been further underlined by the public controversy in the United Kingdom generated by a television commercial for car manufacturer Hyundai showing a man trying, but failing, to complete suicide by filling his car with exhaust fumes because the new model produces only "100% water emissions."

Michael Brennan

See also: Day of the Dead; Public Mourning; Taboo.

Further Reading

Davis, Christie. "Jokes on the Death of Diana." In *The Mourning for Diana*, edited by Tony Walter (pp. 253–68). Oxford: Berg, 1999.

Narváez, Peter (ed.). *Of Corpse: Death and Humor in Folklore and Popular Culture.* Logan, UT: Utah University Press, 2003.

Obrdlik, Antonin J. "Gallows Humor: A Sociological Phenomenon." *American Journal of Sociology,* 47(5) (1942): 709–16.

Rowe, Alison and Cheryl Regehr. "Whatever Gets You through Today: An Examination of Cynical Humor among Emergency Service Professionals." *Journal of Loss and Trauma: International Perspectives on Stress and Coping,* 15(5) (2010): 448–64.

Zackheim, Victoria. *Exit Laughing: How Humor Takes the Sting Out of Death.* Berkeley, CA: North Atlantic Books, 2012.

I

IMAGES OF DEATH

The grim reaper, a black-hooded skeleton with scythe, is the most immediately identifiable image of death, though any skeleton, particularly skull and two crossed bones, is another identifiable embodiment of death. Personifications of death—giving it human forms—from the earliest medieval etchings the "Dance of Death" (*Danse Macabre*) are skeletal figures as a friend, liberator, scourge or foe, holding an hourglass, shovel, crown, or symbol of a profession or station in life, quietly leading their live partners to the grave (see **Dance of Death**). The underlying message is that death is the "great leveler," not at all respectful of accomplishments or social class.

More gruesome images of skeletons brutally and gleefully cutting the throats and sadistically torturing naked men and women are detailed in Peter Brueghel the Elder's *The Triumph of Death.* This panoramic holocaustic horror depiction of hell on earth is replete with animals and strange creatures gnawing at the dead remains of those already slaughtered.

The Vanitas genre of the 16th- and 17th-century Flemish artists use skeletons, but add mirrors, hourglasses, clocks, candles and often symbols of decadence, earthy pleasures, and achievements to remind us of the transience of life and the certainty of death for us all. *Three Ages of a Woman and Death with Skeleton,* by Hans Balding Gruein, is a classic example of *memento mori* ("remember you will die") and continues to be reworked even into the 21st century by such artists as James Hopkins (see **Memento Mori**). Using *trompe l'oeil* illusionism (an artistic technique that literally "deceives the eye" so as to create the illusion that an object exists in three dimensions), a realistic still-life painting by Hopkins, called *Vanitas Skull,* of items on shelves (champagne bottles, disco balls, and technological gadgetry), is transformed into the huge face of a grinning skull, the ultimate symbol of impending death.

Less macabre are the medieval woodcut illustrations of *Ars Moriendi* ("the art of dying"). Neither human suffering, nor decaying bodies, or the ravaging of illness are depicted though these images. Instead, angels and devils are prominent, portrayed as vying, at the moment of death, for our souls. These often cartoon-like, picture sermons are Christian depictions of the last judgment, directing our attention to the eternal afterlife (heaven or hell) and the importance of being pious, attentive to the moral life, absolved, confessed, and spiritually prepared at the moment of death (see also **Ars Moriendi**).

In contrast to ashes placed on the foreheads of Christians in church, on Ash Wednesday, the solemn reminder that from dust we come and to dust we will go, the

Day of the Dead (*Dia de los Muertos*) is a joyous holiday. Parades and decorations—larger-than-life paper-mache whimsical skeletons performing everyday activities like riding a bike, eating, and dancing—are intended to be humorous. This Mexican and Latin American tradition of families honoring their deceased by bringing their favorite foods and sweet candy sugar skulls, picnicking on their graves, though mindful of the fate that awaits us all, reflects an understanding and acceptance of death as a natural part of life (see also **Day of the Dead**).

Sandra L. Bertman

Further Reading

Ariès, P. *The Hour of Our Death.* Oxford: Oxford University Press, 1981.
Ariès, P. *Images of Man and Death.* Cambridge, MA: Harvard University Press, 1985.
Bertman, S. *Facing Death: Images, Insights and Interventions.* New York: Taylor & Francis, 1991.

IMMORTALITY

Immortality is the inability to die or, conversely, the ability to live, or at least exist in some form, forever. The concept of immortality is one that has existed across time and cultures. It has played a role in religious thought, philosophy, history, culture and the arts, and increasingly science and medicine. Discourse about immortality has focused on the soul, the body as a whole, body parts or cells, procreation and family, the collective consciousness, and intellectual, artistic, or business endeavors. Immortality may or may not involve "antiaging" (conceived as eternal youth or eternal health). Related to but somewhat different from immortality, is the pursuit of longevity, also sometimes labeled life extension, life prolongation, or life preservation. For some scholars and scientists working in this field, the goal of longevity is the attainment of a longer and healthier life; that is, a longer life that, while still finite, is one of higher quality with less age-related morbidity (illness and disease). For others, however, life extension or preservation is an attempt to employ modern biotechnologies to enable human beings, or the neurological essences of human beings, to escape illness and death and survive indefinitely. Thus, these terms may be used differently by various proponents, in particular contexts, and for divergent purposes; for example: the scientific study of aging, the invention of medical treatments that alleviate age-related ailments, the pursuit of immortality through techniques such as cloning, cryonics, nanotechnology, and regenerative medicine, or the development of youth-enhancing products by the cosmetic antiaging industry.

In Ancient Civilizations

Notions about immortality have existed since ancient times and perhaps even earlier. In ancient China, for example, the eight Ba Xian sages associated with Taoism were considered immortal, and the practice of Taoism itself, with its emphasis on breathing, dietary, physical, and meditational techniques, was and still is thought to lead to longevity and spiritual immortality. Moreover, the Chinese believed that an "elixir of life" existed and was discoverable either in nature or through alchemy.

The ancient Egyptians, who practiced mummification or the preservation of dead bodies for travel through, and judgment in, the afterlife, also believed in a form of immortality. The god Osiris, after being murdered and dismembered by his brother, was thought to be restored to life by his wife and sister, Isis; he then became god of the underworld and presided over the deceased's journey into eternal life. Associated with both Egyptian gods and people were special elements of being or personhood that endured beyond death, including the *ka* (the life-force), the *ba* (the soul), the *akh* (the immortal union of the *ka* and *ba*), the name, and the shadow. Ancient Egyptians, particularly those of the ruling classes, also achieved immortality in the tombs and other cultural artifacts left to history. The pyramids, intentional symbols of immortality, have perhaps proven the most successful, still erect several millennia later and the object of scientific and popular captivation to this day

Some of the most well-known immortals are the gods and goddesses of Greek and Roman mythology, who often were thought to assume human form, exhibit human emotions, and live among and interact with mortal human beings. The offspring of deities and mortals resulted in demigods, such as Aeneas, Heracles, Perseus, and Theseus, who were half mortal and half divine. While they typically enjoyed certain superhuman abilities due to their parentage, demigods could be wounded or killed.

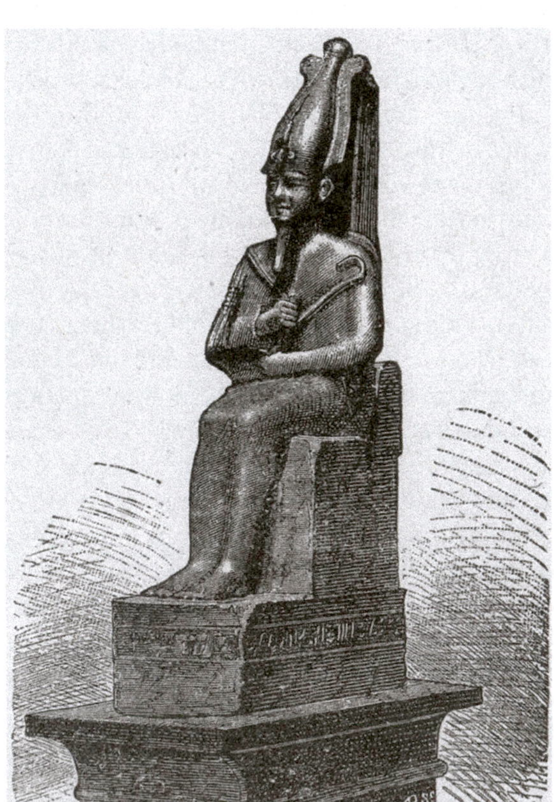

Egyptian god of the underworld, Osiris. (John Clark Ridpath, *Ridpath's History of the World*, 1901)

In Folklore

Many narratives concerning the pursuit of immortality are cautionary tales about its elusiveness or the perils of living forever. For example, the epic of Gilgamesh, the Sumerian king of Uruk in ancient Mesopotamia, speaks to the human desire for, but inability to attain, immortality. In the poem, this semifictional demigod, upset over the untimely death of a friend, is forced to recognize his own mortality and, consequently, sets out to uncover the secret to eternal life. He is told he can find immortality if he can conquer sleep (a sort of "mini-death") for seven days. When he fails, he is offered one more chance and is given a plant that purportedly has special powers of rejuvenation. A serpent steals the plant, however, along with any hope for cheating death.

Conversely, in the Greek myth of Tithonus, problems arise with the acquisition of immortality. When Eos, goddess of the dawn, falls in love with the mortal Trojan, she asks her father, Zeus, to bestow upon Tithonus the gift of living forever. Eos, however, forgets to also ask for eternal youth. Thus, Tithonus is doomed to grow old in body and in mind. Another well-known tale comes from Jonathan Swift's *Gulliver's Travels,* where the hero of this 18th-century novel journeys to the nation of Luggnagg, home of the immortal Struldbrug people. Like Tithonus, however, the Struldbrugs possess eternal life, but do not enjoy eternal youth. Upon the age of 30, they begin to interminably age and decline, and they are declared legally dead at the age of 80 and stripped of their worldly possessions and positions in society. As these stories warn, immortality without eternal youth may be a fate worse than death.

The existence of a fountain of youth is another near-universal theme that can be found in the Bible, the Koran, Greek and Roman writings, the Hindu fable of Cyavana, legends about Alexander the Great, and the reimagined biography of Spanish explorer Juan Ponce de León.

The Immortality of the Soul and the Rise of Antiaging

In Greek philosophy, Plato's *Phaedo,* a dialogue about Socrates's death, purported the immortality of the soul, a concept Aristotle continued in *De Anima.* While Plato identified the soul as a godlike element imprisoned in the body that enables humans to perceive eternal ideas such as Truth or goodness, Aristotle's *anima* was not as distinguishable from the body (and perhaps similar to the ancient Egyptians' concept of *ka*). Platonic and Aristotelian ideas influenced early and later Christian thought, about the soul and immortality, respectively. Early Christian writers, who did not focus much attention on the exact nature of the soul, emphasized the promise of eternal life via salvation. Understandings of this resurrection often included both the body and the soul.

By the late Middle Ages and Renaissance, amid a cultural rebirth following the horrors of the Black Death pandemic, philosophers and theologians returned to contemplating the nature of the soul. This coincided with the invention of the printing press, advances in painting techniques, transoceanic exploration, and the rise of humanism. The shift away from the divine and greater focus on the dignity and achievements of humans contributed to a new sense of immortality through writing, art, and worldly exploits. Moreover, the publication of French mathematician, scientist, and philosopher René Descartes's *Meditations on First Philosophy* in 1641, which lays out a reasoned argument for the separation of body and soul (or mind), elevated the importance of the individual. This further opened up the body, and the physical world, as objects of science, ushering in the Enlightenment and a kind of immortality through unlocking the mysteries of nature.

On the other hand, in response to the human costs of colonialism and the Industrial Revolution, mortality in terms of death, destruction, and decay became a subject of interest during the Romantic and Victorian Gothic periods of the 18th and 19th centuries (which included writers such as William Blake, Mary Shelley, Edgar Allan Poe, and Bram Stoker). Death and disease during the 1800s were medicalized (see **Medicalization**) and transferred from the public and religious arenas to the private and increasingly professionalized spaces of doctors and coroners. Advances in medical science and social reforms around the turn of the 20th century, as well as the increasing secularization of society, heralded a new era focused on personal health and, increasingly, youthfulness or antiaging.

The quest for actual immortality emerged in the mid-20th century in conjunction with developments in, and the popularization of, the science of cryonics (see **Cryonics**). Although science has yet to succeed in extending the life of a human being indefinitely, immortal cell lines have been created, the first of which occurred in 1951 at Johns Hopkins Hospital using the cervical cancer cells of Henrietta Lacks.

Antiaging and the Quest for Techno-Immortality

More modern versions of the quest for eternal youth have centered on the discovery or invention of tonics, elixirs, vitamins, and pharmaceutical medicines or dietary management, physical activity, hygiene, and other behavioral recommendations. While behavioral modifications and some drugs have been shown scientifically to reduce the risk of certain diseases or treat their symptoms—and thus increase longevity and reduce morbidity—these do not change or reverse the underlying processes of aging itself. Moreover, many antiaging products historically and today have often proven to be little more than "snake oil."

Some people are optimistic that scientific advances in biotechnologies, such as stem cell research, genetic engineering, cloning, cryonics, and nanotechnology, will lead to true antiaging and life-extension therapies. While this is theoretically possible, such achievements have not yet transpired.

One of the most public proponents of long-term life extension through biotechnology is Aubrey de Grey, a British computer scientist and self-trained biomedical gerontologist who is the editor in chief of the journal *Rejuvenation Research* and chief science officer of the Strategies for Engineered Negligible Senescence (SENS) Foundation in California. According to de Grey, while many gerontologists focus on the study of aging and the health care of older persons, he rejects the idea that aging is a normal part of life and is primarily interested in delaying or "fixing" aging.

There are several avenues of thinking regarding why the body deteriorates and dies. In general, cell aging and death are thought to be programmed in the body or due to accumulated damage from living. De Grey classifies the causes of aging into seven categories that correlate with his proposed SENS and claims that such biotechnical therapies will eventually be developed faster than age-related damage occurs in human beings. He labels this idea "escape velocity" and believes it will provide the foundation for human life extension and immortality.

Other leading scholars of aging and geriatric medicine such as Leonard Hayflick, Stuart Jay Olshansky, and Bruce A. Carnes, while supportive of such biotechnologies and research on the processes of aging, caution against scientific discourse focused on the idea of humans living forever. They also emphasize that no significant progress has yet been made in any of de Grey's seven SENS areas.

Leigh Rich

Further Reading

Brown, Guy. *Living End: The New Sciences of Death, Aging and Immortality.* Houndmills, Basingstoke, Hampshire and New York: Macmillan, 2008.

Carnes, Bruce A. and Stuart Jay Olshansky. "A Biologically Motivated Partitioning of Mortality." *Experimental Gerontology,* 32(6) (1997): 615–31.

de Grey, Aubrey and Michael Rae. *Ending Aging: The Rejuvenation Breakthroughs That Could Reverse Human Aging in Our Lifetime.* New York: St. Martin's Griffin, 2007.

Fossel, Michael B. *Cells, Aging, and Human Disease.* New York: Oxford University Press, 2004.

Gray, John. *The Immortalization Commission: Science and the Strange Quest to Cheat Death.* New York: Farrar, Straus and Giroux, 2011.

Gruman, Gerald Joseph. *A History of Ideas about the Prolongation of Life.* New York: Springer, 2003.

Hayflick, Leonard. *How and Why We Age.* New York: Ballantine Books, 1994.

Overall, Christine. *Aging, Death, and Human Longevity: A Philosophical Inquiry.* Berkeley and Los Angeles: University of California Press, 2003.

Weiner, Jonathan. *Long for This World: The Strange Science of Immortality.* New York: HarperCollins, 2010.

INFANT MORTALITY

Infant mortality is the death of an infant at any time during the first year of life. This topic deserves special consideration for at least two reasons: first, few human experiences are more emotionally devastating than the death of an infant; and second, the death rate in the first year of life is much higher than in most of the later years of life.

The infant mortality rate (IMR) is the most common measure of infant death and is the number of deaths in a year of persons under age one per 1,000 babies born in the year. Infant mortality rates of 200 or more per 1,000 live births characterized much of human civilization up to around 1800. This means that for most of human history around one of every five babies born were dead before they reached their first birthday. As late as the 1870s, the IMR in European countries varied from 100 in Norway to nearly 300 in Southern Germany. The IMR in China in the early 1900s was around 300. China did not reduce its IMR to around 200 until the founding of the People's Republic in 1949. During the latter part of the 19th century and into the 20th century, almost all countries in the world experienced decreases in their IMRs. The transition to lower levels of infant mortality in the Western countries was due mainly to reductions in infectious and parasitic diseases and to socioeconomic development and modernization.

High IMRs led to the cultural practice in China, Korea, and in many other Asian societies of forgoing the naming of a newborn baby until it had lived for several months and showed signs of continued life. In Korea for instance, even to this day, a small feast is prepared on the 100th day after a baby is born. Rice, red bean cakes, and wine are served. This day was originally celebrated as a feast in honor of the child surviving the first few months of life. A child would not be given a name until the 100th-day celebration. It made little sense to invest emotionally in a newborn by assigning it a name if the chances were only around 2 in 5 that it would survive. In China, parents usually do not take the new baby outside until one month after the baby is born. Then, the family will hold a feast to celebrate the survival of the baby.

In the United States in 2011, the IMR was just under 6 deaths per 1,000 live births. In earlier years, the IMR was much higher; it was over 100 in 1915–1916, and dropped to 26 by 1960 and to 13 by 1980. The IMR has dropped in the United States from 11 in 1983 to 6 in 2011. African Americans have IMRs twice those of non-Hispanic whites. Black infant mortality is the highest of all the racial/ethnic groups in the United States (see also **African Americans**). The IMRs of Hispanics are the lowest.

Infant mortality in the world today varies considerably from country to country. The more modernized the country, the lower its IMR. The IMR of the world in 2011 was about 44, meaning that on average about 1 baby died before reaching the age of one year for every 23 babies born. The IMR was 5 in the more developed countries and 48 in the less developed countries.

Afghanistan had the highest IMR in the world in 2011 with 131 infant deaths per 1,000 live births. The country of Chad was not far behind at 125; the next highest IMRs were in Mali and Congo, higher than 110. Four more countries had IMRs higher than 100 (Somalia, Guinea-Bissau, Angola, and Central African Republic) (Population Reference Bureau, 2011). These are astoundingly high levels of infant mortality (Table 1). Although great success has been achieved in most of the world in the last century in lowering infant mortality, these benefits have not yet been realized by the countries just mentioned.

The countries or regions with the lowest infant mortality rates in the world in 2011 were Hong Kong, San Marino, and Singapore, all with 2 or less infant deaths per 1,000 live births, and there are seven more countries with infant mortality rates less than 3 (see Table 1). IMRs of 2 and 3 are about as low as will ever be attained.

The IMR in the United States in 2011 was 6. Although this is a low level compared to those in many other countries, it is higher than the average IMR of 5 for the developed world. Indeed, most developed countries in the world and many developing countries (48 countries in all) had infant mortality rates in 2011 lower than the IMR of the United States.

Why is the U.S. IMR higher than those of nearly 50 other countries? Part of the reason is statistical. The United States counts as a live birth an infant showing any sign of life, while many other countries are not as stringent in their definitions. However, statistical adjustments that take into account the differences in definitions of live births still do not move the U.S. IMR to the very low IMR levels of

Table 1 Countries or Regions with the Highest and Lowest Infant Mortality Rates, 2011

Country	Location	IMR
The highest:		
Afghanistan	South Central Asia	131
Chad	Middle Africa	125
Mali	Western Africa	116
Congo, Demographic Republic of	Middle Africa	111
Somalia	Eastern Africa	107
Guinea-Bissau	Western Africa	103
Angola	Middle Africa	102
Central African Republic	Middle Africa	102
The lowest:		
Hong Kong	East Asia	1.6
San Marino	Southern Europe	2.0
Singapore	Southeast Asia	2.0
Iceland	Northern Europe	2.2
Slovenia	Eastern Europe	2.5
Sweden	Northern Europe	2.5
Finland	Northern Europe	2.6
Japan	East Asia	2.6
Czech Republic	Eastern Europe	2.7
Norway	Northern Europe	2.8

Japan and Sweden. Also, if one only used the IMR for the U.S. non-Hispanic white population, the IMR would still be almost twice as high as the IMR of the low-IMR countries.

Another reason for the relatively higher IMR in the United States compared to other developed countries is the mother's socioeconomic status. The leading cause of infant mortality in developed countries such as the United States is congenital malformations, a cause of infant death that can be reduced, if not eliminated, with good nutritional intake and prenatal vitamins. However, poor mothers often lack the socioeconomic resources necessary for obtaining these benefits. Many countries in the developed world provide universal health care to the population; and most of these countries have lower IMRs than that of the United States.

The further reduction of infant mortality in the United States is a major goal. In fact, one of the objectives of *Healthy People 2010*, a set of health initiatives being pursued in the United States by several federal agencies, was to reduce the U.S. infant mortality rate in 2010 to 4.5 infant deaths per 1,000 live births. This goal, unfortunately, has not yet been achieved.

Dudley L. Poston Jr., Qian Xiong, and Demetrea Nicole Farris

Further Reading

Frisbie, W. Parker. "Infant Mortality." In *Handbook of Population*, edited by Dudley L. Poston Jr. and Michael Micklin (pp. 251–82). New York: Kluwer Academic/Plenum Publishers, 2005.

Population Reference Bureau. 2011. *2011 World Population Data Sheet*. Washington, DC: Population Reference Bureau.

Poston, Dudley L., Jr., and Leon F. Bouvier. *Population and Society: An Introduction to Demography*. New York: Cambridge University Press, 2010.

INFANTICIDE

Infanticide is the killing of an infant or child under one year of age, usually at the hands of a parent (though the English Infanticide Act of 1938 limits the definition to killing by the mother of the child; and in some, especially Asian societies, infanticide results from communal decisions taken by the husband, village, or extended family). The term infanticide includes *infant murder* (requiring criminal intent or malice aforethought) and *infant slaughter* resulting from willful neglect or violence exercised against the child. More typically, and although the practice today commonly elicits widespread revulsion, infanticide has been employed by almost all societies from the earliest of times as a means of disposing of unwanted, abnormal, or deformed infants.

The practice has been most widespread in societies where famine, poverty, and overpopulation have posed a serious threat to the family unit's ability to sustain itself and to the survival of the wider community more generally. In other instances, and at various times throughout history, the custom of infanticide has also been used to conceal illegitimate births resulting from extramarital affairs, incestuous relationships, and underage sex. Infanticide, especially of the first-born child, has also been used as part of ethno-religious sacrifice in order to appease the gods, secure an abundant harvest, and express gratitude for victory in war. It was used by the Incas to enhance fertility; by the Senjero tribe in East Africa to ensure a plentiful crop yield; and by the Aztecs to placate all manner of deities, from the god of fire (by which children would be ritually burned), the god of rain (whereby children would be ritually drowned), and the god of hunting (whereby children would be shot with arrows). While these will outrage current public sensibilities, it should be remembered that the concept of "childhood" (as protectively distinct from adulthood) is both culturally specific and relatively recent in origin.

The practice of infanticide remains relatively commonplace in Polynesia, China (where government policy aimed at restricting population growth has, since 1979, mandated a "one-child policy"), and in parts of the Canadian northern territory inhabited by the Inuit. The social problem of sex-specific female infanticide (whereby female infants are perceived as a financial burden unable to contribute family earnings, continue the family name, inherit land, and often requiring a costly dowry upon marriage) has been recognized as such by the United Nations, especially in Asian societies such as rural parts of India and China, in which infanticide can be seen as a legacy of their cultural heritage. In the Abrahamic religious traditions of Judaism, Christianity, and Islam, there are strict prohibitions on infanticide, though not on abandonment, which is sometimes erroneously conflated with infanticide (to suggest that those who abandoned their children did so with the intention of them dying is an inference that cannot necessarily be supported, for there is a paucity of evidence for accurately knowing their exact intentions).

In the United States, infanticide occurred among slaves who felt it was better to kill their children than have them live as slaves, though the relatively recent discovery of sudden infant death syndrome (SIDS), and its greater incidence among slave mothers as a result of poor diet and sanitation, has cast some doubt on the established belief that infanticide was rife among slave mothers. It does nevertheless occupy a prominent place in Toni Morrison's novel *Beloved,* which, set after the American Civil War, was inspired by the real-life story of Margaret Garner, who killed her daughter rather than have her captured into slavery.

In Europe, the abandonment of children was relatively common and foundling hospitals (dedicated to receiving infants who had been deserted) were established in Milan as early as AD 787. In the Middle Ages, hospitals and foundling homes established by the Catholic Church were devoted to eliminating infanticide and caring for abandoned babies, and by the 14th century these were extended as municipal institutions where they became the main agencies of adoption. As the centuries wore on, and in circumstances in which unmarried mothers lacked proper support and faced social disapprobation, the practice of overlaying (in which mothers suffocated their children in the blankets of their own beds) became increasingly common. These were often passed off as tragic accidents, though the Catholic Church eventually intervened, describing overlaying as a "sin" and providing the basis for nascent child protection advocacy.

Many societies do not have specific legislation designed to deal with infanticide (in the United States, for example, it is subsumed within the general category of homicide). In English law, there was, until the introduction of the Infanticide Act of 1938, a failure to properly distinguish gratuitous acts of child murder from tragic instances in which infants had been killed by mothers who, because of a lack of social support and poverty-stricken circumstances, could no longer cope and had resorted to infanticide. Sympathetic to the circumstances they faced, juries of the time often refused to convict mothers of murder. Today, judges and juries often look more leniently upon cases of "shaken baby syndrome" when, under pressure of acute tiredness, stress, and postpartum depression, some mothers sometimes temporarily lose control in ways that have tragic and devastating consequences by causing fatal neurological injuries to their offspring. In many societies, notions of "diminished responsibility," and of being mentally incapable of criminal intent through assessments of an unsound mind, serve to limit the charge to that of manslaughter.

Michael Brennan and Gerry R. Cox

See also: Homicide; Sudden Infant Death Syndrome.

Further Reading

Kilday, Anne-Marie. *A History of Infanticide in Britain: c1600 to the Present.* Basingstoke: Palgrave Macmillan, 2013.

King, Michelle. *Between Birth and Death: Female Infanticide in Nineteenth-Century China.* Palo Alto, CA: Stanford University Press, 2013.

Morrison, Toni. *Beloved: A Novel.* New York: Alfred Knopf, 1987.

INFORMED CONSENT

Informed consent is a core principle of modern medical care. As a guide to action, it is underpinned by three key assumptions: (1) that the patient is competent, (2) that the patient's consent to any proposed course of treatment is given freely, and (3) that the patient's consent is based on an adequate understanding of the risks involved in a particular procedure or treatment regimen, including death. A reflection of Western values such as freedom, autonomy, and individual choice, informed consent is important in all medical treatment, but is especially critical in new or experimental procedures where health outcomes are less predictable.

One particular dimension of informed consent pertaining to issues of death and dying is that of disclosure of information by medical staff to a patient with a terminal condition that he or she is dying. Until fairly recently, it was common practice for medical staff to conceal knowledge of a terminal condition from the patient (and sometimes their families), for fear of the psychological distress that such knowledge might cause. Since the early 1960s, and consistent with much of the evidenced-based knowledge generated by early pioneers of the death awareness movement, something of a "sea change" in attitudes has occurred in medical practice. Where only about 12 percent of physicians freely admitted disclosing information of a terminal condition to patients in 1961, by 1977 this had grown to some 97 percent. Providing informed consent to patients is, however, complicated by two situations in particular: (1) when patients are suffering from conditions which impair their cognitive functioning, such as Alzheimer's disease; and (2) when the family of a patient expresses a desire that knowledge of a terminal illness be withheld to protect the patient from possible harm.

Two further dimensions of informed consent in the context of death and dying are evident. First, in Do Not Resuscitate (DNR) orders given to medical staff by patients or their families in order to spare oneself or a relative, especially elderly or frail patients, from the undue distress of intrusive or aggressive procedures such as cardiopulmonary resuscitation (CPR). Second, in the advance directives by which a person may give his or her informed consent *in advance* for the withdrawal of life-sustaining treatment, in the event that the individual is not capable of communicating his or her wishes, and in circumstances where there are no grounds for expecting a reasonable chance of recovery.

Finally, and in places that legally permit euthanasia or physician-assisted suicide, informed consent forms part of a rigorously enforced protocol designed as a safeguard against error and abuse.

Michael Brennan

See also: Advance Directives; Good Death.

Further Reading

Wear, Stephen. *Informed Consent: Patient Autonomy and Physician Beneficence in Clinical Medicine.* Dordrecht, The Netherlands: Kluwer Academic Publishers, 1993.

ISLAM

Islam is a religion that originated in the Arabian Peninsula some 1,400 years ago, and with more than a billion followers, today it is second only to Christianity in total number of believers. While Islam had its birth in the Arab world, most Muslims now live outside the Arab world in an area extending from the Atlantic coast of North Africa to Asia. Currently, Indonesia is home to the largest Muslim population in the world. Thus, while some may see Islam and Arabic culture as being inseparable, not all Arabs are Muslims and the majority of Muslims are not Arabs. Islam takes its name from the Arabic word for submission and refers to submission to the will of God (Allah), whose final messenger was Muhammad. Nevertheless, it is important to note that, while Muhammad is revered as the last in a long line of prophets, Muslims do not see him as a god and he is not to be worshipped as such.

History of Islam

With its origins in what is today Saudi Arabia in the seventh century CE, Islam is chronologically the third of the three monotheistic Abrahamic religions, after Judaism and Christianity. Muslims believe Islam to be the definitive word of God as revealed to the Prophet Muhammad by the angel Gabriel, completing a succession of prophecies stretching back through Jesus to Abraham. Thus, Muslims see themselves not as replacing Judaism and Christianity but as completing a message only partially revealed previously. The completed written message is known as the Koran (recitation in Arabic) and is believed by Muslims to be the actual words of God as spoken to the Prophet in the Arabic language. For this reason, the Arabic language holds particular spiritual significance for Muslims the world over, regardless of the native language of the faithful.

After the death of the Prophet Muhammad, a conflict arose over the issue of his successor. This conflict eventually led to a split in the Muslim community between Sunni and Shia branches, which, to this day, are the source of much political strife in the Middle East and Southwest Asia. Today, Sunnis make up the majority of

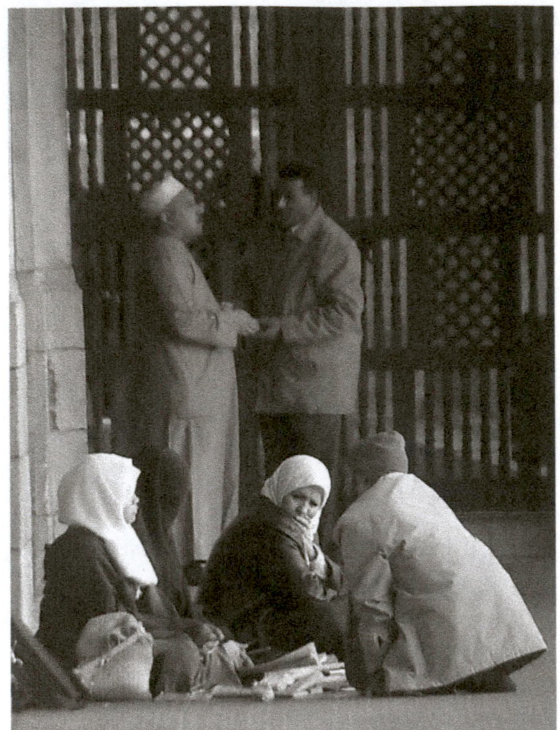

Muslim women and men at Al-Azhar Mosque in Cairo, Egypt, one of the most important of all Sunni Islamic institutions. (AP/Wide World Photos)

the world's Muslims and dominate throughout most of the Arab world, while Shia are a majority in Iran and the Arab countries of Bahrain and Iraq.

The Five Pillars of Islam

Muslim faith centers on five essential practices, sometimes referred to as the "five pillars" of Islam. These are the belief there is but one God and Muhammad is his final messenger; daily prayers; almsgiving; fasting during the month of Ramadan; and for all who are physically and financially able, a pilgrimage to Mecca (*hajj*) at some time in their life.

Islam, Death, and Mourning

Islam, like Christianity, promises its believers reward in the afterlife for having lived a pious life and punishment for having lived an improper one. Islam speaks of heaven, hell, and final judgment. In Islam, death marks the transition from one stage of human existence, in which the spirit resides inside the body within a material world, to another, which is purely spiritual. Following death, the person's spirit begins a journey in which it culminates in eventual reunion with God. During this journey, the spirit undergoes a process of cleansing by which it is removed of the sins committed during a person's life. However, restoration to a state of spiritual purity is only attained via suffering; the more sinful a life one has lived, the greater and more intense the suffering.

Final judgment is determined by weighing a person's righteous deeds against his sinful ones. It is these that determine whether a person will be granted a blissful existence in the afterlife or condemned to a torturous existence in the burning fires of hell. The Hadith (the recorded sayings of the Prophet Muhammad) acknowledges that even those who have sinned and are condemned to hell may still, if they have faith, be eventually admitted to heaven. Unlike in some cultures, death in Islam is not a taboo and Muslims are encouraged to reflect upon death and its meaning for life. Indeed, life on earth is viewed as a test, for which one is ultimately accountable on Judgment Day.

Although there is cultural variation between Muslims regarding the practices and rites following death, there are some key commonalities that appear to be universally observed by Muslims the world over. One such observance is that the dead are buried quickly (usually within 24 hours), so as not to delay spiritual reunion with God. Moreover, because death is perceived as polluting the human body, the body of the deceased is ritually washed, before being buried wrapped in a white shroud, without a coffin, in order to allow decomposition of the body into the original four elements (earth, air, water, and fire). After the prayer leader has recited the fundamentals of the Muslim faith to the congregation, mourners at the burial participate in the funeral by filling the grave with handfuls of soil. In many Muslim communities, the 3rd, 7th, and 40th day following death are marked by ritual and commemorative events, including visits to the deceased's grave. In Islam, providing care and support to the bereaved by way of comforting them, offering condolences, and sharing the burden of grief are an important part of the way Muslim communities deal with death and its aftermath.

Death in Islam is viewed as an important and inevitable part of the human experience; only in our relationship to death do we come to appreciate and understand the essential issues regarding life, death, and the meaning that each possess for us.

Harry Hamilton and Michael Brennan

See also: Afterlife Beliefs; Jihad.

Further Reading

Esposito, John L. *What Everyone Needs to Know about Islam.* New York: Oxford University Press, 2002.

Gatrad, A. R. "Muslim Customs Surrounding Death, Bereavement, Postmortem Examinations, and Organ Transplants." *British Medical Journal,* 309(6953) (1994): 521–23.

Mortimer, Edward. *Faith and Power: The Politics of Islam.* New York: Vintage Books, 1982.

Sheikh, A. "Death and Dying—A Muslim Perspective." *Journal of the Royal Society of Medicine,* 91(3) (1998): 138–40.

J

JIHAD

Jihad is an Arabic word generally meaning *struggle* and is used by Muslims to refer to a spiritual struggle to purify one's faith or that of one's community of believers. *Jihad* implies a struggle with forces, either internal or external, that are deemed to be impeding one's path to spiritual purification. This difference in the focus of the struggle being either on internal failings or external threats has been the source of discussion and scholarly debate within the Muslim community for centuries and remains so today. Regardless of focus, those who struggle for spiritual purity are referred to as *mujahideen,* the name typically associated today with those who use violence to rid Islam of "contaminating" outside influences.

Understanding Violent Jihad

While there are many explanations put forth to explain the violent form of jihad that has captured today's headlines, theories may be generally categorized by their primary focus—religious, economic, political, or psychological. The religious explanations attribute to Islam characteristics that encourage violence against non-Muslims. To the "true believer," nonbelievers, or infidels as they are often called, represent a threat to Islam, and purification requires that they be converted or destroyed. Explanations based on world economics tend to see *jihad* as a reaction to the impact of global free market capitalism on Muslim traditions and sensibilities, and contrast the material advancement of the West with the Muslim world. Such theories are consistent with the argument that *jihadists* are motivated by jealousy. Politically centered theories, on the other hand, highlight Western influence on the political affairs of Islamic nations, such as in the Arab-Israeli conflict or the basing of American troops in Saudi Arabia—home to Islam's holiest sites. Finally, arguments that take psychology as the starting point emphasize the vulnerability and impressionability of some populations, such as the young or otherwise marginalized. In this view, some feature of individual character or disposition is perceived as the primary cause of jihadist behavior.

Jihad and Death

The most obvious link between *jihad* and the subject of death is that those engaged in spiritual struggle sometimes take their own lives and/or the lives of others in their quest for purity. As might be expected, there is disagreement among Muslim scholars as to whether the taking of life in pursuit of jihad is acceptable.

Nevertheless, there are some Muslims who believe that the taking of life is necessary to accomplish the higher purpose of purifying Islam and harmonizing humanity with the will of God, and it is these people who have focused the world's attention on the subject.

Within the Islamic community, *jihad* is a complex idea about which there is continuous debate, but the specific manifestation of *jihad* that calls for the sacrificing of life for a higher cause is not unique to Islam or to the recent past. Indeed, this particular manifestation of *jihad* may be understood in a larger historical and theoretical context. Ernest Becker wrote in *Escape from Evil* (1975) that our species is fundamentally driven to deny our own mortality by seeking what he calls "mortality defenses," one of the most significant of which is religion. Death is a reality that suggests chaos and the meaninglessness of human existence. Religion provides a "grand narrative" that brings order to the universe and places the believer securely within that order. Destruction of the nonbeliever is a means to solidify the community of believers and affirm the faithful against the threat of chaos and meaninglessness. While religion is not the only vessel for such narratives, it is one of the most common and most powerful means by which human beings create and sustain a common worldview, and the destruction of those believed to threaten that worldview is one of the most dramatic means of affirming one's narrative. Indeed, the sacrifice of human life to further some higher cause may be a fundamental human activity. As Robert J. Lifton (1979) noted, there exists an Ancient Egyptian hieroglyphic that defines an enemy as "one who must die so that I may transcend death." Violent *jihad* committed to the destruction of others, it would seem, is an ancient if not primal human drive.

Harry Hamilton

See also: Islam; Martyrs.

Further Reading

Becker, Ernest. *Escape from Evil.* New York: The Free Press, 1975.

Euben, Roxanne. "Killing for Politics: Jihad, Martyrdom, and Political Action." *Political Theory,* 30(1) (2002): 4–35.

Heck, Paul L. "Jihad Revisited." *Journal of Religious Ethics,* 32(1) (2004): 95–128.

Kepel, Gilles. *Beyond Terror and Martyrdom,* translated by Pascale Ghazaleh. Cambridge, MA: The Belknap Press of Harvard University Press, 2008.

Lifton, Robert J. *The Broken Connection.* New York: Simon and Schuster, 1979.

JUDAISM

Judaism is the oldest of the three monotheistic religions, emerging before Christianity and Islam. There are diverse approaches in Jewish rituals involving death and there is no dogmatic acceptance of a theology of a world to come. In the beginning of the Christian century, the Sadducees (a Jewish sect comprising high-ranking individuals, including priests) rejected a belief in an afterlife, while the

Pharisees (a social movement that rejected the traditions championed by the Sadducees) proclaimed there *was* a world to come. Orthodox Jews maintain a conviction of a recompense, immortality, and resurrection in the next world. In the *Olam Ha-ba* (The World to Come) there would be a passage from one stage to another—"a night between two days." In *Tehiyyath Ha-metem* (The Resurrection of the Dead), the remains of body and soul will come before God; the dead would arise and then be judged as to whether they would share in the blessings of the Messianic Era.

The Conservative movement has retained some of this liturgy in their prayer books but may not always regard them literally, but figuratively and poetically. Many recognize the view of the *Nefesh, Neshamah* (The Soul) as a distinct entity with an independent existence. There is wide latitude among the Reform, Reconstructionist, and other movements within Judaism. There is, however, one agreement: death is not viewed as the end of life, not just in terms of another possible world but in paths that transcend death in naturalistic fashion. We are immortal in *body* through our children; in *thought,* through the survival of memory; in *influence,* by virtue of the continuation of our personality as a force to those who come after us; and *ideally* through the identification of the timeless parts or our spirit. The late renowned Orthodox scholar, Rabbi Joseph Soloveitchik believed in directing the mind Heavenward but taking care not to be diverted by the primary task of establishing God's Kingdom right here on earth.

Jewish Mourning Practices

The basic themes of Jewish funeral practices are *Kevod Ha-Met* (Respect for the Dead) and *Kevod Ha-Chai* (Respect for the Living). In ancient days, fragrant flowers and spices were used to offset the odor of decaying bodies. Today, with refrigeration, flowers are generally not part of Jewish tradition. Instead, a contribution is often sent in memory to a hospital, hospice, House of Worship, or medical research foundation. Jewish burial usually takes place as soon as possible after a person's death, as it is considered disrespectful to keep the body unburied for a prolonged period of time.

Since the bereaved are engrossed with myriad details, if there is a visitation, it is usually confined to family members. An ordained rabbi usually conducts the funeral services. Members of the family and friends of different faiths sometimes participate in the sharing of memories. Prayers are recited in English and Hebrew. The eulogy (*Hesped*) recognizes that not only a death has occurred, but that a life has also been lived. Jewish mourners may have a tear in their clothing or a ripped black ribbon (*Keriah*). They wear it to demonstrate their inner anguish, to symbolize "the tear in their heart." When Jacob believed that his son Joseph was killed, the "father rent his garments" (Genesis 37:34).

Burial is the preferred mode of bodily disposal for most Jews. Cremation and autopsy are forbidden for Orthodox and Conservative Jews—which view these practices as a desecration of the body—but are permitted for Reform, Humanistic, and secular Jews. Some of the laws and customs surrounding Jewish funerals and burial include the following:

- It may be a matter of respect and honor not to leave the body unattended. A designated person (*Shomer*) remains with the deceased, reading from the book of Psalms until the start of the funeral. A Holy Society, *Chevra Kadisha*, of trained volunteers may wash, dress, and prepare the body.
- The deceased may be buried in simple shrouds (*Tachricim*) demonstrating that all are equal before God.
- Caskets are usually made of wood so the body naturally returns to the earth.
- Embalming is not permitted for Orthodox and Conservative Jews except when the body is to be transferred a long distance for burial.
- Viewing the body is generally discouraged, but many family members do choose to see the body before the funeral.

The chapel service does not end the funeral. Friends accompany the dead to the grave where brief prayers are recited. Witnessing the burial symbolically emphasizes the final reality of death. The service is relatively brief with Biblical and other texts including the *Kaddish* prayer, which is recited three times for 11 months for the death of a parent, and 30 days for the death of other relatives. The *Kaddish* prayer makes no mention of death but instead praises God and serves as a reaffirmation of a belief in God's will. Friends and family often participate in the actual burial by placing handfuls or shovelfuls of earth on top of the lowered casket, designating the stark reality of their loss.

Following the burial, friends and family may attend the home of the mourners for the *Shiva*, meaning "seven." This custom refers to the first seven days of intensive mourning. *Shiva* has been called "the Habitat of Feeling." There may be a pitcher of water outside the mourner's front door where many will wash their hands as a sign of ritual purity. Upon returning from the cemetery, a memorial candle is lit and kept burning for the entire seven days. Proverbs 20:27 suggests the spirit of humankind is the lamp of the Lord. Mirrors in the home are covered so as to discourage undue attention upon physical appearances and instead utilize the *Shiva* period for recalling memories and spiritual reflection. During this period of mourning, women may refrain from wearing makeup and men from shaving.

Friends and family provide the first food called "The Meal of Consolation" to create an atmosphere of unity and support. It is customary for hard-boiled eggs to be served at the family's first meal after the funeral. The egg, symbolic of renewed life, affirms that life must go on, even during sorrow. It is also customary for visitors to refrain from knocking on the door or ringing the bell of the home of the bereaved; instead visitors just let themselves in.

Following the Shiva, Jews may continue to observe a 30-day period of mourning—*Shloshim*, meaning 30 in Hebrew (this 30-day period is counted from the day of the burial and includes the Shiva). During this period, mourners return to work and resume many normal routines, but may refrain from attending celebratory events. For relatives other than parents, mourning ends at the conclusion of this 30-day period. The family may continue to attend synagogue and participate in the ancient *Kaddish* prayer of condolence. After the 30 days of *Shloshim*, and usually before the first year of mourning is concluded, an unveiling or commemoration of the tombstone or memorial plaque may be conducted at the gravesite for the immediate family and close friends. The deceased are commemorated annually on the anniversary of the person's death and it is customary for persons to mark their visit by leaving a pebble on the gravestone. Through the centuries, Jewish people have practiced time-honored traditions, connecting families and generations. These practices continue to provide comfort and support with the reaffirmation of their faith.

Rabbi Earl A. Grollman

See also: Afterlife Beliefs.

Further Reading

Brener, Anne. *Mourning and Mitzvah.* Woodstock, VT: Jewish Lights, 2006.

Grollman, Earl A. "The Jewish Way in Death and Mourning." In *Concerning Death: A Practical Guide for the Living,* edited by Earl A. Grollman (pp. 119–40). Boston: Beacon Press, 1974.

Grollman, Earl A. *Living with Loss, Healing and Hope: A Jewish Perspective.* Boston: Beacon Press, 2001.

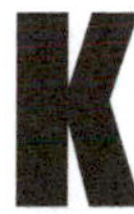

KEVORKIAN, JACK

Jack Kevorkian (1928–2011), a retired pathologist, came to public attention in the 1990s following a series of attempts to convict him of unlawfully helping people to die. In 1999, after four failed attempts to bring a conviction of assisted suicide, Kevorkian was charged and subsequently found guilty of second-degree murder and of delivering a controlled substance to Thomas Youk, a 52-year-old man with advanced amyotrophic lateral sclerosis (commonly known as ALS or Lou Gehrig's disease). Kevorkian was sentenced to 10–25 years in prison for murder and 3–7 years for the supply of a controlled substance. His trial, and the publicity it generated, raised assisted dying as an issue of public debate. Kevorkian became a high-profile advocate of assisted dying and champion of the individual's right to choose a dignified, peaceful death over a life characterized by intolerable pain and suffering.

From the time of his residency as a doctor at Detroit Receiving Hospital in 1956, Kevorkian had a long-standing interest in issues of death and dying: first, in the status of the eye as accurate means of determining death and detecting signs of life in patients considered to be clinically dead (see **Definitions of Death**); and second, in proposing giving murderers condemned to death the option of being executed with anesthesia so that their bodies could be used for medical experimentation and their organs harvested for use in transplantation. Neither was particularly well received by the medical establishment.

Kevorkian went to great lengths to ensure that he took no active part in the action by which individuals ended their own lives, inventing a "suicide machine" (which he first called the "Thanatron" and later the "Mercitron") that was prepared by the physician, but the button of which was pushed by the individuals themselves to release the lethal supply of drugs. Despite this, it was Kevorkian himself who provided prosecutors with the material they needed to bring a conviction by videoing his own part in hastening the death of Thomas Youk and inviting the CBS show *60 Minutes* to screen it.

While Kevorkian, like others within the death awareness movement, was a pioneer who challenged prevailing beliefs in society about death and dying, he distanced himself from the hospice and palliative care movement, inviting accusations that he was not sufficiently informed about new developments within the field of pain relief. Kevorkian, who acknowledged his involvement in some 130 deaths over an eight-year period between 1990 and 1998, was the focus of the 2010 HBO movie *You Don't Know Jack,* starring Al Pacino as Jack Kevorkian.

Michael Brennan

See also: Dignitas; Physician-Assisted Suicide.

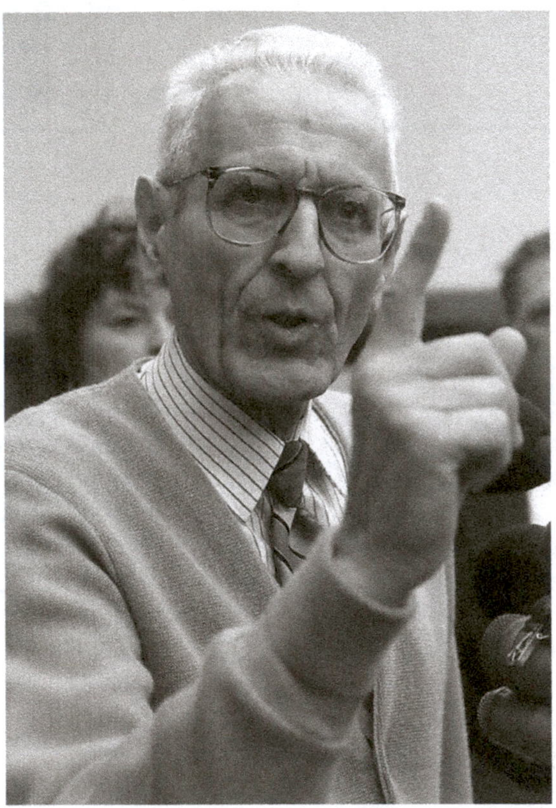

Jack Kevorkian, a retired pathologist and advocate of physician-assisted suicide, helped more than 130 people end their lives during the 1990s. Kevorkian was convicted of second-degree murder in 1999 and sentenced to 10–25 years in prison. (Jeff Kowalsky/AFP/Getty Images)

KÜBLER-ROSS, ELISABETH

Elisabeth Kübler-Ross (1926–2004) was a Swiss-born psychiatrist and advocate for compassionate care at the end of life. She was a pioneering and influential figure in bringing awareness to issues of death and dying in the medical profession and encouraging improved treatment for dying patients. Born one of three triplets, Kübler-Ross was highly influenced by her early experiences as a relief worker in Poland following World War II. During a visit to the Maidanek concentration camp, Kübler-Ross was especially struck by carved butterflies on the camp walls left by children there. As she commented in a 1995 interview with Dr. Daniel Redwood, "It was incomprehensible to me. Thousands of children going into the gas chamber, and this is the message they leave behind—a butterfly. That was really the beginning."

Committed to a career path that would allow her to examine issues of life, death, and the human spirit, Kübler-Ross began her medical training in 1951 at the University of Zurich. It was there that she met her American-born husband, Emanuel Ross, and she eventually moved to the United States with him, where she completed her internship and residency training in psychiatry. In 1965, she secured a teaching position at the University of Chicago Medical School and taught seminars there on death and dying, which involved extensive interviews with terminally ill patients. Based on these interviews, Kübler-Ross wrote her seminal work, *On Death and Dying,* and introduced her now-famous five-stage model of approaching death. Although her first book is the most widely read, Kübler-Ross was a prolific writer, authoring more than 20 books dealing with subjects related to death, grief, and the afterlife.

Using the proceeds from her books, workshops, and talks, in 1977 Kübler-Ross left academia and founded *Shanti Nilaya* (Final Home of Peace) in Escondido, California, which was intended as a healing center for terminally ill patients and their families. Shortly afterward, she and her husband divorced. Kübler-Ross eventually moved her healing center to a farm in Head Waters, Virginia, in 1990, and attempted to create a hospice there for children with HIV/AIDS. However, progress was stifled by opposition within the local community, opposition that ultimately prevented her vision from being fully realized.

Stage Theory

According to Kübler-Ross's five-stage model, terminally ill patients tend to experience five reactions to their impending loss, often proceeding through denial, anger, bargaining, depression, and then finally acceptance. In the *denial* phase, patients may feel shocked or stunned and have a difficult time grasping the reality of their situation. As the reality of their impending death begins to sink in, disbelief can sometimes be replaced by feelings of *anger*, characterized by bitterness, a feeling that life is unfair, and/or a questioning God. In the subsequent *bargaining* stage, patients long to postpone death, in some cases attempting to "make a deal" with God for more time, often in exchange for a reformed lifestyle. This stage may also involve a desire to change the past (e.g., "If only I had taken better care of myself"), which is accompanied by feelings of guilt and regret. Realizing the certainty of death, dying patients may also go through a period of *depression* and experience feelings of despair, hopelessness, and isolation. In the final stage of *acceptance*, individuals acknowledge their mortality and are better able to make preparations for their death, perhaps by attending to any perceived "unfinished business" in their life.

Although Kübler-Ross's five-stage model was initially intended for patients with a terminal illness, she later broadened her focus and suggested that it had applicability for anyone who has experienced a catastrophic loss (e.g., following bereavement, job loss, or divorce). Since the birth of Kübler-Ross's theory, the notion of distinct stages of grief has, to a significant extent, become a conventional wisdom that is ingrained in our cultural beliefs about loss. These models of grieving are still routinely taught as part of the curriculum in medical schools and nursing programs.

Criticism and Controversy

A number of end-of-life theorists and researchers have sharply criticized Kübler-Ross's model, noting that individuals who experience a loss do not necessarily proceed through a linear set of stages and that reactions to loss are often as diverse as the people experiencing them. Others have also pointed to the inconsistency between stage theory and more contemporary research, which suggests that most individuals who experience the loss of a loved one are fairly resilient and report minimal depressive and grief symptomatology.

In her final book, *On Grief and Grieving*, coauthored with David Kessler, Kübler-Ross responded to these criticisms thus:

> The stages . . . have been very misunderstood over the past three decades. They were never meant to help tuck messy emotions into neat packages. They are responses to loss that many people have, but there is not a typical response to loss, as there is no typical loss. Our grief is as individual as our lives. (p. 7)

Although stage theories of loss continue to permeate popular culture, in academic settings alternative models have largely replaced stage theory. For example, Margaret Stroebe and Henk Schut's Dual Process Model, as well as meaning-oriented models (largely popularized by Robert Neimeyer), have been researched extensively and enjoy a strong base of empirical support.

Empirical Findings

Although Kübler-Ross's model has not been researched as extensively as some other models, two recent studies have been conducted that yielded findings that were both consistent and inconsistent with stage theory. In a 2007 study conducted by Paul Maciejewski and his colleagues, the grief experiences of bereaved individuals were found to reach peak levels in a sequence that was consistent with Kübler-Ross's model. However, acceptance was found to be the dominant response throughout the first two years of loss. In another study of stage theory conducted by Jason Holland and Robert Neimeyer in 2010, sharp differences were found for individuals who experienced losses by natural and violent causes. Specifically, acceptance was found to be the dominant response for those bereaved by natural causes regardless of how much time has passed since the loss occurred. In contrast, in the early aftermath of loss by violent means, disbelief and depression were most prominent, which then seemed to be largely replaced by acceptance for those bereaved for 10 months or longer, a finding somewhat more consistent with Kübler-Ross's model.

Jason M. Holland

See also: Death Awareness Movement; Hospice Movement; Palliative Care.

Further Reading

Holland, Jason M. and Robert A. Neimeyer. "An Examination of Stage Theory of Grief among Individuals Bereaved by Natural and Violent Causes: A Meaning-Oriented Contribution." *Omega: Journal of Death and Dying*, 61(2) (2010): 103–20.

Kübler-Ross, Elisabeth. *On Death and Dying*. New York: Macmillan Publishing, 1969.

Kübler-Ross, E. and David Kessler. *On Grief and Grieving: Finding the Meaning of Grief through the Five Stages of Loss*. New York: Scribner, 2005.

Maciejewski, Paul K., Baohui Zhang, Susan D. Block, and Holly G. Prigerson. "An Empirical Examination of the Stage Theory of Grief." *JAMA*, 297 (2007): 716–23.

Redwood, D. (Interviewer). *On Death and Dying: Interview with Elisabeth Kübler-Ross* [Interview transcript], 1995. http://www.healthy.net/scr/interview.aspx?Id=205

L

LIFE EXPECTANCY

Life expectancy is the average additional number of years a person of a given age can expect to live. For example, there is life expectancy at birth or the number of years an individual 60 years of age can expect to live. The word expectancy implies average, so when it is said that someone aged 60 can expect to live 20 more years, this does not apply to any one individual, but rather it means that *on average* someone 60 years old today can expect to live an additional 20 years. Life expectancy is defined mathematically and is one of the elements of the life table, which models the mortality experience of a defined population. The methods used to calculate life expectancy apply current age-specific mortality rates: thus today's rates are used to estimate additional years lived in the future. It is important also to recognize that life expectancy is not the same as *life span,* which is the longest someone has lived. Furthermore, life span is a measure of length of life, and is not necessarily indicative of the quality of life or the amount of life lived relatively free of disability and pain due to illness or accident.

Uses of Life Expectancy

Life expectancy has at least two important uses. First, numerous organizations, including insurance companies, health care payers, the Social Security Administration, Centers for Medicare and Medicaid Services, as well as public and private pension funds, use life expectancy for planning and budgeting purposes, including computing the anticipated distribution of payments to be made in the future. Knowing how long people will live is critical for estimating the dollars needed to fund these programs.

Second, life expectancy is frequently used to compare countries with respect to overall well-being. Poorer, less developed countries tend to have lower life expectancy than nations in the developed world. Among the developed countries, the United States ranks lower than many nations, including Canada, Japan, Norway, Sweden, Monaco, and Greece. Population size and diversity, among other characteristics, should be considered when assessing country rankings based on life expectancy.

Trends in Life Expectancy

One of the most dramatic changes of the past 100 years has been the increase in life expectancy at birth from 49 years at the turn of the 20th century to 78 years in

2009. For men the increase has been 28 years, from 48 to 76, and for women it has been 30 years, from 51 to 81. These specific numbers are for the United States, but this general trend applies to all countries in the developed world. This increase in life expectancy was a continuation of the significant declines in mortality that occurred during the 19th century in both Europe and the United States. This decline in mortality and the consequent increase in life expectancy was part of the demographic transition that began in the late 18th century and continued into the 20th century. For most of human history, both birth and death rates were high, but as death rates began to decline, population increased and eventually stabilized due to declining birth rates. This transition has resulted in more individuals living longer; and thus, especially in countries of the developed world, in an aging (or "graying") and ever older population. There is evidence that the demographic transition also applies to countries in the developing world, although these nations are not as far along in the process.

In the 19th century, the decline in mortality was associated with reductions in deaths due to infectious diseases, including tuberculosis, typhus, typhoid, scarlet fever, cholera, and smallpox (see **Disease**). In particular, infants, children, and young adults were the beneficiaries of these declines.

There are three general explanations for the decline in mortality due to infectious diseases, although the historical data for establishing distinct causes are limited. First, medical therapy in the form of vaccination was most likely responsible for the decline in mortality due to smallpox. Second, in the case of tuberculosis, change in the balance between the lethality of the microbe and the resistance of the host was a likely reason for the decline. Third, and of most significance, changes in the environment were responsible for the decline in numerous infectious diseases, including tuberculosis. For example, public health measures to ensure clean water and food were most likely responsible for reducing the deadly impact of such waterborne diseases as cholera, dysentery, and diarrhea. Improvements in the standard of living, which accompanied economic development, included improved nutrition, particularly for mothers and infants, as well as better housing.

These declines in infectious diseases continued into the early 20th century and were responsible for much of the improvement in life expectancy for individuals of all ages, especially infants under one year. Despite two world wars, and loss of countless lives due to violence, and the fact that impressive gains had already been made, life expectancy continued to increase in the latter half of the 20th century. During this time, there were significant decreases in deaths due to chronic diseases such as cardiovascular disease, stroke, and lung cancer. Nevertheless, cardiovascular disease is still the leading cause of death in the United States, and lung cancer remains the most deadly cancer (see **Cardiovascular Disease**). Improved medical therapy and changes in personal health behaviors are likely reasons for the continued improvement in life expectancy in the latter half of the 20th century. A distinct decline in cigarette smoking has been a major contributor to the reduction in deaths due to cardiovascular disease, stroke, and certain cancers. Again, improvements in living conditions, including safer vehicles and roads, may have also contributed to the decline. For older Americans, income and health security provided by the Social Security and Medicare programs may too have contributed to improved life expectancy.

Factors Associated with Life Expectancy

Life expectancy varies according to a number of individual and structural factors, such as sex, race, socioeconomic status, occupation, heredity, personal behaviors, availability of health care, geographic region, and extent of inequality. For most of human history, women, due in part to superior biology, have lived longer than men, and in the United States, African Americans, due to relative social disadvantage, have not lived as long as their white counterparts. People with higher incomes generally live longer, as they have better nutrition, housing, and access to health care, and are less likely to smoke or drink alcohol excessively, two behaviors that are associated with premature death. In addition, those with higher incomes have occupations that provide more control over when and how they work. There is evidence that having such control is associated with longer life. All of this is not to deny the importance of heredity, particularly for those who, due to family history, are more likely to develop conditions that result in premature death.

Life expectancy varies not only with respect to individual characteristics, but also differs according to country. There is evidence to suggest that the degree of income inequality within a nation is associated with life expectancy, such that the greater the degree of income equality the lower the life expectancy. Income equality can be defined in different ways; an example is the percentage of a country's total income received by the least well off. For example, a country in which 40 percent of income was received by 60 percent of the least well off would have more inequality than a country in which 50 percent of the income was received by 60 percent of the least well off. In 2010, Japan ranked first in the world with an overall life expectancy of 83 years and had one of the most equal distributions of income of any country in the world. The United States with a less equitable distribution of income ranked somewhat lower with a life expectancy of 79 years. While population size and diversity should be considered when comparing national differences in life expectancy, income inequality most likely plays an important role in that those with less see themselves as worse off than those who are relatively better off. This relative deprivation has effects on health and ultimately length of life.

Future Trends in Life Expectancy

Given that life expectancy has increased nearly 30 years in the past 100 years, it is possible but not highly probable that another 30 years will be gained during the 21st century. If this were to be the case, life expectancy would be nearly 110 years in the United States at the end of the current century. The theory that there is an inherent biological limit as to how long most people can live makes achieving such a life expectancy unlikely. What that age is or is likely to be is difficult to estimate, but most likely, 110 years exceeds the age that most people can expect to live. Such a large increase in life expectancy on top of the one already experienced would have profound effects on the structure of society and also have implications for retirement and health insurance programs. The possibility of such long life also raises questions about the nature of work and how rapidly aging societies can sustain themselves when many of their members are not able to work and/or pay taxes.

Alternatively, it is more likely that the gains in life expectancy experienced in the 20th century will not be sustained in the 21st century. There are significant reasons why this may be the case. First, there is an obesity epidemic in the Unites States today and the result has been more diabetes and chronic diseases, resulting in poorer health and reduced life expectancy. Obesity in childhood has become commonplace, and it is likely that obese children will not live as long as their parents. Second, while most of the gains in life expectancy were made possible by the decline in infectious diseases, new infectious diseases have arisen and old ones have resurfaced. The human immunodeficiency virus/acquired immune deficiency syndrome (HIV/AIDS) pandemic has been particularly devastating for countries in the developing world (see **HIV/AIDS**) Life expectancy is less than 50 years in many African countries where the epidemic has been difficult to control and where life-saving drug therapy is not available to all who need it. Even in the developed world, select groups of individuals have experienced reductions in longevity due to HIV/AIDS. Tuberculosis has also resurfaced and there are concerns about antibiotic-resistant diseases as well as pandemic influenza.

Due to this uncertainty, it is challenging to project future life expectancy. Life expectancy could increase if levels of obesity were significantly reduced; yet doing this will require effective public health campaigns as well as improved medical therapies. While it may be possible to reduce the prevalence of obesity, the ability to control a worldwide influenza epidemic, such as the one in 1918, is another matter. An epidemic of this kind could wipe out gains in life expectancy, although improved disease surveillance and treatment may lessen the effects of such a disaster.

In conclusion, given the current situation with respect to obesity, it is likely that life expectancy will not increase but may in fact decrease in the 21st century. While it is seemingly a simple number, increases in life expectancy over the past 200 years have had profound impacts on the structure and function of human societies. What effects a decrease in life expectancy will have in the future remain to be seen.

Charles Maynard

See also: Aging; Infant Mortality; Mortality Rates.

Further Reading

Marmot, Michael. *The Status Syndrome.* New York: Henry Holt and Company, 2012.

McKeown, Thomas. *The Modern Rise of Population.* New York: Academic Press, 1976.

Murphy, Sherry L., Jiaquan Xu, and Kenneth D. Kochanek. "Deaths: Preliminary Data for 2010." *National Vital Statistics Reports,* 60(4) (2012). http://www.cdc.gov/nchs/data/nvsr/nvsr60/nvsr60_04.pdf

Olshansky, S. Jay, Douglas J. Passaro, Ronald C. Hershow, Jennifer Layden, Bruce A. Carnes, Jacob Brody, Leonard Hayflick, Robert N. Butler, David B. Allison, and David S. Ludwig. "A Potential Decline in Life Expectancy in the United States in the 21st Century." *New England Journal of Medicine, Special Report,* 352 (2005): 1138–1145. http://www.nejm.org/doi/pdf/10.1056/NEJMsr043743

Preston, Samuel H., Patrick Heuveline, and Michael Guillot. *Demography.* Oxford, UK: Blackwell Publishers, 2001.

Shrestha, Laura B. Life Expectancy in the United States. *Congressional Research Service Report for Congress,* 2006. http://aging.senate.gov/crs/aging1.pdf

Wilkinson, R. G. "Income Distribution and Life Expectancy." *British Medical Journal,* 304 (1992): 165–68. http://www.ncbi.nlm.nih.gov/pmc/articles/PMC1881178/pdf/bmj00056-0043.pdf

LIFE SUPPORT THERAPIES

The term "life support therapy" is generally used to refer to a group of mechanical devices that replace the biological function of a vital organ that has failed. Such measures may be short term (hours to days) or long term (days to years).

Short-term therapies are used when a failing organ will recover function with treatment. They include: ventilator therapy, kidney dialysis, temporary pacemakers, cardiac ventricular assist devices (VADs), cardiopulmonary bypass machines (CPB), and extracorporeal membrane oxygenation (ECMO). Long-term life support may be instituted when organ failure is permanent, including prolonged or lifelong ventilator therapy, kidney dialysis, pacemakers and other cardiac rhythm devices, and artificial hearts. VADs are occasionally used for longer, though generally not permanent therapy.

Mechanical life support such as VADs and/or artificial hearts may also be instituted as a "bridge to transplant," if a patient is a reasonable candidate for organ transplant and is likely to survive for a time on mechanical therapy until an organ can be found.

History and Technology

The prototype of "iron lungs," or negative-pressure ventilators, was first developed in 1832 at the Harvard Medical School, but not used clinically until 1928. They were large machines that surrounded the entire patient except for head, and created a vacuum around the thorax that expanded the chest, pulling air into the lungs. As of 2008, approximately 30 patients in the United States were still on "iron lungs." "Positive-pressure" ventilation was developed in the mid-20th century during the polio epidemic by Bjorn Ibsen in Denmark. In these patients, a breathing tube was placed in the patient's trachea and air was "forced" cyclically into the patients' lungs by a person or machine. In the 1970s, smaller, quiet mechanical machines were introduced into intensive care units. Subsequent refinements allowed patients to undergo home ventilator therapy.

CPB was first used in 1953 as a means of supplying blood and oxygen to the body during heart surgery. With CPB, blood is pumped from the patient through tubes to pass over a membrane that allows oxygen to enter the blood, and is then

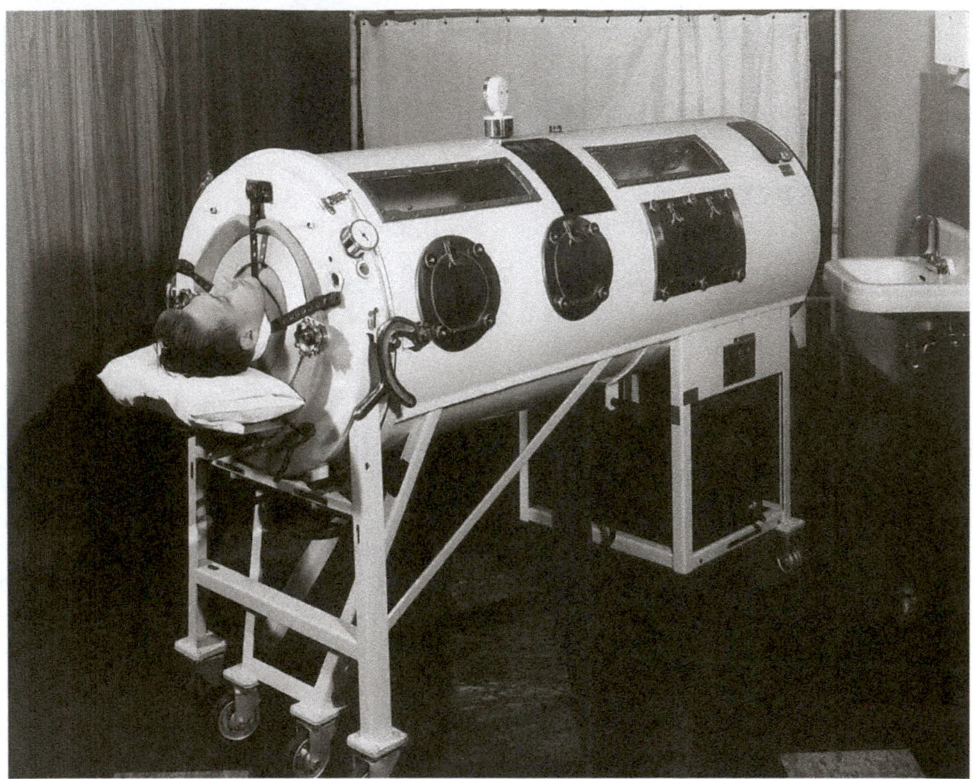

The negative pressure ventilator, or iron lung, was first widely used around 1930 for victims of coal gas poisoning and polio. Positive pressure ventilation has mostly replaced the use of iron lungs. (SuperStock/Corbis)

returned to the body. CPB requires medications to prevent blood clots, as well as control of bleeding in the surgical patient when such medications are administered. CPB technology advanced dramatically during the 1960s and 1970s with more refined methods to oxygenate the blood within the machine. CPB is generally restricted to short-duration life support during surgeries involving the heart, lungs, and great vessels. ECMO is a technology developed from CPB in the 1970s. It is used to supply temporary heart and lung support outside of the operating room for damaged or diseased organs, or as a bridge to transplant if damage to the heart and/or lungs is permanent. Bleeding and clotting complications limit the duration of ECMO to a few days.

During hemodialysis, blood passes through tubes via membranes that filter out solutes and excess fluids from the blood that would normally be eliminated by the kidneys. It was first used clinically in 1945. Long-term hemodialysis depended on the development of means to establish long-term access to the patient's veins, since frequent placement of dialysis tubes (every other day) caused damage that eventually prevented further dialysis. Belding Scribner developed the first such permanent implantable "shunt" in the 1960s and also established the first outpatient dialysis facility, the Seattle Artificial Kidney Center, in 1962.

Pacemakers and implantable cardioverter defibrillators are small devices that deliver electrical stimulation to the heart to either maintain heart rhythm or to convert the heart out of a life-threatening rhythm. The first clinical use of an external pacemaker was in 1932. The first long-term pacemaker was implanted in 1958 in Arne Larsson, who survived more than 40 years. Progressive improvements lead to smaller devices with long battery life, allowing pacemakers to become a mainstay in cardiac therapy.

The first external mechanical heart was implanted by Denton Cooley in 1969, in a patient awaiting heart transplant. An implantable artificial heart was used by Robert Jarvik in 1982. Widespread use of VADs (pumps that support but do not replace the patient's native heart function) and mechanical hearts awaited the development of materials and medications to reduce blood clotting and excessive bleeding. The first total artificial heart implantation was performed in Taiwan in 1996, as a bridge to transplant.

Current Statistics

Statistics on mechanical life-support therapies are summarized in Table 1.

Ethical Issues

Mechanical life support raises issues of cost and fair distribution, since there are usually not enough devices to serve everyone who needs them, and such devices are very expensive. How patients should be prioritized to receive such therapies, and who should bear the cost are issues that are still subject to debate. Should only

Table 1 Life Support Systems

Therapy	**Number of Patients in the U.S Receiving Therapy (Year of Report)**
Mechanical Ventilation (in hospital only)	790,000 (2010) (Wunsch, 2010) *Note: 30 patients were reported to still be using iron lungs in 2008*
Kidney hemodialysis	398,861 (2009) (National Kidney Urologic Diseases Clearing House)
Pacemakers and other cardiac rhythm devices	0.5–1 million people in the U.S have devices, 100,000 new devices are implanted each year (2004) (American Heart Association)
Ventricular-assist devices	Approximately 100 annually as a bridge to transplant (2009)
Artificial hearts	Approximately 1,000 total implanted to date of report (2009) (American Heart Association)
ECMO	No comprehensive statistics available

the sickest patients receive life-supportive therapy, although they are less likely to survive? Should there be an age limit? Should patients with self-inflicted organ damage (e.g., smokers needing mechanical ventilation) be put lower in the priority list? Should society cover the cost of such therapies, which are out of the economic reach of most individuals?

Additional ethical questions arise when a patient is nearing the end of life and requests that therapy be discontinued. Many health care workers and family members often feel uncomfortable with discontinuing life-sustaining therapy when it will result in the rapid death of the patient, since there are both ethical principles and laws against "killing" people or patients. In the United States, laws give patients the right to require that such therapy be discontinued upon request (see **Advance Directives**). Medical ethicists, leaders of most major religions, and legal experts agree that discontinuing such therapies amounts to letting the patient die a natural death, and is not the same as "killing," thus morally and legally permissible.

Gail A. Van Norman

See also: Bioethics; Euthanasia; Physician-Assisted Suicide.

Further Reading

American Heart Association: http://www.heart.org

Beachamp T. L. and J. F. Childress. *Principles of Biomedical Ethics,* 7th edition. New York: Oxford University Press, 2012.

Bynum, W. and H. Bynum. *Great Discoveries in Medicine.* London: Thames and Hudson, 2011.

Fox, Margalit. "Martha Mason, Who Wrote Book about Her Decades in an Iron Lung, Dies at 71." *New York Times,* May 10, 2009. http://www.nytimes.com/2009/05/10/us/10mason.html?_r=0

National Kidney and Urologic Diseases Information Clearing House: http://kidney.niddk.nih.gov

Vincent, J. L., E. Abraham, F. A. Moore, P. Kochanek, and M. P. Fink (eds.). *Textbook of Critical Care Medicine,* 6th edition. Philadelphia: Elsevier Saunders, 2011.

Wunsch, H., W. T. Linde-Zwirble, D. C. Angus, M. E. Hartman, E. B. Milbrandt, and J. M. Kahn. "The Epidemiology of Mechanical Ventilation Use in the United States." *Critical Care Medicine,* 38(10) (2010):1947–53.

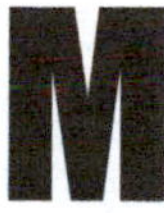

MAKE-A-WISH FOUNDATION

The Make-A-Wish Foundation is a not-for-profit organization whose goal is to help grant the wishes of severely ill children. Since it was founded in 1980, the foundation has helped grant more than 148,000 wishes, funding vacations, facilitating meetings with celebrities, and helping realize the dreams of children whose lives have been blighted by serious illness. The story of the foundation's beginnings can be traced to Christopher Greicius, a seven-year-old boy with leukemia who dreamed of becoming a police officer. After befriending Christopher and his mother, Linda Bergendahl-Pauling, U.S. customs officer Tommy Austin had promised Christopher a ride in a police helicopter. When Christopher's condition worsened, Austin contacted Ron Cox, an Arizona Department of Public Safety (DPS) officer, and together they planned a day to help raise Christopher's spirits. The day included a helicopter ride across the city of Arizona to the DPS headquarters, where Christopher was sworn in as the state's first ever honorary patrolman.

Today, the Make-A-Wish Foundation has 69 chapters across the United States and an affiliate organization, Make-A-Wish International. To qualify, candidates must be aged between two and a half and eighteen years old and have a life-threatening, degenerative, or malignant medical condition, though it need not be terminal. The foundation relies upon the support of some 25,000 volunteers and the financial support of donors in order to help make the wishes of children come true. Grounded in a philosophy of bringing happiness, and of providing respite and relief from the stresses of living with serious illness for children and their families, the Make-A-Wish Foundation grants a wish every 38 minutes, the most popular of which include a trip to a theme park, the desire to meet someone famous, the wish to be someone (such as a firefighter) for a day, and to be given a special gift.

Michael Brennan

Further Reading

www.wish.org

MARTYRS

A martyr is one whose life is sacrificed to further some cause, usually one of a religious or spiritual nature. Whether one dies in the name of Christianity, Hinduism, or any other "ism," there are those who will view them as martyrs. Indeed, all of the major monotheistic religions—Judaism, Christianity, and Islam—have recognized martyrs among their coreligionists, as have other nontheistic religious traditions, including Hinduism and Buddhism. Furthermore, adherents to more secular beliefs, such as communism or nationalism, might also view those sacrificed for their cause as martyrs. That is, the label is somewhat subjective, inviting people to claim martyrdom for those who die for a cause with which they identify, while denying that claim for groups holding a different set of beliefs. One's identification as a martyr is, therefore, a subjective process. Martyrdom, it seems, is in the eyes of the beholder.

While martyrdom may have been a part of many religious traditions over the years, it is its place in some contemporary Muslim thought and practice that has most focused attention on the subject today. Islam has had a long tradition of martyrdom (*shahadah*), but support for the practice is far from universal in the Islamic world, and it is a subject riddled with moral complexity. For example, there is disagreement as to whether it is acceptable to simply offer one's life as a sacrifice for the greater cause, or to intentionally take one's own life, as well as the life of others. There has been, and remains, considerable disagreement among Muslim scholars regarding these and other issues. Nevertheless, there has obviously been enough support in some Muslim circles for significant numbers of mostly young men and a few young women to embrace the practice. Indeed, although the phenomenon was all too familiar in some parts of the world prior to the attacks on the Pentagon and the World Trade Center of September 11, 2001, interest in martyrdom among Western analysts rose dramatically when the twin towers fell. Such horrific acts of death and destruction beg for an explanation.

Numerous explanations have been put forward and these are inevitably shaped by the perspective of the observer: what one observer perceives as martyrdom, another sees as murder/suicide. That is, attempts to explain and understand this phenomenon tend to be clouded by subjectivity. Nevertheless, one sociological approach to the subject has the potential to transcend subjectivity and it is anchored in the works of writers such as Ernest Becker, who in 1975 wrote *Escape from Evil*, and Otto Rank, author of *Psychology and the Soul* (1930). Both of these writers argued that human beings are fundamentally driven by a fear of death. This fear, however, is not primarily of physical death but of psychic or spiritual death. Human awareness of physical death allows the contemplation of our total psychic annihilation. Death awareness allows us to comprehend the possibility that life may be utterly meaningless, and given this state of affairs we seek means of defending ourselves psychologically from this conception of death. One such defense is the embrace of a narrative that places us and "our kind" at the center of the universe. Whether a tribe, a nation, or an ideology, we adopt or construct a worldview that gives meaning to our existence. As Peter Berger observed in *The Sacred Canopy* (1967), we create "all-encompassing fabrics of meaning," and this meaning sustains us against what might otherwise be a chaotic and meaningless existence.

One way of understanding martyrdom, then, is as a "mortality defense," in that the actions of one willing to make the ultimate sacrifice for a belief, provide a powerful affirmation for those who share that belief. Indeed, self-sacrifice not only reinforces the *sacred* narrative in the minds of the believers (using *sacred* to include a broad array of "isms"), but also the martyr ensures for himself or herself a revered place in the cosmos, and by extension for family, friends, and cobelievers. Furthermore, when martyrdom includes the intentional deaths of nonbelievers, the narrative takes on even greater significance and power. For as Robert J. Lifton noted in *The Broken Connection* (1979), the Ancient Egyptians may have formulated "the most fundamental of all definitions of an *enemy: a person who must die, so that one may oneself transcend death*" (304). The taking of the life of someone who does not share in our "mortality defense" holds the promise of weakening theirs and strengthening ours.

Martyrdom is unique to no particular historical period or religion. The identification of one as a martyr gives legitimacy to all who share the martyr's narrative as a defense against mortality. Thus, to label one a martyr is a political as well as a religious act, since it grants legitimacy, and therefore power, to one set of beliefs over others. As such, the concept of martyrdom will likely continue to be controversial and a source of conflict. Furthermore, because martyrdom is so closely linked to what some social scientists have identified as a core human drive, the practice should be expected to continue undeterred or to increase. As populations grow and splinter, the potential number of competing narratives grows, and along with that growth comes an increasing need to legitimize those narratives. Martyrs can provide that legitimacy.

Harry Hamilton

Further Reading

Becker, Ernest. *Escape from Evil.* New York: The Free Press, 1975.
Berger, Peter. *The Sacred Canopy.* New York: Anchor Books, 1967.
Lifton, Robert J. *The Broken Connection.* New York: Simon and Schuster, 1979.
Rank, Otto. *Psychology and the Soul.* Translated by Gregory C. Richter and E. James Lieberman. Baltimore: The Johns Hopkins University Press, 1998/1930.

MEDIA AND DEATH

In modern and highly mediated societies, in which face-to-face encounters with death and dying have been largely sequestered and removed from public life, many people's first encounter with death, dying and bereavement is, perhaps not surprisingly, via the media. These vicarious encounters appear in many different guises (in news reporting; fictional and documentary film and television; as well as in a whole genre of videogames and even children's animated cartoons). The media's impact and influence in this respect is hugely significant, helping both communicate and shape our cultural attitudes and perspectives about death, dying, and bereavement, including our firsthand experiences of it.

In early and classic accounts of the role played by the media, a general assumption appeared to be that death, dying, and violence were portrayed wholly unrealistically (in comic books, popular novels, and film) in ways that served a "narcotizing dysfunction" by derealizing the experience and desensitizing us to

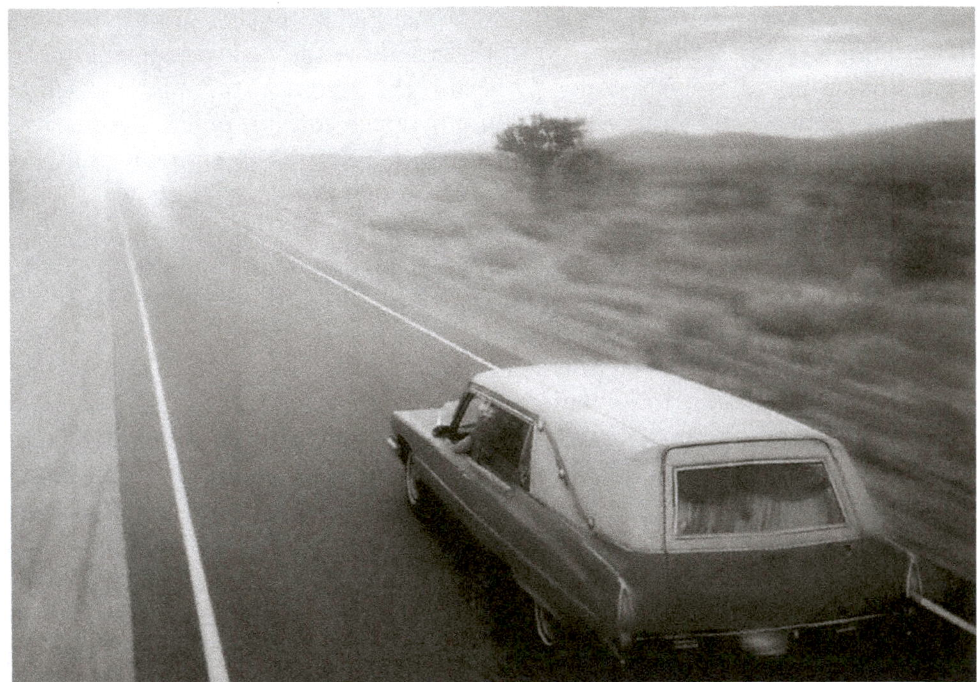

The hearse from *Six Feet Under*, an American drama that ran for five seasons on HBO (2001–2005). The show centered on a family who owned a funeral home. (Photofest Digital Library/HBO)

the suffering of others. In his now classic essay, "The Pornography of Death," Geoffrey Gorer was among the first to argue that portrayals of death in popular culture had become commodified, reduced to a cheap source of titillation that bore little resemblance to reality, and were akin to a kind of pornography. More recently, others, including journalists and academics, have continued and extended this argument by suggesting that modern media (from YouTube, to videogames such as *Call of Duty* and *Grand Theft Auto*) have accelerated and ratcheted up a tendency toward highly graphic and voyeuristic portrayals of death in ways that are less likely to provide genuine insight and understanding of death and dying than they are psychological maladjustments, including a likelihood that viewers of such imagery may themselves be influenced to commit heinous acts of violence resulting in death.

Particular examples that we could point to in order to illustrate unrealistic media portrayals of death include a whole genre of animated children's cartoons (including timeless favorites like *Tom and Jerry* and *Roadrunner*) in which characters are repeatedly killed, flattened by an oncoming steamroller, or shot at close range, only to magically spring back to life again and again in ways that are likely to give the false impression that death is reversible and nonpermanent. That death has now "come out of the closet" and is now seemingly in vogue within popular culture (witnessed by the popularity of shows like *Dexter, CSI,* and *Six*

Feet Under) is not, for some, *prima facie* evidence of a more mature relationship with death and dying, but rather of a new fetish and fascination for death and the human corpse in ways that have transformed it into the new "porn star" of popular television.

In contrast, there are those who argue that the media's treatment of death and dying at the end of the 20th and the beginning of the 21st century is markedly different from when Gorer was writing in the 1950s. While many would acknowledge that there are significant strands within the media that continue to sensationalize death (especially the news media's fascination with dramatic rather than mundane deaths), there are increasingly sensitive and nuanced portrayals of death and dying that have the potential to be genuinely insightful, educational, and enriching. Television documentaries, such as the 2007 PBS Frontline production *The Undertaking*, about the Lynch family undertakers, or the 2011 BBC film, *Choosing to Die*, about assisted suicide, are but two recent examples. Further examples might include media reporting of celebrities who have chosen to publically narrate their experiences of dying (such as Farrah Fawcett or former *Big Brother* contestant Jade Goody in 2009) in the hope that others might gain insight into the experience of dying and greater awareness about the benefits of early screening for conditions, such as cervical cancer, from which Goody died (see also **Public Dying**).

In other ways, the media have the potential to distort our perception of reality, as some commentators suggested following the death of Princess Diana in 1997 (see also **Public Mourning**), by appearing to amplify the extent of people's grief; while at the same time allowing unprecedented access to images and eye-witness accounts—often in real time, as was the case in the terrorist attacks of 9/11 and others since, in ways that contribute to the shaping of public memory.

In an age that has witnessed the purported decline in organized religion, it is the media rather than religious leaders who are charged with providing meaning and making sense of events that appear meaningless. Recent developments in the portability and functionality of hand-held media suggest that ordinary individuals will continue to narrate their own experiences of death and dying in ever greater numbers (in blogs and social networking sites), and to serve as "citizen journalists" by recording and reporting their own images and accounts of accidents and disasters as and when they occur.

Michael Brennan

See also: Facebook; Sex and Death; Video Games.

Further Reading

Foltyn, Jacque Lynn. "Dead Sexy: Why Death Is the New Sex." In *Making Sense of Death, Dying and Bereavement: An Anthology*, edited by Sarah Earle, Caroline Bartholomew, and Carol Komaromy (pp. 47–51). London and Thousand Oaks, CA: Sage, 2008.

Kitch, Carolyn and Janice Hume. *Journalism in a Culture of Grief*. New York: Routledge, 2008.

McIlwain, Charlton D. *When Deaths Goes Pop: Death, Media and the Remaking of Community.* New York: Peter Lang, 2005.
Weber, Tina. *Drop Dead Gorgeous: Representations of Corpses in American TV Shows.* Frankfurt and New York: Campus Verlag, 2012.

MEDICALIZATION

Medicalization is the process by which a behavior or condition becomes defined and viewed as a medical problem requiring medical treatment or intervention. As social conditions, scientific understanding, and cultural attitudes change, the perception of certain behaviors and conditions may also change to reflect advances in our awareness and understanding of these phenomena. For example, activities previously viewed as sinful, immoral, or criminal, such as homosexual activity, heavy drinking, or stealing have come to be viewed and defined as illnesses (whether of body or mind). While homosexuality is no longer considered a mental disorder by mainstream psychologists and psychiatrists, heavy drinking may be indicative of alcoholism, and stealing may be a manifestation of kleptomania. Similarly, natural conditions and processes have also been medicalized. Conditions such as aging, balding, childbirth, and shortness, have all come to be viewed as medical ailments that can be "corrected" or "improved" through medical intervention.

Medicalization also refers to the process by which the definition of an illness is expanded. For example, in 2003, blood pressure guidelines were revised, adding a new category called "prehypertension" for individuals with a systolic blood pressure between 120 and 139 millimeters of mercury. Previously, systolic blood pressure in that range was considered normal. Similar changes in the definition and diagnosis of conditions such as osteoporosis, prostate cancer, and attention-deficit hyperactivity disorder (ADHD) have led to dramatic (and often controversial) increases in the number of persons being treated for these conditions.

Factors Impacting Medicalization

While the general trend in contemporary, Western societies is toward greater medicalization, it is not inevitable for every behavior or condition. In order for medicalization to occur, it is essential that three factors be present: (1) one or more influential groups in society have a vested interest in defining the behavior or condition as a medical concern; (2) the group(s) is sufficiently organized with ample power and resources to enact a change in the existing perception of the behavior or condition; and (3) the group(s) must be able to convince the appropriate professional/regulatory bodies to accept the new definition. Typically, doctors, the general public, pharmaceutical companies, insurance companies, and professional organizations (such as the American Medical Association and the American Psychiatric Association) are involved in the process of medicalization. Doctors usually play a prominent role due to the fact that their power, scope of practice, client base, and revenue can be increased substantially. Pharmaceutical companies can profit from the development of drugs to help treat a newly defined medical ailment. In recent years, the Internet has also played a significant role in helping bring individuals together to reaffirm each other's perception of a condition, and thereby help unite them to lobby for the medicalization of particular conditions.

Medicalization and Dying

Parallel to other domains of social life, the process of dying has also become increasingly medicalized. Prior to the late 19th century, the realm of death and dying was largely very private, personal, and often spiritual. Individuals generally died at home, surrounded by friends and family. Death was viewed as an inevitable and natural part of life, often framed by religious discourse. Instead of friends, family, and priests helping prepare a person for death, the medicalized approach to death and dying centers on resisting death by attempting to prolong life for as long as possible. Death came to represent a failure for the medical community; a problem that might be solved, or at least avoided, by appropriate medical intervention and technology. Advances in the fields of human anatomy, pathology, and probability analysis, helped drive increasing medical involvement in the process of dying.

Medicalization is not an inherently positive or negative phenomenon. The primary focus is rather on the degree of medicalization. In many ways, medicalization has undoubtedly played a positive role, bringing greater awareness to a condition, destigmatizing certain conditions, improving the quality of life, and extending life by promoting research for effective treatments. One of the greatest triumphs of science, and the medicalization of disease, has been the development of vaccines that have saved the lives of millions of people and contributed to the considerable increase in life expectancy over the last 100 years (see **Life Expectancy**). The length and quality of life have thus been greatly improved by medical science. However, in the areas of death and dying, there are numerous counterexamples where medicine has become *too* invasive and pervasive, fostering new problems known as overmedicalization.

Overmedicalization

Overmedicalization refers to the point at which medical treatment and intervention become a major threat to health. Medicalization in this context exceeds what is in the best interests of the public in general, and of patients in particular. Such threats to health include unnecessary medical interventions (with their associated risks), as well as psychological and emotional harm to patients resulting from ineffective medical treatment. In the areas of death and dying, one can find numerous examples of the use of invasive technology with little regard for the physical and emotional well-being of the patient and his or her family, as well as medical interventions that are in direct contradiction of the patient's wishes.

Debates about euthanasia focus on medicine's ability to prolong life, but frequent inability to improve the *quality* of life. Death and dying are viewed as compartmentalized and "bracketed off" from everyday life, whereby individuals are segregated from larger society, increasingly dying in institutionalized settings (such as nursing homes and hospitals), in which they are isolated, disempowered, and largely dehumanized. Medicalization in this context is viewed as contributing to prolonging individuals' pain and suffering, rather than allowing them to die with peace and dignity (see **Hospice Movement**). As a result of the problems associated with overmedicalization, organized groups have fought to actively reverse the process, known as demedicalization.

Demedicalization

Demedicalization refers to the process of redefining an existing medical condition as no longer a medical problem. The previous medicalization of the condition or behavior would thus be reversed. Examples in the areas of death and dying include natural death movements, hospice, and palliative care, all of which reflect opposition to overmedicalized approaches to the process of dying. This form of resistance to the medical field is likely to continue to expand in late-modern societies, opening up the possibility of a shift in the balance of power between the medical profession and the general public. The challenge for the future will be to find an appropriate balance in order to enjoy the benefits of medicalization while avoiding the negative consequences of an overmedicalized society.

Tim Thornton

Further Reading

Conrad, Peter. *The Medicalization of Society: On the Transformation of Human Conditions into Treatable Disorders.* Baltimore: Johns Hopkins University Press, 2007.

Foucault, Michel. *The Birth of the Clinic: Archaeology of Medical Perception.* New York: Vintage Books, 1973.

Howarth, Glennys. *Death and Dying: A Sociological Introduction.* Cambridge, UK: Polity Publishing, 2007.

Illich, Ivan. *Limits to Medicine: Medical Nemesis, the Expropriation of Health.* London: Marion Boyers, 2000.

Szasz, Thomas. *The Medicalization of Everyday Life: Selected Essays.* Syracuse, NY: Syracuse University Press, 2007.

Woods, Simon. *Death's Dominion: Ethics at the End of Life.* New York: McGraw-Hill, 2007.

MEGADEATH

Megadeath is a term originally used to describe a death toll of over 1 million people caused by a nuclear explosion. It is also referred to as "megacorpse" or "mass death." The term "megadeath" was first used by Herman Kahn, a military strategist with the RAND Corporation. In his book, *On Thermonuclear War,* Kahn spoke of the deaths from nuclear war measured in units of "megadeaths." The term was one used by analysts of both the United States and the Soviet Union during the

Cold War. Since that time, the term has taken on additional meaning and is now used to refer to mass deaths of a million or more caused by any weapon of mass destruction. Such weapons include nuclear, biological, and chemical weapons (see **War**).

The term "mass death" can also be used to describe such casualty figures. However, since mass death is commonly used when referring to animal or insect deaths, the term megadeath appears to be more limited in scope and is used to refer only to human deaths, typically to such human deaths that occur as a result of weapons of mass destruction.

If one looks only at the final death toll, the megadeath unit can be applied to some conventional wars. World War II is estimated to have resulted in the deaths of 60 to 72 million people. Almost 2 million people may have died from the two nuclear explosions in Japan, but the greatest number of deaths was caused by conventional weapons and disease. World War II was not the first war to have taken millions of lives. Some other wars with death tolls in the millions include China's An Shi Rebellion of the 8th century (over 30 million deaths), the Mongol Conquests of the 13th century (30 to 60 million deaths), The Tai Ping Rebellion of the 19th century (over 20 million deaths) and, in the 20th century, World War I (15 to 20 million deaths) and the Second Sino-Japanese War (20 million deaths). There is a wide range in numbers of deaths caused by many of these events because some studies do not include deaths from epidemic diseases. For example, if deaths from the Spanish Flu are included, some estimates put the death total for World War I (1914–1918) as high as 65 million.

Technological advances have increased the ability of a single conventional weapon to take increased numbers of lives. However, such deaths do not run into the millions unless weapons of mass destruction are employed. Cruise Missiles can be launched from ground, air, or sea. Their conventional payloads can cause thousands of deaths from a variety of high explosives. However, if armed with nuclear, chemical, or biological weapons of mass destruction, the death toll can reach over a million from a single explosion or discharge. All of this can be done with little or no risk to the personnel who launch the missile, since it is typically mobile, can be fired from long range, flies at low altitude, and presents only a small signature to missile detection radar.

Megadeath in Popular Culture

The term megadeath has become a part of popular culture. The American metal band *Megadeth* took its name from the term. They formed in the 1980s and their albums and lyrics reflect nihilistic themes of death and destruction, featuring such titles as "Killing is My Business . . . and Business is Good" and albums entitled *Peace Sells, but Who's Buying* (1986); *Youthanasia* (1994); and *United Abominations* (2007).

The term megadeath was used in the classic film *Dr. Strangelove or: How I Learned to Stop Worrying and Love the Bomb* (1964). When a deranged military officer ordered an attack on the Soviet Union, one of the characters, General Buck

Turgidson (played by George C. Scott), described in detail the aftermath of a nuclear war and calmly discusses the anticipated megadeaths that would result. He saw 20 megadeaths as a "better" outcome than 150 megadeaths.

There was also a character in the Transformer cartoon series named Megadeath. His character was one of the groups known as Decepticons. He was presented as insane and wanted to end all life through the use of neutron bombs. There is also a Megadeath PlayStation 3 game in which megadeath is the objective of the game. The enemy is alien zombies but the game does provide a way to release stress and does show how the word is moving into many levels of society (see also **Video Games**).

Psychological Effects

It was Joseph Stalin who once said "One death is a tragedy, a million deaths is only a statistic." He also saw death not as a problem but a solution when he said, "Death solves all problems . . . no man, no problem." Death on such a large scale is difficult for humans to process and comprehend to the extent that some people may shut down psychologically and emotionally as a result, and behave as if the event is finished and forgotten rather than dwell on its effects.

When it attacked Iraq in 1998 in an operation now called Operation Desert Fox, the United States said that the invasion was to locate and destroy Iraq's weapons of mass destruction. Ten years earlier in 1988, the Iraqi regime under the leadership of Saddam Hussein, had killed thousands of Kurds with poison gas. However, when no weapons of mass destruction were found in Iraq following the operation, and again following the second Iraq War of 2002, that "cause" no longer carried as much weight as it once had. Initially, the belief that such weapons *did* exist and that Iraq had shown a willingness to use them was a legitimate factor when war was considered. The mere possibility and belief that weapons of mass destruction did exist in Iraq may itself have been cause enough to start a war.

Some deny that there is any real danger of weapons of mass destruction being used. They point to the fact that research on neutron bombs has ceased and that, as far as is known, no such weapons have ever been deployed. Neutron bombs differ from other nuclear weapons because their destruction is limited to living tissue, causing relatively minimum damage to technology or a nation's infrastructure. As was the case with poison gas after World War I, there is widespread agreement that the use of such weapons would be immoral given the probability of mass death.

In the mid-20th century, operators at nuclear missile silos were, as an exercise, directed to fire their rockets in order to judge their individual responses. The missiles had been previously deactivated without the knowledge of the soldiers being tested. To launch the missiles—each carrying multiple nuclear warheads—two keys on opposite sides of the room had to be turned simultaneously. The result was that many of the soldiers refused to turn their keys. For them, the possibility of causing megadeaths was quite real and they made a conscious decision by refusing to participate in that action. Despite the availability of weapons of mass destruction, and because of the accompanying likelihood of megadeath, there seem to be some things that people, even members of a nation's military, simply will not do.

As was the case during the Cold War, civilians are once again worried about the possibility of mass death. This time, however, the fears stem not from attacks by other nations but from possible terrorist acts. The symptoms of post-traumatic stress disorder (PTSD) may also be found in anticipatory feelings of people who fear the possibility of megadeath. These symptoms include bad dreams, frightening thoughts, apathy, and hyperarousal (the sense of being easily startled, feeling tense or "on edge," and difficulty sleeping and/or outbursts of anger). As nuclear proliferation intensifies (especially among less-stable nations of the developing world) and as fears continue to grow about the possibility of a terrorist organization acquiring a "dirty bomb," these effects are likely to be experienced more frequently.

There was, however, one positive effect provided by the possibility of megadeath. During the most dangerous periods of the Cold War, the stockpiles of nuclear weapons held by the Soviet Union and the United States could have ended life on this planet. The very thought and possibility of catastrophic devastation wrought by mass death and destruction may well have been the reason that the Cold War never exploded into actual, violent conflict. This idea, in which each party to a conflict would be effectively annihilated by war, was referred to as the doctrine of Mutual Assured Destruction (MAD). If one side initiated a nuclear attack, it knew that the response from the other side would inevitably result in its own destruction and that any such attack would therefore be irrational. Ironically, it may thus have been the thought of MAD that in the end preserved peace.

Robert G. Stevenson

Further Reading

Kahn, Herman. *On Thermonuclear War.* Westport, CT: Greenwood Press, 1978.
Levine, Robert A. *The Arms Debate.* Cambridge, MA: Harvard University Press, 1963.
Rummel, R.J. *Death by Government.* New Brunswick, NJ: Transaction Publishers, 1997.
Snyder, Timothy. *Bloodlands: Europe between Hitler and Stalin.* New York: Basic Books, 2010.

MEMENTO MORI

The term *memento mori* is Latin and means "remember, you must die!" In Europe during the late medieval and early modern period, reminders that death was a universal and inescapable event affecting everyone—regardless of status or wealth—became extremely widespread and could be found in an array of symbolic imagery: from the visual arts (in paintings and woodcuttings), to decorative and practical items (such as in jewelry and silverware), as well as in architecture and sculpture. In this imagery, death was personified, often as a skeleton (as in the Dance of Death), or represented in the macabre symbolism of skulls, bones, and coffins, which appeared not just on gravestones but in a range of household and personal items, such as pocket watches, candlesticks, and clocks. Together with a genre of devotional Christian literature (see **Ars Moriendi**), which emphasized that the path to salvation lay in leading a virtuous life, this *memento mori* imagery and paraphernalia served a moralizing purpose by confronting the individual with stark reminders of his or her own mortality.

From the late 18th century onward, however, such imagery became less explicit and was represented metaphorically through the use of urns, cut flowers, and downturned torches, as well as in the form of watches and hourglasses, symbolizing the passage of time. It is unclear whether this shift marked simply a change in fashion or was reflective of a much deeper trend toward the avoidance and denial of death characteristic of the modern mind-set.

During the Victorian era, *memento mori* imagery assumed a more sentimental tone reflective of the Romantic Movement in literature and art. Now, rather than serving a moralizing function by reminding everyone of death in general, *memento mori* objects served a memorializing function, reminding individuals not necessarily of their own deaths but of cherished loved ones who had died. This reflects what French historian Philippe Ariès calls the shift in concern from *my death* (about what will happen to the fate of the individual's own soul on judgment day) to *thy death* (the anxiety about how the individual will cope without a loved one who has died). *Memento mori* imagery of this period can be found in linking objects that provide a memory of the lost beloved, such as postmortem photography of the deceased and in brooches containing portraits of the deceased that were worn upon the flesh or close to heart.

In the late 20th and early 21st centuries, *memento mori* commemorative practices reflective of the Victorian tradition have been revived in the form of memorial tattoos and the use of postmortem photography among parents of stillborn babies, where photos provide a material object to help families construct an identity for the child and serve as a vehicle of grieving and remembrance.

Michael Brennan

See also: Ariès, Philippe; Ars Moriendi; Dance of Death; Memorial Tattoos; Photography.

MEMORIAL DAY

Memorial Day is an annual day of remembrance observed in the United States, honoring deceased members, or former members, of the U.S. military, particularly those who died in battle. In 2000, President Bill Clinton clarified the meaning of Memorial Day as a "day of national awareness and reverence, honoring those Americans who died while defending our Nation and its values. While we should honor these heroes every day for the profound contribution they have made to securing our Nation's freedom, we should honor them especially on Memorial Day."

Honoring the noble and military dead has been a long tradition in human history. The ancient Chinese, Japanese, Greek, Roman, and Druid civilizations honored the graves of their dead with flowers and rituals to stimulate remembrance. Citizens of modern nations honor their military dead through ritual, narrative, statues, and sacred burial sites. Whatever the design, the intent is to remember the sacrifice, particularly of young lives, for a cause. Ebersole (2005, 2243) insists that "religious calendars are punctuated with festivals and observances related to the dead, but so are secular calendars."

Historically, May 30 was called "Decoration Day," given the tradition in many communities immediately after the Civil War of decorating the graves of "the heroic fallen" with fresh flowers. Waterloo, New York, is credited with holding the first documented local "memorial day" observance in 1866, although many communities claim to have originated Memorial Day. Some identify the placing of flowers on the graves of Union and Confederate dead in Arlington National Cemetery on May 30, 1868, as the first official observance and the antecedent of today's commemoration.

In 1967, Waterloo's claim was recognized by Lyndon Johnson's presidential proclamation and Congressional legislation as "the birthplace of Memorial Day" for its century-long celebration of the war dead that began on May 5, 1866.

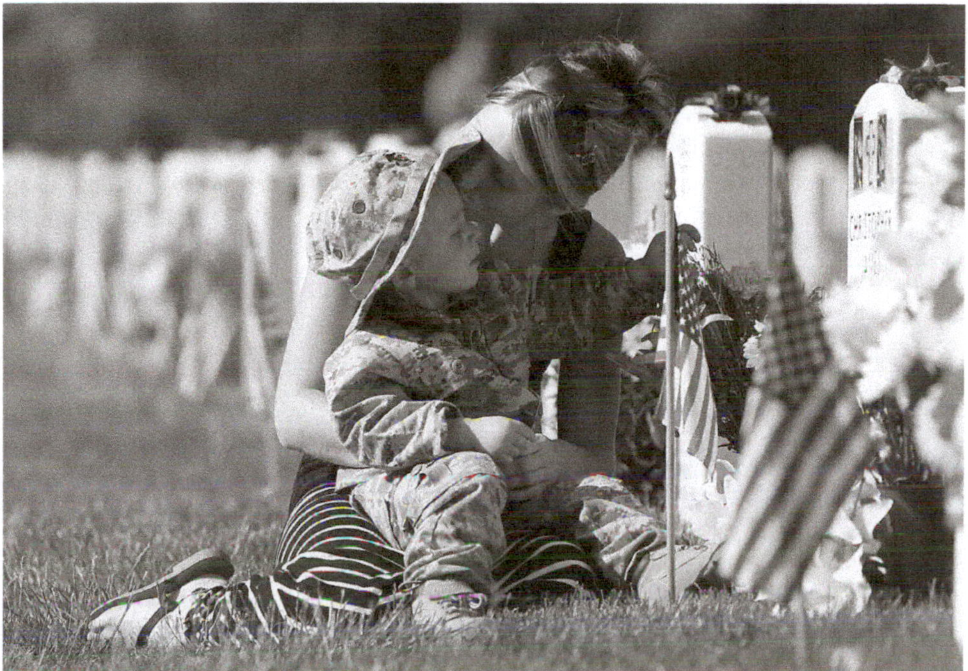

Brittany Jacobs kisses her son Chris at the grave site of her late husband, Christopher Jacobs on Memorial Day at Arlington National Cemetery in Arlington, Virginia, May 27, 2013. (AP Photo/Molly Riley)

Boalsburg, Pennsylvania, claims, however, that its observation began two years earlier in 1864.

In the years immediately following the Civil War, given the collective grief of the nation following 600,000 deaths in the conflict, numerous periodic local observances were organized. George John A. Logan, commander in chief of the Grand Army of the Republic, a veteran's organization, issued General Order 13 in 1868, establishing May 30 as a day to decorate the graves "of comrades who died in defense of their country."

By 1890, all of the states that made up "the Union" of 1861–1865 recognized May 30 as a day of commemoration. Former Confederate states preferred memorial celebrations on April 23, April 26, April 30, or May 10. Many Southerners decorated graves on June 3, the birthday of Jefferson Davis, the president of the Confederacy. The common date of May 30 emerged after World War I as the commemoration was expanded to honor Americans who had died in all wars.

Generally, on Memorial Day, the president of the United States (or his representative) places a floral tribute at the Tomb of the Unknown Soldiers during ceremonies at Arlington National Cemetery. The president delivers a speech on the importance of intentional remembrance of the sacrifice of the fallen dead and recognition of the day for the American people. This tradition was enhanced on Memorial Day, 1958, when bodies of unknown service members from World War II and the Korean War were interred in graves alongside the Unknown Soldier from World War I.

The Uniform Holiday Bill signed by President Lyndon Johnson on June 28, 1968, mandated four three-day weekends for federal employees with official celebrations on Mondays, beginning in 1971: Washington's Birthday, Memorial Day, Veterans Day, and Columbus Day. Legislators were then convinced that that these extended weekends would encourage travel, recreational and cultural activities, and stimulate the economy. Many states, however, preferred to celebrate Memorial Day on its original date, May 30.

In 1971, the U.S. Congress designated the last Monday in May as a day of commemoration and authorized a three-day holiday. The federal government and most states mark the day as a legal holiday so that banks, schools, post offices, and government offices are closed.

Critics contend that providing a three-day weekend defused public awareness on the focus of the holiday. For many citizens and businesses, Memorial Day is now the official start of the summer vacation season. Responding to this reality, President Bill Clinton in 2000 called for a "National Moment of Remembrance" on the afternoon of Memorial Day. Clinton insisted, "This memorial observance represents a simple and unifying way to commemorate our history and honor the struggle to protect our freedoms." At 3 P.M. local time on Memorial Day, Americans are asked to observe a moment of silence "to remember and reflect on the sacrifices made by so many to provide freedom for all" (Clinton, 2000, May 2).

In rural areas with church-owned graveyards, Memorial Day offers an opportunity for individuals to clean cemeteries and provide maintenance repairs, particularly in cemeteries without provisions for perpetual care (see also **Cemeteries**).

Memorial Day is a parallel celebration with Veterans Day, a November holiday honoring *all* service members. Canada observes both traditions on Remembrance Day, November 11. Although a federal holiday, individual provinces honor different traditions. Across Europe, where the day is called Armistice Day, November 11 officially commemorates the end of World War I, as hostilities ended on the "eleventh hour of the eleventh day of the eleventh month."

Harold Ivan Smith

Further Reading

Clinton, W. J. Memorandum on the White House Program for the National Moment of Remembrance. Office of the President, May 2, 2000.

Ebersole, G. L. "Death." In *The Encyclopedia of Religion,* 2nd edition, Vol. 6, edited by L. Jones (pp. 2235–45). Detroit, MI: Thomson Gale, 2005.

MEMORIAL TATTOOS

Memorial tattoos are tattoos that commemorate and represent an individual after he or she dies. Tattoo artist Vince Hemingson explains that memorial tattoos often commemorate a dead child, friend, or family member, and enable individuals to both grieve and honor the dead. Many individuals also choose to memorialize pets with tattoos, wanting to remember a deceased dog or cat in the same way a dead family member is remembered.

The word tattoo is a Polynesian expression, from the Samoan *tatau*. The British explorer James Cook and his men first encountered Polynesian tattooing during their 1769 expedition. Memorial tattoos are found in many ancient and contemporary cultures, often representing not just one specific relative but *all* deceased relatives. The Māori people of New Zealand practice Tāmoko, which is a tattooing/body marking practice often used to commemorate and memorialize all family relations.

Memorial tattoos come in many different shapes, styles, and sizes. They are an extremely personal form of memorialization, so many individuals will select designs that defy quick recognition. Contemporary memorial tattoos often use the following forms:

- The name of the deceased, in an ornate or other nontraditional script, near both a death and birth date. Sometimes only the date of death will be used for the memorial tattoo. It may also include the letters RIP (Rest in Peace).
- A tattoo portrait taken from a photograph of the deceased individual and/or a pet which holds special meaning for a grieving individual. Names, significant dates, and specific sayings are often added to portrait memorial tattoos.

- Abstract and/or concrete symbols that represent the deceased individual are also common. The concrete symbols can be religious, such as a cross, or designate public service; for example, a police force badge. Some abstract memorial tattoos might include the deceased's favorite color or a flower. Parents may choose to take the footprints of a recently deceased newborn and use either one or both feet as the tattoo memorial image.
- Some people now mix a very small portion of cremated remains into the ink used for a memorial tattoo. The amount of cremated remains used is so minimal that it does not alter the tattoo's overall appearance or healing.

Within the broader history of memorialization for the dead, the memorial tattoo represents an ancient form of body marking merged with a popular, contemporary form of artwork. As tattooing has become more socially accepted, so too has the choice to permanently remember a deceased individual with a memorial tattoo.

John Troyer

Further Reading

Death Reference Desk, "Memorial Tattoos." http://deathreferencedesk.org/tag/memorial-tattoos

Hemingson, Vince. "Memorial Tattoo Designs." http://www.vanishingtattoo.com/tattoos_designs_symbols_memorials.htm

Hemingson, Vince. *Tattoo Design Directory: The Essential Reference for Body Art.* New York: Chartwell Books, Inc., 2009.

Riemschneider, Burkhard and Henk Schiffmacher (eds.). *1000 Tattoos.* Los Angeles, CA: Taschen Books, 2005.

MEMORIALS AND MEMORIALIZATION

The famous New York newspaperman and writer Damon Runyon (1880–1946) once said: "You can keep your things of bronze and stone, just give me one person who will remember me once a year." This quotation gives us a broad understanding of memorialization. The goal of all memorials is to help us remember (literally *re-member* or *reconstitute*) the person who has died. For some, it is a marked place in a cemetery, for others it is the naming of an institution, foundation, or a business to honor an individual that will outlive and help future generations to "remember" the contributions of a person who has died. Following Runyon's death from cancer, his friend and fellow journalist, Walter Winchell, appealed on his radio program for contributions to help fight cancer. This appeal eventually led to the establishment of the Damon Runyon Cancer Memorial Fund, which supports scientific research into cancer and provides a lasting memorialization of Damon Runyon.

The most traditional method of providing memorialization is the memorial stone, grave marker, or head stone in a cemetery, usually consisting of the name of the individual and his or her dates of birth and death. Sometimes, these stones are engraved with religious symbols, a picture of the person who has died, the words

RIP or other messages to the dead, and/or other information about the deceased (such as spouse, parent, occupation, hobbies, etc.) that the living would like remembered about the person who has died.

Another very different method to memorialize a loved one is the current trend of creating an RIP tattoo (see also **Memorial Tattoos**). The most basic of these tattoos is the wrist tattoo, where the name of the individual to be memorialized is tattooed on the inside of the wrist so that a person can be remembered as often as the person wishing to memorialize them can view this very visible part of the body. A date can also be placed on the body as powerful reminder of the significant person to be remembered. This might include a birth or death date or even a significant date in the life of the person to be remembered, such as a marriage anniversary. Another important RIP tattoo can be a religious tattoo such as a cross, an angel, or a Buddha image. Finally, the facial image of a loved one can be a significant RIP tattoo which assists one to memorialize or remember a significant loved one.

Public memorials are also employed in the cause of memorializing the dead for wider society. This would include the 9/11 Memorial in New York City and war or veterans memorials, such as the Vietnam Veterans Memorial in Washington D.C. The latter is a memorial wall consisting of the 58,195 names of American soldiers who died or were missing in action during the U.S. War in Vietnam and Southeast Asia. The wall is maintained by the U.S. National Park Service, and receives around 3 million visitors each year.

Another public memorial, but of more personal or family significance, is the roadside memorial that often commemorates a site where a person died suddenly and unexpectedly, away from home (see also **Spontaneous Shrines/ Roadside Memorials**). Unlike a gravesite headstone, which marks where a body is laid, the memorial marks the last place on earth where a person was alive. Usually the memorial is created and maintained by family members or friends of the person who died. A common type of roadside memorial is a cross or plaque with an inscription, decorated with flowers (real or plastic) or wreaths. Handwritten messages and personal mementos may also be included.

Social or societal meanings are another way of memorializing the life of an individual or groups of people. Temporal interpretations of death provide a means for protecting social order and personal meanings in the face of death. Such interpretations tend to emphasize the empirical, natural, and "this world" view of death. But more importantly, these memorials provide an immortality of the deceased that is related to the activities and accomplishments of the individual during his or her lifetime—including biological offspring and social relationships that the individual has created.

There is a strong temptation to view a person who has a secular or temporal orientation as being very different from a person who finds comfort in a religious interpretation of death. In fact, both will attempt to restore the order in their personal lives, and societal order, by placing death into the context of a higher order that will transcend the person who has died.

For the individual with religious commitments, comfort for anxiety and protection from anomie (the absence of shared norms governing social behavior) are to be found by being in a relationship with the supernatural. For the person with a secular or temporal orientation, these same benefits are found in becoming involved with other people, projects, and/or causes. These involvements, although not pertaining to the supernatural, still provide a frame of reference that transcends the finite individual—a person may die, but his or her concerns will continue after death and they will be remembered or memorialized into the future.

From an existentialist perspective, the creative efforts that comprise one's life can provide individuals with personal meaning for both life and death. One way this is accomplished is through the creation of a symbolic immortality, which actually includes surrogate forms of immortality—such as the continuity of history, the permanence of art, or even the biological force of sex. Symbolic immortality (Lifton and Olson, 1974) refers to the belief that the meaning of a person can continue after he or she has died. From a religious standpoint, symbolic immortality often relates to the concept of a soul, which may return to its preexistent state, move on to an afterlife, be reincarnated in another body, or be united with the universe. From a secular standpoint, symbolic immortality may be attained via remembrance by others, by the creation of something of an enduring quality (either in terms of its beauty of usefulness), or by being part of a cause or social movement that outlives the individual. It is this memorialization that keeps the meaning of the deceased alive (see also **Immortality**).

Following her death, Mother Teresa was beatified by Pope John Paul II and given the title "Blessed Teresa of Calcutta." Beatification, the third of the four steps in the canonization process that declares a deceased person to be a saint, is a recognition accorded by the Catholic Church of a dead person's accession to heaven and capacity to intercede on behalf of individuals who pray in his or her name. A parallel perspective can be found in non-church-based civil religion. Civil religion is concerned with the transcendent meanings that support the state and provide it with a super-empirical or supernatural identity. Governments may grant pardons to convicted persons years after their deaths. Meaning is a flexible, yet powerful, thing. Furthermore, from the perspective of American civil religion, only the dead can be honored and memorialized by having their images appear on U.S. postage stamps and coins.

Investing oneself in relationships with others also ensures that one will be remembered after death. Some argue that if we have influenced the lives of others, something of us will continue in their lives after we die. Organ donations supply a tangible method for providing this type of symbolic immortality (see also **Organ Donation/Transplantation**). In this way, one can even ensure that a part of his or her physical self can continue in another person. Currently, there is an increasing tendency for individuals to donate their organs and tissues upon death to the living. In many urban areas, kidney foundations, eye banks, and transplant centers will supply donor cards and, when death occurs, will arrange for transplants. So if one's organs live on in another, the memory of that person continues in a living person even though the organ donor is dead.

One of the reasons why people write books is to promote their own symbolic immortality and provide a memorial to the life they have lived. As long as their books can be read, their influence will outlive their biological body. The same is true for television and motion picture stars. Each year, the youthful Judy Garland is resurrected from the dead as *The Wizard of Oz* is shown on television. The movie becomes a memorial to the people who were in it when it was filmed in 1939, more than 70 years ago.

Great inventors, political leaders, and athletic "hall of famers" are also memorialized or given immortality when we use their products, remember their accomplishments, and celebrate their achievements. In the case of medical practitioners and bionic inventors, not only do the living remember their accomplishments, but also these accomplishments extend the lives of those who provide the dead with immortality.

The search for meaning and symbolic immortality is a task that all people share. In many respects, memorials, and the meaning they have for those who have died, turn out to be meaningful for the group or society itself. Symbolic immortality and memorials are something that only the living can give the dead. People live with the faith that their survivors will remember or memorialize them and perpetuate the meaning of their lives after they die. Like religious interpretations of death, temporal meanings enable individuals to protect themselves and their social order from death.

Michael R. Leming

See also: Memorial Day; Monuments.

Further Reading

Anderson, E., A. Maddrell, K. McLoughlin, and Alana Vincent (eds.). *Memory, Mourning, Landscape.* Amsterdam: Rodopi, 2010.

Andrews, M., C. Bagot Jewitt, and Nigel Hunt (eds.). *Lest We Forget: Remembrance and Commemoration.* Stroud, England: The History Press, 2011.

Gobel, David and Daves Rossell. *Commemoration in America: Essays on Monuments, Memorialization, and Memory.* Charlottesville, VA: University of Virginia Press, 2013.

Lifton, R. J. and E. Olson. *Living and Dying.* New York: Praeger, 1974.

MONUMENTS

Monuments symbolize a given culture's "death system" by acknowledging the existence of someone who has lived and died. They commemorate the dead, and typically reflect the birth and death dates of the deceased individual. Monuments are often personalized, reflecting something that is important to the person left behind by expressing some aspect of his or her relationship to the individual who has died. Monuments are quite diverse in nature, and range from church monuments and individual grave markers intended to commemorate the dead, to mounds, Mosques, statues, temples, war memorials, or triumphant arches. Monuments may not only have personal significance, but they also have historical significance in reflecting the unique aspects of a city's or a country's growth and development, in that they may reflect events or symbolize entire cultures (e.g., the USS *Arizona* memorial at Pearl Harbor, the Tomb of the Unknown Soldier, the Eternal Flame marking the death of John F. Kennedy, the Wall commemorating the Vietnam War, the Parthenon, the Eiffel Tower, the Great Pyramids of Egypt, and the Great Wall of China). Some monuments reflect a culture's response to issues of the time, as with that commemorating the French heroes of the Bastille or American Civil War dead. Monuments are often legally protected as they have historically valued significance, and become more worthy of such protection as a society or culture grows and ages. In such cases, the symbolic value of the monument increases, as the essence of a culture's identity and political power rests and is bound up with the monument. Culturally speaking, monuments create a physical reference point for rituals of commemoration, as with Arlington National Cemetery, and thus help to reinforce core beliefs and assumptions that cultures themselves help create and maintain over time. These moments can come to assume a sacred quality that itself becomes part of a national or "civil religion" that both celebrates and reflects the collective memory of a community.

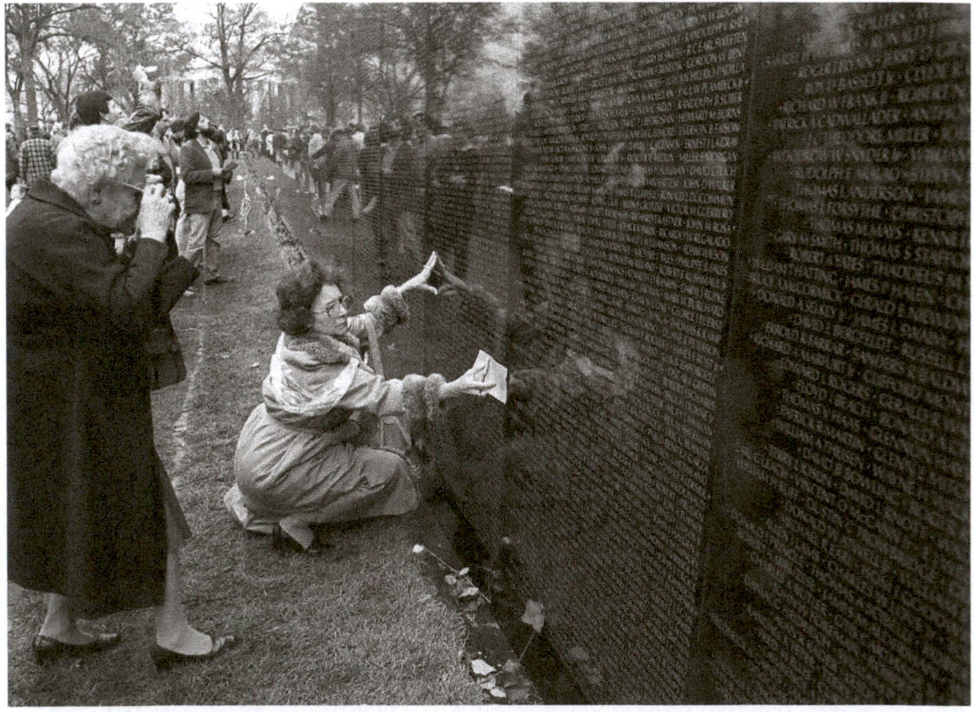

Visitors at the Vietnam Veterans Memorial on the day before its official dedication, November 12, 1982. Located in Washington, D.C., and today the capital's most visited monument, the Vietnam Memorial is inscribed with the names of the more than 58,000 American men and women killed or missing in the Vietnam War. As is fitting for a war that was so controversial, the unconventional design of the monument, done by then 21-year-old Yale student Maya Ying Lin, is both loved and hated. (Department of Defense)

As manifestations of either personal or collective memories, monuments and memorial structures help give meaning to people's individual lives, just as they give meaning to the cultural events that symbolize an entire community or nation. They enable the living to make sense of things that are difficult or impossible to understand, such as why do people die? Why do people wage war against one another? In many cases, it seems to be the very *process* of creating a monument or memorial structure that is the most important, as was the case with events surrounding the assassination of John F. Kennedy or the events of September 11, 2001. The creation of such memorials represents an attempt to understand death and to heal the feelings of loss that accompany it. Such monuments convey the grief that many people feel in acknowledging the loss of people who are important to us in both a personal and collective capacity. They may also come to represent myriad other losses, such as the loss of a way of life, and perhaps most poignantly, the loss of the taken-for-granted assumption that our loved ones will always be there or that we will always be safe and secure. The monument in general therefore becomes less important than the idea or feeling that it represents. In order to retain the monument's value in eliciting important memories, it is important that we periodically engage with it. For example, visiting the grave of a father who fought in the Second World War once a year on Memorial Day or on that father's birthday serves to symbolize our feelings about the man and the war that he fought in. These ideas and feelings transcend the event that the monument or memorial structure was constructed to represent. They give it meaning that lasts much longer than the time it takes us to visit. As memorials themselves change (as when names are added to the list of people dying in war), our relationship to them also changes. This is the real value that monuments have for us, helping to symbolize our grief and our attempts to struggle with what a particular death or event means to us.

Further Reading

Kastenbaum, Robert J. *Death, Society, and Human Experience,* 10th edition. Boston: Allyn & Bacon, 2009.

Palkovich, Ann M. and Ann Korologos Bazarrone. "Monuments in Motion: Gravemarkers, Cemeteries, and Memorials as Material Form and Context." In *Handbook of Death and Dying,* edited by Clifton D. Bryant (pp. 730–39). Thousand Oaks, CA: Sage, 2003.

Peelen, Janneke. "Monuments." In *Encyclopedia of Death and the Human Experience,* edited by Clifton D. Bryant and Dennis L. Peck (pp. 743–45). Thousand Oaks, CA: Sage, 2009.

Winter, Jay. *Sites of Memory, Sites of Mourning: The Great War in European Memory.* Cambridge: Cambridge University Press, 1998.

Bert Hayslip Jr.

MORTALITY RATES

Every life on earth will ultimately end with death. As human beings, death is a certainty for every one of us. Demographers use the mortality rate to measure the degree of death in a population. The mortality rate is calculated by taking the number of deaths in a given period of time (typically one year), divided by the mid-year population, and multiplied by 1,000. Death will not occur at the same time for everyone. Death varies considerably by age; the likelihood of death is greater at the beginning and end of life. In general, death will come earlier to males than to females, and earlier to people from racial and ethnic minorities than to those who are members of the dominant group. There are a variety of social, behavioral, environmental, political, and economic explanations for the differences in causes of death.

Global demographic trends can help to explain mortality. The theory known as Demographic Transition Theory (DTT) is one of the most important explanations of population and mortality change. DTT proposes four stages or levels of fertility and mortality. During the first stage (preindustrialization stage), the world was characterized by high birth and high death rates and had stable population growth. The second stage (first transitional stage) was characterized by declining mortality and thus, lower death rates. However, birth rates were still high and the population grew. The next stage was characterized by decreasing population growth from lower birth rates. The final stage, called incipient decline, is characterized by very low fertility and mortality and stable population change. In more developed countries, the demographic transition has been pretty much completed. In less developed countries, the demographic transition is not yet complete, and while many of these countries do have lower death rates, they still have higher birth rates.

Measurement of Mortality

An easily understood method for measuring mortality is the crude death rate (CDR), or the number of deaths per 1,000 people in a population in a given year. The CDR is referred to as "crude" because its denominator comprises the entire population. And the risk of death varies by age, sex, race/ethnicity, socioeconomic status, and many other characteristics. Thus, crude death rates must be interpreted and used with caution. Because the risk of death varies dramatically with age, demographers prefer to use age-specific death rates (ASDR), or the number of deaths to persons in a specific age group per 1,000 people in that age group.

Infant mortality receives special consideration from demographers because the death rate in the first year of life is much higher than the other years, and the death of a child is a most devastating human experience. Infant mortality rate (IMR) is the number of deaths to persons under age one per 1,000 babies born in a given year. IMR is generally used as one of the most important indicators of social development of a population (see **Infant Mortality**).

Causes of Death

A most distinguished demographer, Donald Bogue, has noted that death is an event led by complicated causes, and it should not be treated as a unitary force. He also noted that a full understanding of mortality requires an understanding of the trends in each of the major causes of death.

Historically, people died mainly of infectious and parasitic diseases (like the flu and plagues). There were short-term fluctuations in mortality caused by famines, epidemics, wars, and natural disasters. Some of those have been controlled by humans but to this day, some continue to influence mortality in certain areas.

The 20th century was characterized by the most rapid decline in mortality in human history. The forces of modernization and industrialization led to a reduction in mortality in both the developed and developing worlds. Developments in medical technology enhanced the ability to control infectious and parasitic diseases. Improvements in medical care and public health, as well improvements in living standards, also indirectly helped to reduce the number of deaths.

The major causes of death today in the United States and most countries of the developed world are heart disease and cancer. In 2008, the World Health Organization reported approximately 57 million deaths in the world. The top cause of death was ischemic heart disease; accounting for 7.3 million deaths, and cerebrovascular disease (disease of blood vessels supplying the brain) and stroke, accounting for another 6.2 million deaths.

However, unlike the situation in the other regions of the world, many countries of Africa have experienced harder times in reducing mortality. Since the late 1980s, mortality rates in Africa have also been high because of the HIV/AIDS epidemic, armed conflicts, economic stagnation, and resurgent infectious diseases such as tuberculosis and malaria.

Mortality: Historically and Globally

While we know that levels of mortality prior to the Industrial Revolution were high, the data are limited and incomplete. In the first to third centuries, data from the census records of Roman Egypt show that average life expectancy at birth was between 22 and 25 years; this finding has been supported by data on tombstones in Roman North Africa. As late as the 18th century, average life expectancy in much of Europe and the United States ranged from only 30 to 40 years. As recently as 1901, in the United States, men had a life expectancy at birth of 47.9 years, while for women it was 50.7 years.

Although many modern countries have set up population registration or death reporting systems, many deaths around the world these days are not officially recorded. In many countries, deaths occur outside the presence of a physician, and the cause is either unknown or incorrectly identified. Often, the cause of death is misrepresented if it is considered socially unacceptable, such as suicide or HIV/AIDS. Furthermore, international comparisons of data relating to the causes of death are problematic because counties frequently differ in their use of terminology, diagnostic techniques, method of certification, and quality of data collection. However, it is still possible to make some generalizations about the general structure of cause of death in contemporary societies.

Socioeconomic Development and Mortality

The chief causes of death for people around the world differ. The differences are largely due to the disparities in the socioeconomic levels of countries. There is wide variation in socioeconomic status (SES) both within and among countries, and this is one reason why people around the world die from an assortment of causes.

An illustrative example is provided by the World Health Organization. Consider an imaginary population of 1,000 people to represent all the women, men, and children around the world who died in 2008. Of these 1,000 decedents (i.e., persons who died), 159 of them would have come from rich countries, 678 from middle-income countries, and 163 from poor countries. The distributions of death for each group of countries are not identical, nor are they ranked in the same way. In the developed and developing countries, most people are expected to live at least 70 years and will most likely die of chronic diseases, such as heart disease, cancer, and stroke. In the less developed countries, located mainly in sub-Saharan Africa, less than one-fifth of the population lives to the age of 70, and more than one-third of all deaths are of children under the age of 15. Lower respiratory infections, diarrheal diseases, and HIV/AIDS are the major causes of death in these countries.

Mortality in the United States

Mortality declines in the United States are consistent with the demographic transition theory. Recent data from the National Center for Health Statistics shows a crude death rate of 8 per 1,000 in the year 2012, and the infant mortality rate reached a record-low level of 6.1 infant deaths per 1,000 live births in 2012.

Despite these advances, there are still substantial differences in the United States among men and women and various racial and ethnic groups. Generally, the higher the SES, the lower the mortality. The gap between male and female life expectancy was 4.8 years in 2011. Additionally, there is a persistent difference in mortality among racial and ethnic groups. In 2011, whites still lived 3.7 years more than blacks, on average. A major reason for the racial and ethnic disparity in mortality is the SES consequences of lifelong poverty. Blacks generally have low birth weight and poor levels of childhood nutrition. In mid-life, blacks tend to lack access to health insurance and are more likely to be engaged in physically demanding work and be exposed to behavioral and environmental toxins. However, the largest minority population in the United States, the Hispanic population, has lower mortality than any other racial/ethnic group. This unexpected pattern is known as the Hispanic paradox.

Dudley L. Poston Jr., Demetrea Nicole Farris, and Qian Xiong

See also: Cancer; Cardiovascular Disease; Disease; Epidemics and Plagues; Famine; HIV/AIDS; War.

Further Reading

Bogue, Donald J. *Principles of Demography.* New York: John Wiley and Sons, Inc., 1969.

Hoyert, D. L. and J. Q. Xu. Deaths: Preliminary Data for 2011. *National Vital Statistics Reports,* 61(6). Hyattsville, MD: National Center for Health Statistics, 2012.

Population Reference Bureau. *2012 World Population Data Sheet.* Washington, DC.: Population Reference Bureau, 2013.

Poston, Dudley L., Jr. and Leon F. Bouvier. *Population and Society: An Introduction to Demography.* New York: Oxford University Press, 2010.

Scheidel, Walter. "Ancient World, Demography of." In *Encyclopedia of Population,* edited by Paul Demeny and Geoffrey McNicoll (pp. 44–48). New York: Macmillan, 2003.

United Nations. "World Population Prospects, the 2010 Revision Highlights and Advance, 2010. Tables." World Health Organization. "The Top 10 Causes of Death," 2011. http://www.who.int/mediacentre/factsheets/fs310/en/index.html

MORTUARY SCIENCE

The term mortuary science refers to various aspects of the disposition of dead human bodies in the context of the professional practice of funeral directing and embalming. Practitioners of mortuary science are typically called "morticians." Morticians serve the living by caring for the bodies of deceased persons in accordance with the wishes of those who have the legal right to control disposition. Morticians also create, conduct, and supervise funeral and memorial services that honor the life of the person who has died. Methods of disposition in the United States today commonly include earth burial (also known as interment), entombment (the placing of a body in a crypt within a building called a mausoleum), and cremation (the process of reducing a body to bone fragments by exposure to intense heat and flame) (see **Burial; Cremation**). Although morticians are most often employed by mortuaries (or funeral homes—the terms are synonymous), some morticians work in allied fields, such as cemeteries, crematories, anatomical bequest programs (i.e., whole body donation), and medical examiner offices.

Licensure

States commonly regulate the disposition of dead human bodies by law, rule, or statute, and a license is typically required in order to practice mortuary science. License types vary across states. For example, in Minnesota, there is only one mortuary science practitioner license, which is "mortician." Minnesota-licensed morticians may practice both funeral directing and embalming. In New York, a mortuary science practitioner is licensed as a funeral director, but may practice both funeral directing and embalming. In contrast, several states, such as Texas and California, have separate "funeral director" and "embalmer" licenses. Sometimes referred to as "bifurcated" or "split" licenses, the academic credentials required to earn these licenses often differ. If one desires to practice embalming in a state with a bifurcated licensing system, it is usually necessary to complete a college-level program of mortuary science accredited by the American Board of Funeral Service Education. However, if one wants only to practice as a funeral director in a state with a bifurcated licensing system, it may be possible (depending on the state) to earn a funeral director's license by completing only an apprenticeship under the supervision of a duly licensed preceptor (a teacher or instructor, who, in this case, is usually a fully licensed and practicing funeral director). Whether or not a person licensed to practice only funeral directing (and not embalming) should refer to their work as "mortuary science" is debatable, for generally speaking "mortuary science" is inclusive of both the practice of funeral directing *and* the art and science of embalming.

Mortuary Science Education

Most states require that mortuary science practitioners complete a college-level academic program of at least two years (60 credits) that is accredited by the American Board of Funeral Service Education (ABFSE). The ABFSE is the only accrediting body in the United States for mortuary science higher education that is recognized by the U.S. Department of Education. The curriculum of accredited programs includes a diverse range of subjects in both the arts and sciences. Funeral service arts coursework includes the study of accounting, business law, communications, ethics, the Federal Trade Commission, funeral directing, merchandising, law, management, psychology, and sociology. Funeral service sciences coursework involves the study of human anatomy, chemistry, embalming, microbiology, pathology, and restorative art.

Since 2004, all mortuary science students must take the National Board Examination (NBE) of the International Conference of Funeral Service Examining Boards (ICFSEB) as a requirement for graduation. The majority of mortuary science programs in the United States offer an associates (i.e., two-year) degree program. These programs are typically found at either public community colleges or private, single-purpose institutions. Of the 56 ABFSE-accredited programs of mortuary science in the United States today, only 4 confer the bachelor of science (BS) degree with a major in mortuary science. Baccalaureate degree programs in mortuary science are typically housed at research universities, but some two-year programs maintain articulation agreements with four-year institutions.

Evolution, Contemporary Practice, and Future Trends

Mortuary science developed in the United States as a distinct occupation following the Civil War (1861–1865). The arterial injection of preservative chemicals into the bodies of the war dead, in order to retard decomposition, was first practiced by battlefield surgeons. This process, known as embalming, reduced the effects of putrefaction and decay, thereby making it possible for deceased soldiers to be transported long distances to their hometowns for burial. Embalming became increasingly popular in America following the Civil War. Chemical companies that manufactured embalming products started educational programs to teach undertakers how to arterially embalm dead bodies.

Historically, mortuary science education programs have emphasized instruction in sanitary care of human remains as a core component of their curricula. Instruction in the sciences was also important because many morticians ran ambulance services and served as coroners. In recent years, however, embalming has declined somewhat in popularity. Fewer morticians serve as coroners, and ambulance services are now handled by other professionals, such as emergency medical technicians (EMTs). Increasingly today, people are also choosing cremation as a way of preparing bodies for final disposition. In some cases, the presentation of an embalmed body for public visitation and funeral ceremonies occurs prior to cremation, and in other cases it does not—funeral preferences will depend on the wishes of the deceased person (in cases of preplanning) and/or the desires of the next of kin. Today, many mortuary science education programs include instruction in cremation procedures and protocols. An emerging mortuary science technology is that of alkaline hydrolysis, a process that involves reducing the body to bones by placing it in an aqueous solution that has a very high pH.

Michael LuBrant

See also: Burial; Cremation; Embalming; Funeral Director; Funeral Industry; Rigor Mortis.

Further Reading

Habenstein, Robert W. and William M. Lamers (eds.). *The History of American Funeral Directing,* 7th edition. Milwaukee, WI: National Funeral Directors Association, 2010.

Harris, Mark. *Grave Matters: A Journey through the Modern Funeral Industry to a Natural Way of Burial.* New York: Scribner, 2007.

Laderman, Gary. *Rest in Peace: A Cultural History of Death and the Funeral Home in Twentieth-Century America.* New York: Oxford University Press, 2003.

Lynch, Thomas. *The Undertaking: Life Studies from the Dismal Trade.* New York: W. W. Norton, 1998.

Slocum, Joshua and Lisa Carlson. *Final Rights: Reclaiming the American Way of Death.* Hinesburg, VT: Upper Access Inc., 2011.

The Undertaking. DVD. Directed by Mira Navasky and Karen O' Connor. Place of Production. PBS Frontline, 2008.

MOURNING

The term mourning encompasses two distinct domains: outward manifestations of loss and the subjective experience of loss. Thus, mourning involves both things one does in public as well as thoughts and feelings. Mourning is usually associated with the death of someone significant. But, one can also mourn the loss of an abstraction like one's country or a previously held ideal. Mourning is likely to be accompanied by grief but has a wider meaning (see also **Grief**).

Public Expressions of Loss

The outward expression of mourning is shaped by cultural norms and is likely to include signs that tell others you have experienced a loss. These signs can

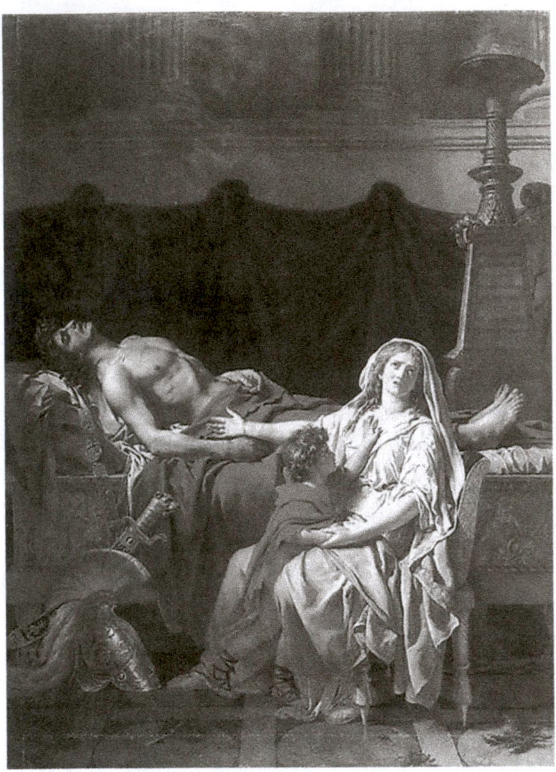

Neoclassical painting by Jacques-Louis David, *Andromache Mourning Hector*. (Carol Gerten-Jackson, http://www.cgfa.florida-imaging.com)

be manifest via undertaking established rituals and following culturally recognizable patterns of behavior, for example wearing garments of a particular color. There may be norms about who is expected to mourn and about appropriate time periods for mourning. There are mourning rituals that are enacted as death is imminent, between the death and the funeral, at the funeral, and following the funeral. These rituals can include very specific tasks, often demarcated by gender and family position. For example, in a Hindu family, a series of mourning and funeral rituals are enacted, ideally from the point where death is clearly imminent, through funeral and then purification rituals. In effect, the bereaved step outside their usual life into a devotional realm. If the death is of a parent, the eldest son has specific responsibilities, culminating in his lighting his parents' funeral pyre, while relatives and other mourners chant sacred mantras. The mourning process here is best understood as a series of rites of passage allowing the deceased's spirit to move on and allowing the mourners to fulfill a religious and a social obligation.

Lamentation

Both the rituals of mourning and the public expressions of loss that accompany them vary over time and from place to place. Consider the practice of lamentation, an aspect of mourning and also a public manifestation of grief. Prior to burial or cremation, often in the presence of the corpse, this is the ritual of mourning the dead through raising collective voices, sometimes accompanied by physical displays of grief. The Hindu ritual of chanting sacred texts is perhaps one end of a spectrum, with King Lear's lamentation for the death of his daughter Cordelia at the other. Shakespeare has Lear entreat a shocked and silent crowd thus, "Howl, howl, howl, howl! O, you are men of stones, Had I your tongues and eyes, I'd use them so, That heaven's vault should crack" (Act 5, scene 3). Here, giving public voice to loss varies from its being an aid to the soothing transition from one state to another, to a cry of anguish and rage.

The Absence and Return of Public Mourning

Lamentation is a practice integral to the experience of loss in many communities in the world today, including communities living within the Christian West. Here, it exists alongside a widely prevalent, less outwardly expressive, private and meditative mourning. Indeed, in the West, what were established mourning rituals have been banished or seriously cut short. For example, the period that a bereaved person is expected to be "in mourning" has got shorter, or disappeared. In the United Kingdom, Queen Victoria remained in mourning after the death of her husband for 40 years until the end of her own life in 1901. Mourning here does not mean being absent from the social world—the bereaved Victorian mill or farm worker did not have a prolonged period off work (and the Queen returned to her royal duties). Rather, it refers to the presence of signifiers of loss—wearing black for example—and to a sense that what this signifies is that one's emotional world is still attached to the deceased; one is not expecting or expected to engage fully with the here and now of ordinary life.

In recent years, it has been argued, that there has been a reappearance of outward signs of mourning. This is manifest in two sorts of activity. First, in forms of quiet expression of loss and public commemoration that includes: leaving flowers in impromptu roadside memorials (see **Spontaneous Shrine/Roadside Memorials**) or outside the home of the deceased, holding vigils, and pursuing routes to create solidarities and avenues for personal expression via social media, for example, using Facebook. These mourning practices are characteristically tailored by individuals or small groups in ways that are meaningful to them and so exhibit a considerable variety of forms. Second, we see mourning as spectacle, where masses of people share in responding to the death of someone they know of, rather than someone they know. In the United Kingdom, such events have been particularly evident in response to the death of celebrities and sports spectators (see also **Public Mourning**).

Continuities in Public Mourning

Throughout the years where there was a decline in public signs of personal loss, there were still examples of mass public mourning. The death of former British prime minister Winston Churchill in 1965 saw thousands standing in silence as his funeral cortege passed through London. In the United States, after the assassination of President John F. Kennedy in 1963, 250,000 people filed passed the coffin lying in state, about a million lined the funeral procession route, and a large proportion of the U.S. population watched on television. Popular reactions to these deaths combined a sense that one had lost someone who shaped one's sense of national identity; a public loss, with a sense of personal grief. The common assertion that one would always remember where one was when President Kennedy was shot reflected a sense that this was a *personal* as well as a communal loss.

This combination of public and private mourning was evident in Great Britain following the death in a road accident of Princess Diana in 1997. The response to this death has been cited as evidence of a new sort of expressive public mourning. After Princess Diana's death, there was mass involvement in public mourning, lining the route to the funeral service and to the burial, in ways that were similar to mourning Churchill, or President Kennedy. What was different was that a series of commemorative rituals both before and after the funeral, including leaving flowers outside her home in London and making statements identifying one's sense of personal loss in remembrance books and in individual testimony to the media, presented a more overt and expressive subjectivity than the more formal, emotionally restrained, public morning evident previously.

There is also some historical continuity in mourning associated with mass death. Two examples that have helped shaped the literature on grief and bereavement are the deaths in Aberfan (1966) and Hillsborough (1989). In the small Welsh village of Aberfan, the collapse of a colliery spoil tip led to the deaths of 116 children and 28 adults. A mass response from across Great Britain and abroad was evidenced by 90,000 individual donations to a disaster fund. These were deaths publically mourned by people who did not know of the deceased and who had not previously heard of the village of Aberfan. Twenty-three years later, at Hillsborough in Sheffield, Yorkshire, 96 soccer supporters were crushed to death in an overcrowded stadium. There was a similar public mourning but, as with the death of Princess Diana, it was accompanied by a more overt expressiveness in which people spoke of personal loss as well as mourning a public tragedy.

The Private Experience of Loss

Philosophers and creative artists have frequently engaged with loss. At their best, their work touches on the universal, often reached via a portrayal of the intensity of personal experience. Tennyson's *In Memoriam* (1850) reflects that the loss experienced by others does not reconcile him to his own loss.

> That loss is common would not make
> My own less bitter, rather more:
> Too common! Never morning wore
> To evening, but some heart did break.

Nor does Tennyson find that there is a time limit to his grief, or that he wishes for one:

> Let Love clasp Grief less both be drown'd,
> Let darkness keep her raven gloss:
> Ah, sweeter to be drunk with loss,
> To dance with death, to beat the ground,
> Than that the victor Hours should scorn
> The long result of love, of boast,
> "Behold the man that loved and lost",
> But all he was is overworn.

Also consider C. S. Lewis in *A Grief Observed* describing how, after his wife's death, grief overwhelmed him: "I not only live each endless day in grief, but live each day thinking about living each day in grief." "The act of living is different all through. Her absence is like the sky, spread over everything."

For the last 100 years, there have been attempts to capture the experience of grief and mourning via discipline-based, systematic approaches. These seek to identify common patterns in grief and mourning, to attribute an idea of factors, in addition to the loss itself, that underlie responses and to suggest ways that problems can be overcome (or the risk of problems arising be reduced). While there is no wish to classify grief and mourning *per se* as problems that need expert intervention, there is a case made that in some circumstances, normal responses to loss develop into pathological responses, for example, clinical depression.

These approaches return to the questions about what solace can be found in the recognition of the shared experience of mourning. They engage with challenges akin to Tennyson's reluctance to forego the intensity of the experience of grief, less, as it fades, the love of the person lost fades also, and they consider how one can sit alongside and assist those, like C.S. Lewis, for whom grief becomes their life.

Some approaches focus on psychological processes, others emphasize the social dimension. Freud observed how the "work" a person does while grieving is designed to disentangle the mourner from the person who has died, not in the sense of forgetting them and moving on, but rather in understanding who *you* really are in a world without that person. John Bowlby's starting point was looking at the behavior of children separated from parents during World War II. These children mourned their separation through three stages: protest, despair, and detachment. Bowlby argued (1969) that if attachment bonds are broken, then bereavement, grief, and mourning are naturally occurring social processes designed to enhance survival.

The social or public aspects of mourning, as well as the psychological, continue to be manifest in a wide range of work that has followed Freud and Bowlby.

Neil Small

See also: Bereavement; Freud, Sigmund.

Further Reading

Bowlby, J. 1969. *Attachment.* London: Hogarth Press and Institute of Psycho-Analysis, 1969.

Brennan, M. *Mourning and Disaster: Finding Meaning in the Mourning for Hillsborough and Diana.* Newcastle upon Tyne: Cambridge Scholars Publishing, 2008.

Freud, S. "Mourning and Melancholia." In *The Standard Edition of the Complete Psychological Works of Sigmund Freud,* Vol. 14 (pp. 237–58). London: Hogarth Press, 1957 (Original work published 1917).

Lewis C. S. *A Grief Observed.* London: Faber and Faber, 1961.

McLean, I. and M. Johnes. *Aberfan: Government and Disasters.* Cardiff: Welsh Academic Press, 2000.

Tennyson, Alfred Lord. *In Memoriam* (1850). In *Poems of Tennyson.* Oxford: Oxford University Press, 1916.

Walter, T. *The Revival of Death.* London: Routledge, 1994.

N

NEAR-DEATH EXPERIENCES

Near-death experience (NDE) is a term coined and first popularized by author, Raymond Moody, in the 1970s. NDEs are typically experiences of body-spirit separation or of "travel" to heaven- or hell-like places that are reported by people who were clinically dead, and were then revived, hence the term "near death." Stories of travel to another place are a defining characteristic of NDEs and are found in all cultures, with travelers reporting glimpses into a scientifically unexplainable (i.e., paranormal) existence. A NDE can be characterized as containing some of the following elements by those people who claim to have had one:

- Learning that she or he died
- Realizing that she or he leaves the body
- Meeting with dead loved ones and/or religious beings
- Returning to the body

A distinction has been made between two types of NDE; chiefly, between NDEs resulting from life-threatening illness and NDEs resulting from near fatal accidents involving a high degree of danger and risk. The latter is believed to involve three distinct stages: (1) resistance (recognizing danger, struggling against it, and then accepting the likelihood of death); (2) life review (as the self leaves the body, accompanied by a panorama of memories of one's life just ended); and (3) transcendence (the cosmic and transcendental awareness that replaces a less enlightened and spiritually conscious self).

Typical sensations involving "good" (heaven-like) NDEs include entering a tunnel, seeing a bright light, hearing beautiful sounds, and having feelings of unconditional love, joy, peace, warmth, levitation, and security. Persons who have "bad" (hell-like) NDEs usually report being tortured by elves, giants, or demons, accompanied with feelings of extreme terror or fear.

Beliefs about NDEs

The earliest accounts of NDEs can be traced to Plato's *The Republic,* which was written around 380 BC. In this story, Plato described a mythical soldier who told of his "afterlife" experience. Many years later, popular interest in NDEs arose following the publication of Raymond Moody's 1975 book, *Life after Life.* Currently, approximately 8 million Americans claim to have had a NDE, but it is likely that the actual figure exceeds this, with many cases going unreported. People who have had a NDE may not be comfortable telling others about it. Nevertheless, following advances in medicine, such as cardiopulmonary resuscitation (CPR), reports of NDEs are increasing.

Some people believe that if the person with the NDE does not die (because it is not his or her "time"), ancestors will "push" the person back to life. A similar thought was typical many years earlier. For example, early Hawaiians believed that their ancestor god would meet a soul who left the body prematurely and would either send it back to be revived or lead it to safety with its ancestors.

Many people view NDEs as proof that people survive death. An ongoing debate exists, however, regarding that proof. For instance, some people argue that these experiences are not evidence of continuing life and are nothing more than a neurological event. Some examples of neurological events include shortage of oxygen in the brain (cerebral anoxia), hallucinatory imagery associated with the brain and nervous system, drug side effects, or seizure-like discharges in the brain (temporal lobe paroxysm).

Don Piper, author of the book *90 Minutes in Heaven,* reported that he was skeptical of the existence of NDEs. That was, until he experienced one. While he was seemingly dead for 90 minutes from being in a terrible accident, he later reported being enveloped by a bright light beyond earthly comprehension. His NDE included standing in heaven and feeling intense joy as he became aware of special people who died in his lifetime. He also gave details about seeing colors that he never believed existed and reported feeling more alive in the NDE than in his life before the event. What he cherished the most, though, was what he described as the most beautiful music he had ever heard. Despite Piper's graphic explanations about his NDE, certainty in general about NDEs is difficult to establish.

Research about NDEs

Albert Heim, a Swiss geologist, is believed to have been the first person to gather data on NDEs. In the early 1900s, Heim, himself a mountain climber, interviewed some 25 skiers and climbers who had suffered an accident resulting in a near-death episode. Another person, Oskar Pfister, reviewed Heim's interview notes and concluded that the described experiences of the skiers and climbers were caused by shock in the face of impending death and, therefore, life after death was not proved. Since that time, research studies on NDEs have come from several academic disciplines, including psychology and medicine, with little or no consensus between them.

In 1981, the International Association for Near-Death Studies (IANDS) was formed. Through this organization, scientific research and education on the physical, psychological, social, and spiritual nature of NDEs is encouraged. The *Journal of Near-Death Studies* is published by this organization. A few years after IANDS was formed, Kenneth Ring constructed a Weighted Core Experience Index to differentiate between people who likely experienced a NDE and those who had not. Ring identified a set of changes associated with people who had NDEs, including physical sensitivity, a feeling that the brain was altered, and a diminished tolerance to light, alcohol, and drugs. In addition, these people often had not adjusted to ordinary life after the NDE.

As recently as 2008, 25 researchers agreed to examine NDEs among 1,500 heart attack patient survivors. In 2010, one of those researchers, Dr. Sam Parnia, reported that the evidence suggested that mental processes may continue for a period of time after death begins, meaning that the brain/mind is lost gradually and therefore that NDEs do indeed exist. Yet, other current researchers continue to argue that NDEs are caused by a surge of electrical activity as the brain runs out of oxygen.

Two main ways exist to interpret NDEs. First is whether NDEs offer definitive proof of an afterlife or whether they are merely a phantom of brain chemistry. Second is the possibility that NDEs are influenced by cultural expectations during life, meaning that what survivors encounter during a NDE may well be filtered through a person's expectations about what he or she believes is indicative of life after death. In the mid-1900s, the English writer, C. S. Lewis, wrote that regardless of what view people have regarding the afterlife, their view is either dead right or dead wrong. Alas, the exact nature of the afterlife remains unknown.

Dixie Dennis

See also: Near-to-Death Experiences.

Further Reading

DeSpelder, Lynne A. and Albert L. Strickland. *The Last Dance: Encountering Death and Dying,* 6th edition. Boston: McGraw-Hill, 2002.

Moody, Raymond A., Jr. *Life after Life.* San Francisco: Harper-Collins, 1975.

Piper, Don. *90 Minutes in Heaven.* Grand Rapids, MI: Revell, 2004.

NEAR-TO-DEATH EXPERIENCES

Near-to-death experience is an umbrella term to describe a range of transcendent experiences—experiences beyond the ordinary—that commonly occur around the time of death. Because these experiences are beyond the ordinary, they are often difficult to describe and explain.

Near-to-death experiences share some common features with the more well-known term, near-death-experiences (NDEs), such as visions of deceased relatives or religious figures and the presence of a radiant light (see **Near-Death Experiences**). They differ from NDEs in that the person having the experience is often, although not always, close to death, thus he or she may not be able to talk about the experience and so these experiences may be difficult to capture.

Deathbed Visions

Deathbed visions have been reported in nearly all cultures and across time. These visions describe the experiences that some people have when they are nearing death—seeing or hearing deceased relatives, or in some cases, religious figures of importance to the dying person. These visions are generally of comfort, as they can bring peace, calm, and joy, but they may sometimes be frightening for the dying person and family members.

A number of studies have been conducted specifically about these visions, such as *Deathbed Visions* by Sir William Barrett—a physician in London—and first published in 1926. Karlis Osis and Erlunder Haroldsson conducted a major cross-cultural study in the United States and India in the late 1960s and early 1970s and there have been a number of small-scale studies conducted since.

Nearing Death Awareness

The dying person may also develop a growing awareness of the time when they will die in the days or weeks prior to their death. This is sometimes perceived through vivid or poignant dreams. Sometimes, a dying person may talk about this in a symbolic or metaphorical way and this has led to misunderstandings about these experiences in the past. An awareness of impending death (in the weeks or days before a person dies) provides the basis for what, Maggie Callanan and Patricia Kelley, U.S.-based hospice nurses, have termed nearing death awareness. Callanan and Kelley recognized that some behavior and speech, often mistaken as confusion or delirium, may in fact be understood as a growing awareness that death is near. For example, a dying person may talk about making preparation for a journey—literally or metaphorically—months or weeks before death, by way of an apparent intuitive awareness of impending death. They observed that patients might have a special awareness that death is near as well as the ability to control when it will happen.

Umbrella Terms

These experiences have been described in several ways. Umbrella terms such as end-of-life experiences (ELE) phenomena; deathbed phenomena (DBE), deathbed experiences (DBE), nearing death awareness (NDA), and death-related sensory experiences (DRSE), among others, have been employed. These terms allow us to group together what might, at first, appear to be isolated events, and in so doing deepen our understanding of these experiences.

Near-*to*-death experiences also encompass a variety of other transcendent experiences such as seeing a radiant light and people waking up from a coma to communicate meaningfully with family and friends before they die. Increasing understanding of these experiences suggests they may occur in the weeks and months before death and not just in the last 72 or 48 hours before death. There is also evidence, presented by Raymond Moody in *Glimpses of Eternity*, that visions and other experiences can be shared by both the person who is dying as well as by family members and friends. As a result, the term near-*to*-death experiences is being used to describe these phenomena. This term better fits the time frame in which these experiences occur and encompasses a wide range of experiences such as shared near-*to*-death experiences.

Una MacConville

Further Reading

Callanan M. and P. Kelley. *Final Gifts: Understanding the Special Awareness, Needs and Communications of the Dying.* New York: Bantam Publishing, 1997.

Moody, Ray. *Glimpses of Eternity: An Investigation into Shared Death Experiences.* London: Rider, 2011.

NECROPHILIA

Necrophilia literally means love (*phil*) of the dead body (*necro*), but more commonly refers to any kind of sexual activity between a living person and a human corpse. The word necrophilia first appeared in the late 19th century and is synonymous with the term corpse abuse. Historically, necrophilia gained broader attention in 1882 when it appeared in Dr. Richard Freiherr von Krafft-Ebing's book *Psychopathia Sexualis.* Krafft-Ebing originally published his book in Germany and subsequent editions were translated into English. Krafft-Ebing also described necrophilia as the "mutilation of corpses," a practice that included any sexually violent act done against dead bodies. In contemporary usage, the American Psychiatric Association (APA) defines necrophilia as a paraphilia and sexual disorder in the *Diagnostic and Statistical Manual of Mental Disorders, Fourth Edition* (*DSM-4*).

Both terms, necrophilia and corpse abuse (sometimes also referred to as "abuse of a corpse"), are used by most American states to define certain kinds of illegal activity. Each state individually defines what constitutes necrophilia, so this often creates variations across the country. The state of Ohio, for example, uses statute *2927.01 Abuse of a Corpse,* to prohibit individuals from treating a dead body in a way that would outrage family or community sensibilities. Hawaii statute *711–1108 Abuse of a Corpse* explicitly outlaws any sexual contact with dead bodies and uses the word necrophilia as an all-encompassing term. The state of Nevada takes a slightly different approach with its law, statute *201.450 Sexual Penetration of Dead Human Body.* Nevada's law explicitly states which kinds of necrophilic sexual acts are prohibited within the state.

In September 2006, Wisconsin authorities dealt with an attempted necrophilia case involving three men: Nicholas Grunke, Alexander Grunke, and Dustin Radtke. The trio attempted to remove a deceased woman's body from its grave in a Cassville, Wisconsin cemetery, for sexual purposes. Local police stopped the men before the body was removed and each of them confessed to the attempted crime. Wisconsin authorities brought attempted necrophilia charges against all three but failed to win the case. At that time, the state of Wisconsin did not have a law explicitly prohibiting necrophilia. After a series of lower court rulings, the Wisconsin State Supreme Court ruled in July 2008 that

Wisconsin's current attempted sexual assault law did include necrophilia, noting that a victim could either be living or dead.

John Troyer

Further Reading

Hawaii, Hawaii Revised Statutes "711–1108 Abuse of a Corpse." http://www.capitol.hawaii.gov

Krafft-Ebing, Richard Freiherr von. *Psychopathia Sexualis.* Translated by F. J. Rebamn. 12th edition. Brooklyn, NY: Physicians and Surgeons Book Company, 1933.

Nevada, Nevada Revised Statutes "201.45 Sexual Penetration of Dead Human Body." http://www.leg.state.nv.us

Ohio, Ohio Revised Code "2927.01 Abuse of a Corpse." http://codes.ohio.gov/orc

Rosman, J. P. and P. J. Resnick. "Sexual Attraction to Corpses: A Psychiatric Review of Necrophilia." *The Bulletin of the American Academy of Psychiatry and the Law,* 17(2) (1989): 153–63.

Troyer, John. "Abuse of a Corpse: A Brief History and Re-Theorization of Necrophilia Laws in the USA." *Mortality,* 13(2) (2008): 132–52.

O

OBITUARY

An obituary is a published notice of death that typically provides information about a person's death, along with a chronological summary of the person's life. Its primary function is to honor the life of the deceased and to announce to the local community and wider public details of the funeral arrangements. "Death notices" are one particular type of obituary and are often placed (in small type and in alphabetized columns next to the classified section) in local newspapers as a legal requirement. Death notices are shorter than obituaries, and often do not contain any biographical information, other than the name and age of the deceased, and the date of their death. Both obituaries and death notices are important in announcing a person's death so that a community (of family, friends, coworkers, etc.) can come together to pay its respects and offer mutual support to one another in a time of grief.

In the past, obituaries were brief and provided only the date of death and the particulars of services being held. Today, we can expect to find more details: marital status, names of children, grandchildren and other significant people (and even pets), hobbies, memberships of clubs and organizations, community involvement, employment details, educational achievements, military service, etc. Details of any funeral or memorial services, if there are any, or arrangements for cremation or place of interment are also included. Obituaries frequently contain instructions for donations to the deceased's charity of choice and may sometimes mention, and thank, caregivers, such as hospice teams. Also noted are the names of those in the family who preceded the deceased in death. Depending upon the wishes of the family, the manner of death may also be included in the obituary.

The obituary may or may not be accompanied by a photograph of the deceased person. In the past, if a photograph was included, it was common to provide a recent one, but today a new trend is to include a photograph of the deceased at an earlier time in their life. In some instances, both past and recent photographs are placed side by side in obituary notices.

Writers/Publishing

In the United States, the obituary is generally written by a funeral director (as part of the paid services) or by a family member. The latter usually focuses on the public life of the individual, whereas obituaries of ordinary members of the public tend to refer more to their everyday character and aspects of their private family life. National newspapers often report the deaths of famous or prominent people in feature-long obituaries, which are written by freelance journalists or staff writers. Many news organizations commission the writing of obituaries for some public figures while they are still alive. These are updated regularly so that when a famous person dies, even if this was sudden and unexpected (as in the case of Princess Diana), news agencies can quickly publish an obituary within hours of their death. Indeed, the passage of time between the death of a famous person and the publication of their obituary has been radically reduced by the advent of electronic media.

Obituaries differ from death notices, the latter of which contain somewhat limited information and are typically free of charge. In smaller cities with local newspapers, and depending on the number of lines and character counts, the publication of the obituary costs several hundred dollars. This fee varies with each newspaper and can differ depending on geographical location. On occasion, the editors of newspapers may request a copy of the death certificate so as to confirm that the person is really dead and that a prank is not being played on a living person.

The obituary in the 21st century has made its way onto Internet websites, courtesy of funeral homes and other social networks, such as Facebook, as well as online genealogy sites such as Ancestry.com. The latter allows registered users to search millions of online obituaries in over 2,000 newspapers. On Facebook, deaths are now being reported and new pages are created for the deceased person in order for people to offer condolences and support to the bereaved (see **Facebook**). These days, funeral homes will often have a homepage for advertisement of their business, on which they provide the obituary, as well as a guest book, where people can share stories and memories of the deceased and offer comfort to the bereaved.

Historical Documents

Reporting of death in earlier centuries focused on the explicit recounting of the cause of death, whereas today the nature of obituaries is typically one of character assessment. On occasion, obituaries may contain euphemisms in which less-direct phrases—describing, for example, how an individual "passed away"—are substituted for explicit mention of death. This itself tells us much about prevailing attitudes toward death and dying and is often reflective of a culture of death denial (see also **Death Denial**). The obituary can also be viewed as a source of historical documentation, providing not only a record of public memory but also information about an individual that may be hard to find and not accessible from other sources. Obituaries connect published memories of individual lives with family remembrance and with American collective memory, while offering a glimpse into American cultural values at a particular moment in history.

Laurel Hilliker

See also: Condolence (and Condolence Books); Epitaphs; Eulogy.

Further Reading

Hume, J. *Obituaries in American Culture.* Jackson, MS: University Press of Mississippi, 2000.

Johnson, M. *The Dead Beat: Lost Souls, Lucky Stiffs, and the Perverse Pleasures of Obituaries.* New York: HarperCollins Publishers, 2006.

Starck, N. *Life after Death: The Art of the Obituary.* Victoria: Melbourne University Press, 2006.

ORGAN DONATION/TRANSPLANTATION

The term "organ transplantation" refers to the removal and transfer of an organ, such as a kidney, from one body or person to another. Organ transplantation can occur between two living beings (i.e., from a "living donor") or from a deceased individual to a living individual (i.e., from a "dead" or "cadaveric" donor). Living organ donation among humans is only morally and legally permissible if the organ donation will not cause the death of the donor.

Organs and tissue that can be donated by living donors include bone marrow, skin, a single kidney, a lobe of the liver, or a lobe of a lung. Those that can be transplanted from dead donors include heart and heart valves, whole livers, whole lungs, kidneys, bone, tendons, corneas, intestines, pancreas, and thymus.

Current Statistics: United States and International

In February 2013, over 74,000 patients awaited organ transplantation in the United States. Between 25,000 and 30,000 transplants occur in the United States annually. Over 2 million people are estimated to need transplants worldwide. The Global Observatory on Donation and Transplantation reported transplants in 96 countries during 2010 provided in Table 1.

These transplants were estimated to meet less than 10 percent of the world's needs.

Survival

Survival after major organ transplantation depends on many factors, including the recipient's age and underlying disease, and whether the organ came from a living or deceased donor. In February 2013, the United Network for Organ Sharing (UNOS) published the ranges for patient survival for the most common organs transplanted between 1997 and 2004 provided in Table 2.

Table 1 Transplants

Kidney	Liver	Heart	Lung	Pancreas	Small Bowel
73,179	21,602	5,582	3,927	2,362	227

Table 2 Survival

	Survival for 1 year	Survival for 3 years	Survival for 5 years
Kidney transplant	91–99%	80–98%	78–96%
Liver transplant	82–93%	69–87%	62–85%
Heart transplant	84–90%	75–84%	65–77%
Lung transplant	78–88%	53–78%	33–76%

History and Origin of Organ Transplantation

A major obstacle to organ transplantation has been overcoming the human body's immune mechanisms that attack and reject foreign substances. Major organ transplantation was not possible until the late 20th century, when advanced surgical techniques and medications to prevent rejection of transplanted organs were developed. The earliest successful kidney transplant in the United States was performed by Joseph Murray and J. Hartwell Harrison in 1954, involving identical twins who did not require immunosuppression techniques. Christian Barnard performed the first successful human heart transplant in South Africa in 1967.

Improved understanding of the human immune system led to the development of drugs such as corticosteroids to reduce transplant rejection. The discovery in 1972 of the immunosuppressive effects of the drug cyclosporine-A brought about a revolution in organ transplantation. In 1981, the first successful heart-lung transplant was carried out at Stanford University using cyclosporine-A to prevent rejection. Following Food and Drug Administration (FDA) approval in 1983, cyclosporine-A became a staple in transplantation regimens, moving transplantation out of the realm of experimental treatment and into mainstream therapy.

Future Directions in Transplantation

There is a widening gap between the number of patients seeking organ transplantation each year and the supply of available organs. This has led to research regarding "xenotransplantation"—the transplantation of organs from animals to humans. Clinical trials using pancreatic cells from pigs to treat diabetes have shown some promising results, but currently xenotransplantation is not an accepted treatment for humans. "Regenerative medicine" is another growing area of research, in which the patient's own cells are extracted and used to grow new tissue in the laboratory, which is then reimplanted into the patient. Because the tissue is grown from the patient's own cells, rejection is reduced or eliminated. In 2008, the first successful tracheal transplant was reported. The transplanted trachea was built in a laboratory from a dead donor's trachea that had been stripped of donor cells and then implanted with the patient's own cells.

Ethical and Social Issues

Organ transplantation raises many tough ethical and social questions. Because it would be unethical for physicians to willfully cause the death of one person to save the life of another, the medical world has struggled with the concept of what "death" is, and therefore when a person can be declared "dead" and donate vital organs such as a heart or liver (see also **Definitions of Death**). In the United States, a person can be declared dead if his circulation has irreversibly stopped functioning (cardiopulmonary death), or if his brain has irreversibly stopped functioning ("brain death").

Measures to improve the organ supply for patients needing transplants have included laws to require everyone to be an organ donor unless they specifically "opt-out"—or "mandated consent" laws. Such laws have not been successful in the United States, where many people belong to cultural or religious groups that do not support organ transplantation under all circumstances. Mandated consent laws raise the issues of both the human right to decline donation, and the potential problem of "forced" donations if such laws are enacted.

It has been suggested that paying for organs would encourage more organ donations. But paying donors beyond reimbursing them for their medical expenses creates the possibility that the poor or uneducated might be unfairly targeted and influenced to donate organs. In addition, a lack of international laws governing organ distribution and transplantation has led to inconsistent organ availability, and has promoted the development of global "black markets" for organs. Unregulated trade of human organs for profit raises concerns about whether some donors are harmed or even killed for their organs, as well as about the quality of the organs obtained. In extreme cases, accusations have been made that some countries, such as China, trade the organs of executed prisoners—who may even be condemned to death for the express purpose of procuring their organs and making a profit.

Lastly, organ transplantation is expensive—both for individuals and society. With decreasing health care dollars available, many question whether scarce resources should be spent on organ transplantation, which benefits a relatively small proportion of the population, when the same dollars could benefit a much greater number of patients if spent on basic healthcare and preventative medicine.

Gail A. Van Norman

Further Reading

Beachamp, T. L. and J. F. Childress. *Principles of Biomedical Ethics,* 7th edition. New York: Oxford University Press, 2012.

Bynum, W. and H. Bynum. *Great Discoveries in Medicine.* London: Thames and Hudson, 2011.

Miller, F. G. and R. D. Truog. *Death, Dying and Organ Transplantation: Reconstructing Medical Ethics at End of Life.* New York: Oxford University Press, 2012.

United Network for Organ Sharing, www.unos.org

OSCAR THE CAT

Since he was adopted by the staff in a New England nursing home, Oscar the cat has had the mysterious and reliable knack of being able to predict when patients are about to die. His presence at the bedside of residents of the Steere House Nursing Home in Providence, Rhode Island, is seen by physicians and nursing staff as an accurate indication that death is imminent, usefully allowing them to notify relatives so that they can be at their loved one's bedside when death occurs. Although not especially friendly or social with people who are not about to die, Oscar the cat is renowned for curling up close to patients who are between two and four hours away from death. Because many of the patients in the nursing home have end-stage dementia that impairs their cognitive functioning, they have little cognizance of the significance of Oscar's visit but are nevertheless comforted by his physical presence. Oscar the cat has presided over some 50 deaths, comforting patients who, because they have outlived their loved ones or have no relatives who live nearby, would otherwise have died alone. Explanations as to Oscar's uncanny capacity for predicting the imminent deaths of patients include a feline's heightened sensitivity to changes in the environment, such as an ability to detect a lack of movement in patients who are less mobile than usual, and an ability to pick up on the biochemical odors (*ketones*) released by cells in people who are dying.

Michael Brennan

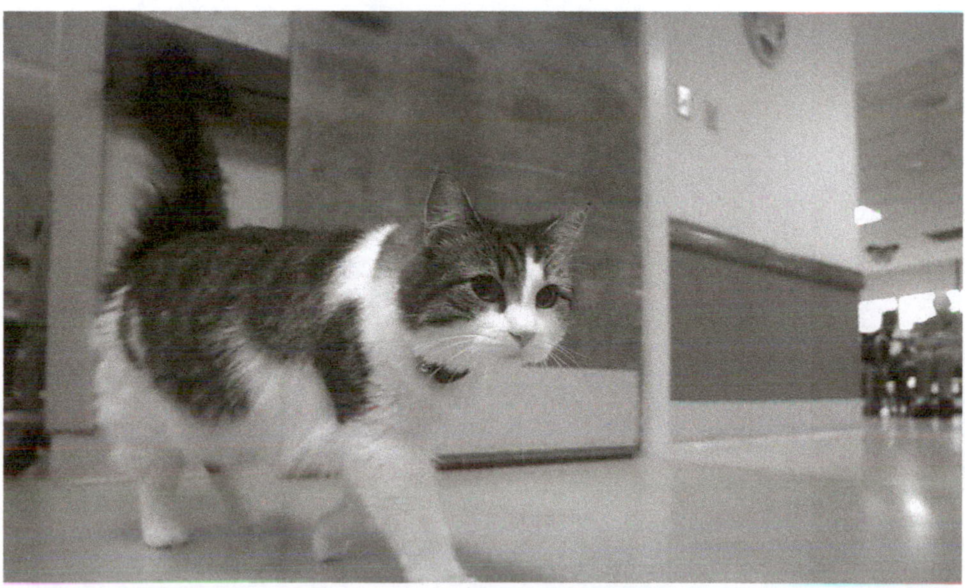

Oscar, a hospice cat at the Steere House Nursing and Rehabilitation Center in Providence, Rhode Island, walks past an activity room at the facility July, 2007. Oscar the cat seems to have an uncanny knack for predicting when nursing home patients are going to die, by curling up next to them during their final hours. (AP Photo/Stew Milne)

Further Reading

Dosa, D. M. "A Day in the Life of Oscar the Cat." *New England Journal of Medicine,* 357(4) (2007): 328–29.

Dosa, David. *Making the Rounds with Oscar: The Extraordinary Gift of an Ordinary Cat.* New York: Hyperion, 2010.

P

PALLIATIVE CARE

Palliative care is a domain of health care that is concerned with the care of people who are in pain and may be facing death. The internationally agreed World Health Organization (WHO) definition of palliative care lays down a comprehensive, ambitious, and multidisciplinary agenda for the care of those facing the end of life. Palliative care, moreover, is an approach that aims to improve the *quality* of life of terminally ill patients (and their families) through the prevention and relief of physical suffering, as well a range of associated issues, be they emotional, psychosocial, or spiritual in nature.

Palliative care, thus

- Provides relief from pain and other distressing symptoms
- Affirms life and regards dying as a normal process
- Intends neither to hasten nor postpone death
- Integrates the psychological and spiritual aspects of patient care
- Offers a support system to help patients live as actively as possible until death
- Provides a support system intended to both help families cope during a patient's illness, as well as in their own bereavement following a loved-one's death
- Uses a team approach to address the needs of patients and their families, including: physicians, nurses, pharmacists, social workers, bereavement counselors, clergy and spiritual care workers, as well as trained volunteers
- Aims to enhance quality of life, and may also positively influence the course of illness
- Is applicable early in the course of terminal illness in conjunction with other therapies that are intended to prolong life—such as chemotherapy or radiation therapy—and includes the relevant medical investigations needed to better understand and manage distressing clinical complications

Social "Charismatic" Movement and Its Origins

Palliative care, and its historical progenitor, hospice care, can also be viewed more broadly as a social movement with a clearly discernible ethos and worldview (see also **Hospice Movement**). This ethos emphasizes that an open acknowledgment of the dying process, together with a preparedness for death, helps ensure the least distressing pathway for patients and their families as they navigate the end of life and the grieving that accompanies it. This ethos, which is also perceived as having intrinsic existential worth, is perhaps attributable to the early religious roots, symbolism, and charisma of the leaders of this pioneering movement (see also **Kübler-Ross, Elisabeth**).

The hospice movement developed as a response to the documented neglect of dying people in the United Kingdom's National Health Service (NHS) in the middle of the 20th century. At this point in time, when technological developments had opened up completely new treatments, modern medicine became preoccupied with a focus on cure. Advances in medical science in an age of scientific optimism led to high expectations by the public that medicine could prolong life in ways that were, and continue to be, out of proportion with reality, especially, for example, in the treatment of cancer. The medical and nursing professions often perceived death as "defeat." In some circumstances, the best contribution of health care professionals to the care of dying people may have been to know when to stop treatment aimed at cure, but staff often felt clinically, morally, and perhaps even legally bound to treat with curative intent, no matter how poor the chances of prolonging life, and often with scant regard for quality.

Palliative care emphasizes the need to be able to "accompany" a dying person on their "journey," to be at ease with the inability to provide a cure, and to help patients and their families cope with the uncertainty that is inherent in terminal illness. In addition, palliative care recognizes that there is a significant medical, and most importantly, multidisciplinary contribution to be made to the care of people who are dying.

The early pioneers in Britain deliberately went outside the mainstream NHS to establish their pioneering hospice and home hospice services. Many of the early leaders and providers of palliative care around the world came from either the Protestant evangelical or Catholic traditions. There was always a strong thread of opposition to euthanasia, as can be seen in the WHO definition, which articulates a position of careful "causal neutrality." While this position has attracted its critics, it is clear that there are many myths about palliative care practice, especially the capacity of opioid and sedative drugs—as well as medical decisions at the end of life—to cause death. Indeed, there is half a century of accumulated international experience to show that palliative care can be practiced without bringing causation into question. The capacity to care for all, regardless of their values and beliefs, is fundamental to medicine and palliative care practice. On the other hand, palliative care is routinely maligned in public debates on euthanasia, where many of its practitioners and leading bodies appear to find themselves out of step with public opinion in many Western countries (see also **Dignitas**; **Euthanasia; Physician-Assisted Dying**).

Emergence of Palliative Care from Hospice Care

From the beginning, palliative care services also had a focus on community care, consultation, advice, support, and education to the public and professions alike. Originally, most new palliative care initiatives around the world attempted replication, to varying degrees, of the early stand-alone British hospice and home-care model, and this happened throughout the United Kingdom (although even there, the coverage was far from complete). It became clear early on that this model did not fit all situations or health systems, and had significant challenges regarding its sustainability. It was British Commonwealth countries, and a few pioneer centers in the United States, which first took up the model in the 1970s and 1980s. Doctor Balfour Mount at the Royal Victoria Hospital in Montreal, Quebec, Canada, is credited with the introduction of the term "palliative care." This allowed for a more secular and "mainstream" branding that reflected the rapid spread of palliative care initiatives around the world, across religious and national boundaries. There are now few developed countries that have no palliative care services at all, and there are many demonstration and mission initiatives in developing countries. Many parts of Europe and Asia that did not initially engage with palliative care have done so with enthusiasm in recent years.

Community Engagement

Despite the fact that palliative care may be perceived as countercultural in many settings, including the British one in which it originated, it has been remarkably successful. Given widespread reticence to contemplate mortality, and make personal preparation for death in Western societies, there is also ample evidence from studies and opinion polls that people are concerned about suffering and compromised dignity at the end of life, as the debate surrounding it has shown.

Community support has been substantial in terms of volunteering, fund-raising, lobbying, and feedback from families following death. This voluntary participation has been a defining quality of services worldwide, ensuring that extra time and support can be offered to patients and their families. Volunteers have also acted as a welcome counterbalance to the increasing medicalization of palliative care (see also **Medicalization**). It is also important to emphasize that the whole hospice and palliative care movement has been a practical response to the needs of dying people, their families, and caregivers, and not primarily an ideological one (although this is certainly present and important). In this lie the seeds of its success—in its "sleeves rolled up" approach, and its human connection at times of greatest vulnerability.

Michael Ashby

See also: Death Awareness Movement; Good Death; Hospice Movement.

Further Reading

Ashby, M. "Death Causation in Palliative Medicine." In *Causation in Law and Medicine,* edited by D. Mendelson and I. Freckleton (pp. 229–49). Aldershot, Hampshire, England: Ashgate/Dartmouth, 2002.

Hanks, G., N. I. Cherny, N. A. Christakis, M. Fallon, S. Kaasa, and R. K. Portenoy. *Oxford Textbook of Palliative Medicine,* 4th edition. Oxford: Oxford University Press, 2009.

Kellehear, A. K. *A Social History of Dying.* Cambridge: Cambridge University Press, 2007.

World Health Organization: www.who.int/cancer/palliative/definition/en/

PERINATAL DEATH

The term *perinatal death* refers to any death of an embryo, fetus, or baby at any time from the conception, during the pregnancy, or birth. Thus, a perinatal death may involve a miscarriage (which is the spontaneous loss of a pregnancy), abortion (the choice to end a pregnancy), stillbirth (the delivery of a baby that has died *in utero*), and neonatal deaths that occur shortly after birth. Perinatal death may also occur as a result of complications from the pregnancy that require immediate surgical intervention, such as an ectopic pregnancy, where the embryo has implanted in the fallopian tube or anywhere outside the uterus, and also in a situation called a molar pregnancy, where the fetus dies, but the placenta that is attached to the mother continues to grow in a cancer-like way.

Prevalence and Cause

It is estimated that approximately 18–25 percent of all pregnancies end in miscarriage. This number is difficult to verify because many women who miscarry were not aware that they were pregnant when the miscarriage occurred, and many women who miscarry do not seek medical treatment. It is often erroneously assumed that the mother "did" something wrong to cause the loss of the baby, such as too much physical activity, working too hard, or lifting something heavy. Social attributions regarding the cause of the loss may imply that the loss was the result of some psychological imbalance or ambivalence on the part of the mother, or from unresolved issues and feelings toward her own mother. These attributions have no merit in the research that has been conducted on this topic. Some women who experience perinatal loss may describe feeling that they are being "punished" for previous choices and attitudes, such as previous abortions, choosing a career, and waiting until they were older to have a family, or "pushing" normal biology by using medical technology to assist them with conception. In reality, most perinatal losses occur from a variety of causes that are usually completely out of the mother's control.

Social Aspects

The historical/popular view of pregnancy loss is that the parents have not experienced the baby as a separate person, and that grief should be minimal. Parents are often told that they can "try again" in the hope of having another baby that will assuage the grief they feel as a result of the loss. In general, the loss is *disenfranchised* (see **Grief**), or not validated, because the pregnancy may not have even been known by others, the fetus is generally not seen as a "full" human being, and the mother (and/or father) have not had an opportunity to create shared memories or life experiences with the baby. In addition, there are no formally established rituals for acknowledging the loss of an unborn baby, and there is usually no tangible evidence of the baby's existence after the loss occurs. Recent understanding of the grief experienced by parents following a perinatal loss has resulted in efforts on the part of some hospitals and clinicians to provide a way to acknowledge the reality of the lost baby, and to validate the significance of the parent's grief. In the past, stillborn babies were taken away quickly from the parents, presumably to spare them pain. However, it is now recognized that parents often want to see and hold their stillborn babies, and that doing so helps them in their grief process later down the road. Some hospitals now have photographers available to take sensitively arranged pictures of the baby and the family. Locks of hair may be cut and framed, memory boxes may be created, and plaster casts of hands and feet may also be taken and given to the parents to provide a tangible way to acknowledge their loss.

Current research indicates that women tend to form attachment bonds with their babies while they are *in utero*, often very early in the pregnancy. The unwanted ending of a pregnancy at any point during the gestation period is repeatedly demonstrated to be a profound loss to most individuals. It is important to note that grief after such a loss is not necessarily related to the gestational age of the baby, but more to the psychological attachment to the developing fetus and the meanings associated with the pregnancy. With the rise of routinely used medical technology, such as ultrasonography that allows prospective parents to hear the heartbeat of their baby or to "see" their unborn child at an early time in the pregnancy, there is higher likelihood for the development of stronger attachment to the baby at an early gestational age. This can have implications for the grief response in the event of the loss of a baby. There also does not appear to be a correlation between the specific nature and circumstances of the loss and the extent to which parents grieve in its aftermath. For instance, mothers who lost one of twins typically experience grief that is no different from mothers who lose a single baby. It is also clear that many women who choose to terminate a pregnancy, for whatever reason, can still experience significant grief over the loss of their baby.

In the past, perinatal death was viewed as a commonplace event that occurred with regularity. However, with the current reliance upon, and belief in, medical technology, there are often unrealistic expectations regarding the delivery of a healthy baby. The loss of a pregnancy often therefore comes as a profound shock, dashing these expectations, and parents frequently experience feelings of shame or failure afterward.

Implications for Grief

The loss of a baby typically occurs as a sudden event, without warning to the parents. Women may describe traumatic symptomatology surrounding the event, with the pain, bleeding, and feelings of powerlessness and helplessness that can accompany a spontaneous pregnancy loss. Women typically describe feelings of intense grief, most likely due to the presence of prenatal attachment that has developed through the pregnancy experience. The mother's losses may center on profound grief over the loss of the baby, with expressions of emotional distress and physical symptoms; whereas, the father's losses may focus more upon the loss of their plans and dreams for the baby (see **Grief**) and for their family, and their inability to alleviate their partner's distress.

While not every individual grieves in the same way, it is important to validate the loss for its significance to both the mother and the father, allowing opportunity for each to share their grief as they experience it. It is also important to keep in mind that a choice to end a pregnancy does not necessarily mean that there will not be grief after the loss. Research has also demonstrated that the experience of perinatal loss can have an impact upon prenatal attachment in subsequent pregnancies.

Darcy Harris

See also: Infant Mortality.

Further Reading

Covington, Sharon N. "Pregnancy Loss." In *Infertility Counseling: A Comprehensive Handbook for Clinicians,* 2nd edition, edited by Linda Hammer Burns and Sharon N. Convington (pp. 290–304). New York: Cambridge University Press, 2006.

Glazer, Ellen S. "Miscarriage and Its Aftermath." In *Infertility: Psychological Issues and Counseling Strategies,* edited by Sandra R. Lieblum (pp. 230–45). New York: Wiley, 1997.

Harris, Darcy L. and Judith C. Daniluk. "The Experience of Spontaneous Pregnancy Loss for Infertile Women Who Have Conceived through Assisted Reproduction Technology." *Human Reproduction,* 25(3) (2010): 714–20.

Kalb, Claudia. "A Vast and Sudden Sadness." *Newsweek,* February 9 (2009): 54–56.

Lang, Ariella, Céline Goulet, and Rhonda Amsel. "Lang and Goulet Hardiness Scale: Development and Testing on Bereaved Parents Following the Death of Their Fetus/Infant." *Death Studies,* 27 (2003): 851–80.

PETS

Quotes and expressions describing humans' relationships with pets note that a pet can be "man's best friend" and that pets provide unconditional love, ask no questions, and never complain or criticize. Not surprisingly, people often experience intense grief when a pet dies, mourning the loss of a close personal relationship that may have spanned many years. For many pet owners, the death of a cherished pet signals not just the loss of a trusted companion, but it is also experienced as a loss of "part of the family." And while in the past there has been a tendency to trivialize the death of a pet and its emotional impact on humans, there is today a growing recognition that the loss of a pet can be grieved every bit as intensely as the loss of another human being.

Memorialization of Pets

A variety of options are available to bereaved owners following the death of a pet: burial, cremation, and preservation (see **Taxidermy**). Home burial is an option if local law permits and pet cemeteries provide owners with a gravesite away from one's home. Traditional options for cremated remains include burial or keepsake pet urns for display. Innovative options include "art from ashes" and "life gems," in which pieces of jewelry, such as diamonds, can be fashioned from the carbonated remains of loved ones, including beloved pets. This increasingly popular practice is reminiscent of the *memento mori* tradition of Victorian and earlier times, when jewelry was created using the enduring parts of a deceased loved one such as their hair or teeth. In an increasingly electronic and digital age, virtual memorials of pets on websites such as www.petsremembered.com provide a useable place for online remembrance and commemoration that can be (re)visited whenever and wherever one is in the world.

Because grief is unique for everyone, the online resource www.petthinktank.com suggests honoring the memory of one's pet in whatever way is meaningful, with ideas ranging from having a funeral or memorial service, through creating a memorial garden, to purchasing a children's book on coping with the loss of a pet and donating it to a local library in the pet's memory. Participation in a communal ritual with other bereaved pet owners is another option made possible through the Rainbows Bridge Monday Night Candle Ceremony, which has been held every week since 1993, and National Pet Memorial Day, which is held annually on the second Sunday in September. Since non-pet owners may have difficulty validating another's grief following the loss of a pet (see **Grief**), a bereaved pet owner may want to affirm the right to grieve by reading the Bill of Rights for Grieving Animal Lovers (www.griefhealing.com/article-bill-of-rights-for-grieving-animal-lovers.htm).

A Teachable Moment for Death Education

The death of a pet is frequently a child's first encounter with grief, providing parents with a "teachable moment" to help their children learn to cope with loss. Numerous books are available to help parents support children through their grief following the death of a pet, as well as to help adults cope with the grief of losing a beloved companion.

Pet Therapy

Therapy animals are increasingly being used to assist people who are coping with physical or psychological trauma and grief. Residential hospices and end-of-life care centers may have pets to provide comfort to the dying and bereaved. One such cat has received international media attention for his ability to predict the impending death of residents at the Steere House Nursing Home in Providence, Rhode Island, curling up on the bed of a resident until he or she died (see **Oscar the Cat**).

Animals Grieve Too

While the presence of emotions among animals remains a controversial subject, genuine grief and mourning behaviors have been documented among domesticated companion animals, as well as in the wild. Domesticated pets demonstrate behavioral changes following the death of an owner or the death of a fellow companion animal. Grieving rituals have been observed in the wild (and in captivity) among elephants, dolphins, gorillas and chimpanzees, wolves, llamas, mole rats, magpies, and social insects (i.e., insects that exhibit social behaviors), to name only a few. Grief reactions among animal species may facilitate "reshuffling" of status relationships, fill the reproductive vacancy left by the deceased, or foster group cohesion among the survivors.

After tearlessly giving orders that brought death to thousands of soldiers, Napoleon Bonaparte was reportedly stirred to tears by the grief of a dog that refused to leave the side of his deceased master on the battlefield. More recently, in September 2012, various media outlets reported a news story of a dog in Argentina that refused to leave the grave of his dead owner, remaining there and rarely leaving the spot for six years. As this story and others like it illustrate, pets have been known to remain by the side of a dying owner and to remain with a deceased owner's casket until burial (and beyond), giving new meaning to the phrase "faithful until the end."

Carla Sofka

Further Reading

Alderton, David. *Animal Grief: How Animals Mourn.* Dorchester: Hubble & Hattie, 2011.

Angier, Natalie. "Do Animals Grieve Over Death Like We Do?" *New York Times,* September 2, 2008. http://www.nytimes.com/2008/09/02/health/02iht-02angi.15827535.html

Dosa, David. *Making Rounds with Oscar: The Extraordinary Gift of an Ordinary Cat.* New York: Hyperion, 2010.

Katz, Jon. *Going Home: Finding Peace When Pets Die.* New York: Villard, 2010.

Stump, Scott. "Dog Mourns at Casket of Fallen Navy SEAL." *Today MSNBC,* August 25, 2011. http://today.msnbc.msn.com/id/44271018/

Walker, M. "Birds Hold 'Funerals' for Dead." *BBC News,* September 1, 2012. http://www.bbc.co.uk/nature/19421217

PHILOSOPHY

In its direct, literal sense, the term philosophy means "love of wisdom." The term is used to refer to our efforts to develop wisdom in order to try and make sense of our world. This has traditionally involved asking such questions as:

- Does life have any meaning?
- Is there a purpose to the universe?
- What really exists, and what do we mean by "existence"?
- What do we mean by "mind"? How does it relate to "matter"?
- What do we know? Do we know anything, or is it just all hypothesis?
- Do we have free will, or is what we do determined by prior causes and circumstances?
- Is the question of "right" and "wrong" just a matter of opinion?

While science tries to answer the kinds of questions that can be resolved by experimentation (i.e., by "empirical" means,), philosophy is concerned with more abstract but nonetheless important questions. Many people put their faith in science to provide us with the knowledge we need and therefore disregard philosophy and its concerns. However, to do so is itself a philosophical position that can be questioned and challenged; the study of knowledge is known as epistemology, and science as a way of making sense of how knowledge is developed and used is but only one form of epistemology. Science is therefore an important source of knowledge, but it is no substitute for the learning and understanding that can be gained from philosophical study, debate, and inquiry.

When the term philosophy is mentioned, people often think of the ancient Greek philosophers, such as Plato, Aristotle, and Socrates, whose works have been very influential over the centuries. However, we should also recognize that there is also a long tradition of Eastern philosophy, for example, Confucianism, Daoism, and Buddhism. In addition, we need to be aware that the work of the ancients has been developed over time, in both East and West. So, philosophy is not limited to ancient history nor to Western thinking.

Death and dying have been important topics of study for many philosophers. For example, Martin Heidegger wrote about "being-towards-death," by which he meant that death defines life to a certain extent, insofar as the fact that we will all die one day makes us finite beings (see **Existentialism**). While many people may live their lives as if mortality is not an issue for them, this is a form of self-deception that prevents us from living an authentic life. Acting as if we are not finite beings (often referred to as death denial), in effect, distorts the reality of our existence (see **Death Denial**).

Philosophy is also relevant in terms of the perennial debate about whether or not there is an afterlife. Can a soul exist independently of a body? Is there such a thing as the soul in the first place? When we talk of spirit, are we speaking metaphorically or is there literally a spirit? These are important philosophical questions that reflect the longstanding relationship between philosophy, as an academic discipline, and death and dying as key aspects of what it means to be human.

The question of meaning is particularly important, insofar as philosophy can be seen as a matter of exploring meanings and trying to develop systems of understanding that enable us to make sense of human experience. Meaning is also relevant to our understanding of death and dying, as it can be argued that grieving is a form of, what psychologist Robert Neimeyer has labeled, "meaning reconstruction," that is, a way of developing new ways of making sense of our lives after a major disruptive loss. From this point of view, grieving can be understood as a painful process of developing a new sense of what our life is all about after a significant loss has prevented us from continuing as before (see **Bereavement; Grief Counseling**).

Philosophy can also help us to cast light on what are known as "death systems" (a term coined by Robert Kastenbaum and Ruth Aisenberg). This refers to the different ways in which different societies and cultures portray, define, and respond to death and dying. As Leenaars (2009) suggests, death systems not only *describe* matters relating to death and dying, but actually *prescribe* them, exerting pressure on people to behave in established ways when they encounter a bereavement. This may take the form of expected rituals or other established patterns of behavior and/or emotional expression. Where people do not conform to such expectations, there may be informal sanctions in the form of stigma or other forms of social disapproval. Trying to understand how and why different societies respond to death in different ways raises many philosophical questions about how cultures (as frameworks of meaning) differ in the ways they conceptualize death and how they create expectations about what are appropriate ways of reacting to such a loss.

Philosophy can help us make sense of the complexities of death and dying and, while not providing definite answers (that is not what philosophy is about), can provide important and fascinating insights into important aspects of human existence. An appreciation of philosophy can significantly enrich our lives. As Socrates put it over 2,000 years ago: the unexamined life is not worth living.

Neil Thompson

Further Reading

Choron, Jacques. *Death and Western Thought.* New York: Collier, 1973.

Craig, Edward. *Philosophy: A Very Short Introduction.* Oxford: Oxford University Press, 2002.

Kastenbaum, Robert and Ruth Aisenberg. *The Psychology of Death.* New York: Springer, 1972.

Leenaars, Antoon A. "Death Systems and Suicide around the World." In *Death and Bereavement around the World, Volume 5: Reflective Essays,* edited by John D. Morgan, Pittu Laungani, and Stephen Palmer (pp. 103–38). Amityville, NY: Baywood, 2009.

Neimeyer, Robert A. (ed.). *Meaning Reconstruction and the Experience of Loss.* Washington, DC: American Psychological Association, 2001.

Stokes, Philip. *Philosophy: The Great Thinkers.* Royston, UK: Eagle Editions, 2007.

PHOTOGRAPHY

Although opinions about, and levels of comfort with, images of death vary significantly from person to person, photographs related to accidents, murder, war, and natural disasters are displayed in the news and social media on a daily basis, serving as a constant reminder of our own mortality. Reactions to death-related imagery range from those who believe these images portray a truth that needs to be told, to those who view images of the dead and dying as exploitative and voyeuristic. Some of these images—of emaciated bodies piled high following the liberation of Nazi concentration camps at the end of World War II; of the self-immolation by a Buddhist monk in protest at the Vietnam War; of the Vietcong prisoner being shot in the head at close range also during the Vietnam War—are so powerful and arresting that they are irreversibly seared into our imagination; indelible images that are an inescapable part of the 20th- and, and if we include images from 9/11, 21st-century history.

During the first 40 years of photography (ca. 1840–1880), professional photographers advertised taking likenesses of the deceased. In the 19th century, postmortem photography (sometimes known as thanatography) became especially common, replacing the tradition of death masks and deathbed portraiture, especially among those who could not afford such memorializing practices that were, hitherto, the preserve of the wealthy elite. Due to high infant mortality rates, postmortem photographs of children were frequently the only photographs available to a working-class family due to the prohibitive cost of early daguerreotypes. Unlike today, where photographs are taken as part of everyday life, in the past they were reserved (because of their expense) for extraordinary and momentous events, such as birth and death. Casket photos of a deceased child or adult (often taken as if they were asleep) were quite common, taken in the parlor of the deceased's home and often including floral displays (see also **Wake**). Postcard photos of gravestones and cemetery shots including mourners can also be found in family albums from this era and were sent to not only confirm the death, but also to offer consolation to those who were unable to pay their respects in person.

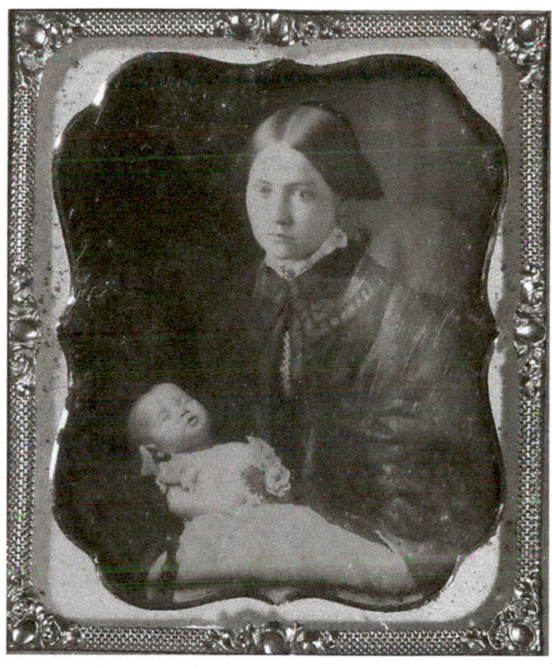

A post-mortem daguerreotype portrait shows a woman holding her baby, circa 1855, United States. (George Eastman House/Getty Images)

The practice of taking post-mortem photographs continues, and has been revived, particularly following a stillbirth or live birth of a child with a fatal genetic disorder; and has been used increasingly to document the final hours and days of those dying at home or in institutional hospice care. In the case of perinatal deaths, some professional photographers offer their services to capture the image of the deceased child and to document the family's interactions with that child. The not-for-profit organization, *Now I Lay Me Down to Sleep,* which is made up of volunteer photographers, provides remembrance photography to bereaved parents based on the assumption that these images serve as an important part of the healing process: honoring the child's memory, allowing parents to document a final farewell, while providing a material reminder of a life ended before it had begun (see also **Perinatal Death**). Following the stillbirth of their 21st child in December 2011, the posting of a photo of the tiny hand of the Duggar family's baby ignited a debate between those who felt it was inappropriate and sensationalistic behavior by a reality TV family, versus those who applauded the decision to publically acknowledge the loss of a child and validate a type of loss that is frequently disenfranchised within our society (see **Grief**). Today, videographers also record wakes and funerals, which may be webcast to those unable to attend in person (see also **Cyberspace**).

Controversy and debate regarding death-related issues are also prompted by the strategic placement of death-related images in the public eye. Public discussion about "right-to-die" issues has been fueled by the prominent display of photographs of specific cases, such as that of Terri Schiavo, while images depicting war and the aftermath of military conflict are also a source of significant debate. The "coffin controversy" involved debate about the appropriateness and effect of showing photographs of American soldiers' coffins returning from Iraq during the first

Gulf War (where it was believed by some, following the experience of the Vietnam War, that such images would be bad for public morale and add support to the arguments of antiwar protesters). The ban on publishing these photos placed in 1991 by President George H. W. Bush was lifted in 2009, on the condition that permission from a soldier's family had first been given.

After 9/11, individuals tended to either avoid television and newspapers or felt themselves unable to stop viewing images and stories about the events. A photograph of a man plummeting to his death from the North Tower of the World Trade Center on 9/11 became a point of fierce debate among news editors as to whether to publish an image that some might perceive as voyeuristic and distasteful. The image was eventually published in newspapers around the globe, including the *New York Times,* producing an angry and passionate response from readers, some of whom were offended by the image, while others felt that this was part of the story of 9/11 that needed to be told. The story of the falling man, and subsequent attempts to identify him, were made into a television documentary (*The Falling Man*) first broadcast in 2006.

On another level, there can be seen to be a profound and intimate relationship between death and photography. Photographs, as cultural theorists Susan Sontag and Roland Barthes have observed, are "melancholy objects" that attempt to freeze and fix in place the objects of a mortal and disappearing world (be they people, places, or events). The photograph, in this way, is an attempt to protect the object being framed by the camera from the ravages of time; to materialize something that is temporal and finite. "All photographs," Sontag writes, "are *memento mori.* To take a photograph is to participate in another person's mortality, vulnerability, mutability" (Sontag, 1977, 15).

Carla Sofka and Michael Brennan

Further Reading

Barthes, R. *Camera Lucida: Reflections on Photography.* New York: Farrar, Straus and Giroux, 1981.

Gibson, M. *Objects of the Dead: Mourning and Memory in Everyday Life.* Victoria, Australia: Melbourne University Press, 2008.

Linkman, Audrey. *Photography and Death.* London: Reaktion Books Ltd., 2011.

Ruby, J. *Secure the Shadow: Death and Photography in America.* Cambridge, MA: MIT Press, 1995.

Sontag, S. *On Photography.* New York: Doubleday, 1977.

PHYSICIAN-ASSISTED SUICIDE

Physician-Assisted Suicide (PAS), as the name implies, is a practice that involves a physician facilitating a patient's desire to end their own life. As opposed to euthanasia, a practice in which a *physician* (or another person) administers a lethal medication to a *patient,* PAS involves a *patient* who administers a lethal medication to himself or herself. The role of the physician is to provide the patient with a prescription for the lethal medication. (There is disagreement concerning the issue of whether this practice ought to be called physician-assisted suicide or physician-assisted death. The former, some claim, implies irrationality on the part of the patient and is too value laden.)

PAS is a controversial practice. As of December 2011, only 2 of the 50 states have passed statutes permitting PAS: Oregon, which was the first state to legalize PAS, and Washington. Although Montana has not passed a statute permitting PAS, the Montana Supreme Court (in *Baxter v. Montana*, 2009) ruled that there is "nothing in Montana Supreme Court precedent or Montana statutes indicating that physician aid in dying is against public policy."

Oregon's Death with Dignity Act (DWDA), which was passed in 1994 and survived subsequent legal challenges, allows physicians to prescribe medication to terminally ill patients for the express purpose of taking their own lives. Oregon's DWDA allows patients, who have been diagnosed with a terminal illness and are expected to die within six months, to request a prescription for a lethal dose of a medication that the patient can ingest to terminate his or her own life. All requests for a prescription under this act must originate with the patient, and physicians are not required to comply with, or participate in, patient suicide. Requests must be written, and they must be witnessed by two people, one of whom is not a relative of the patient, not the patient's physician, not a beneficiary of the patient's estate, and not a health care worker employed by the facility in which the patient is receiving care. Finally, a second physician must examine the patient after she requests a prescription for a lethal dose of medication. The role of this second physician is to ensure that the patient is terminally ill and free from mental conditions impairing her judgment.

In 2008, the state of Washington passed its own DWDA. Washington's legislation is, for all intent and purposes, no different from Oregon's DWDA.

Laws regulating or pertaining to PAS vary throughout the world. In 2002, the Netherlands became the first country in Europe to legalize (or depenalize) PAS. Shortly thereafter, Belgium passed legislation legalizing PAS.

Arguments in Favor of Physician-Assisted Suicide

A variety of arguments can be deployed to support and oppose PAS. Perhaps, the most common argument in support of PAS is one based on compassion or the physicians' right/duty to relieve pain. According to this argument, a physician's professional duties extend to limiting or alleviating severe pain and suffering. There are some situations in which the only way a physician can alleviate a patient's pain and suffering is by helping this person terminate his own life. Since a physician's duty is to reduce or alleviate pain, it follows that in those situations in which the only way to relieve pain is to help the patient terminate his own life, a physician has a duty (or is permitted) to help a patient terminate his own life. Hence, physicians ought to be permitted to write prescriptions for lethal medications.

A second argument in support of PAS is grounded in patient autonomy. According to this argument, human beings have the right (or ought to have the legal right) to decide what medicines they want to take or not take. This right includes the right to take medicines that would lead to one's own death. Since physicians are the only ones who can provide a person with a prescription that would lead to one's own death, it follows that if we take this right to patient autonomy seriously, a patient must have the right to obtain from a physician a prescription that would lead to her own death.

The argument in support of PAS that is grounded in patient autonomy can also be articulated in terms of a person's right to end her own life. If a person has this right (and we take this right seriously), it follows that a patient ought to have the right to obtain medicine that will allow or help him to take his own life. Since physicians control a patient's access to medication, they ought to prescribe to patients lethal doses of medicine when requested to do so. Or, at the very least, physicians ought to be permitted to do so.

Arguments against Physician-Assisted Suicide

One argument marshaled against PAS centers around the "sanctity of life." A key assertion is that human life is valuable in and of itself. Accordingly, one should not intentionally terminate or help another terminate a human life, even if the life consists of extreme pain and suffering. Prescribing lethal medicines to terminally ill patients involves helping one terminate a human life. Hence, physicians ought not to prescribe lethal medicine to one intending to terminate her own life (or the life of another).

Another argument commonly deployed against PAS is the "slippery slope" argument. Many of those opposed to the passage of the Oregon and Washington DWDAs relied on this argument. Essentially, the "slippery slope" argument against PAS states that if we legalize PAS, we begin walking down a path that will eventually lead to the legalization of (voluntary) euthanasia. Those who advance this argument fear that judges, or the public, may come to find (voluntary) euthanasia—which is now classified as homicide in most states—as being morally equivalent to PAS. Hence, if we legalize PAS, people will, in the not too distant future, support the legalization of (voluntary) euthanasia. Furthermore, some claim that if physicians become comfortable with, or inured to, PAS, they may eventually become comfortable with, or inured to, euthanasia. David Souter, while sitting as a U.S. Supreme Court Justice, made such an argument in *Washington v. Glucksberg:*

> Whether acting from compassion or under some other influence, a physician who would provide a drug for a patient to administer might well go the further step of administering the drug himself; so, the barrier between assisted suicide and euthanasia could become porous.

This argument can be countered with a further explanation of the qualitative differences between PAS and euthanasia: A physician who gives a patient a prescription to buy a lethal dose of medication is *not* participating in the patient's suicide. Administering a lethal dose to a patient is very different.

The "slippery slope" argument against PAS is sometimes articulated differently, focusing not on how PAS will lead to euthanasia, but rather asserting that if we pass laws permitting PAS in cases in which a patient is terminal, it will not be too long before physicians prescribe lethal doses of medicine for nonterminal patients, such as patients in chronic pain.

Both of these "slippery slope" arguments were advanced by opponents of Oregon's DWDA. Most people agree that the predictions, at least up to this point in time, did not, in fact, come to pass.

Further arguments against PAS revolve around the potential decline in the quality and availability of palliative care. These arguments were also advanced by some of the opponents of Oregon's DWDA. Some claimed that the field of palliative care and a patient's opportunity to obtain palliative care would suffer if PAS were to be legalized. They claimed that patients would be urged (or even pressured) to utilize PAS as opposed to palliative care.

A final argument against PAS is grounded in a claim concerning the traditional role of a physician. Those who advance this type of argument assert that the role of a physician is limited to improving the health of his or her patients. PAS, they claim, is inconsistent with this role and should, therefore, be prohibited. A different way to articulate this type of argument is to rely on the Hippocratic Oath, which states: "I will neither give a deadly drug to anybody if asked for it, nor will I make a suggestion to this effect." PAS may violate this injunction. Whether PAS does, in fact, violate this oath depends on what is meant by "*give* a deadly drug." Does *give* mean "administer" a drug to a patient or "hand" medicine to a patient? Nevertheless, some argue that the original wording of the Hippocratic Oath, which is over 2,000 years old, does not bind contemporary physicians. In fact, the original oath, which has been modified many times over the past 2,000 years, prohibits surgery. Hence, some claim, if one believes that PAS is wrong because the Hippocratic Oath prohibits it, consistency dictates that one should also believe that physicians should not practice surgery.

Scott Gelfand

See also: Euthanasia; Good Death; Hospice Movement; Kevorkian, Jack; Palliative Care.

Further Reading

Battin, M. P., R. Rhodes, and Anita Silvers (eds.). *Physician-Assisted Suicide: Expanding the Debate,* New York: Routledge, 1998.

Callahan, D. "Organized Obfuscation: Advocacy for Physician-Assisted Suicide." *Hastings Center Report,* 38(5) (2008): 30–32.

Emanuel, E. "Euthanasia and Physician-Assisted-Suicide: A Review of the Empirical Data from the United States." *Archives of Internal Medicine,* 162(2) (2002): 142–52.

Foley, K. M. and Herbert Henden. *The Case against Assisted Suicide: For the Right to End-of-Life Care.* Baltimore: Johns Hopkins University Press, 2002.

Quill, T. E. and M. P. Battin (eds.). *Physician-Assisted Dying: The Case for Palliative Care and Patient Choice.* Baltimore: Johns Hopkins University Press, 2004.

Wolf, Susan. "Gender, Feminism, and Death: Physician-Assisted Suicide and Euthanasia." In *Feminism and Bioethics: Beyond Reproduction,* edited by S. Wolf (pp. 282–317). New York: Oxford University Press, 1996.

POPULAR CULTURE

There are numerous ways by which researchers have approached death's role in popular culture. For instance, researchers have analyzed the death themes developed within various mediums. Rock and roll, for instance, the coming-of-age music of "baby boomers" and later generations, has long had an intimate relationship with death. The connections begin with the very name of the groups, such as *Grateful Dead, Megadeth, Dead Kennedys, Morbid Corpses, Cannibal Corpse, Terminal Mind, Youthanasia,* and *Dark Funeral*—as well as the messages of their songs. A popular performer's death can mean a financial windfall. For instance, in the week before he died, Michael Jackson's catalog was selling less than 10,000 albums a week; during the three weeks following his 2009 death, more than 1.1 million were sold.

Given the importance of the artists' role in molding a culture's orientation to dying and grief, considerable social attention is often given to how artists die. Rock and roll has produced a surfeit of premature deaths (i.e., Buddy Holly, Jimi Hendrix, Brian Jones, Duane Allman, John Lennon, Kurt Cobain, Michael Jackson, and Amy Winehouse), typically victims of drug overdose, auto- and aircraft crashes, suicide, and murder. The "27 club" is the name that has been given to the uncanny phenomenon of singers who have died, often as a result of drug and alcohol abuse, at the age of 27 (including Janis Joplin, Kurt Cobain, Brian Jones, Jim Morrison, and most recently in 2011, Amy Winehouse). Facing old age and diminishing powers, Ernest Hemingway took his own life with the blast of a rifle. Yukio Mishima, a Japanese author and Nobel Prize contender, ritually disemboweled himself before being decapitated by his chief lieutenant following the failure of his radical militarist movement.

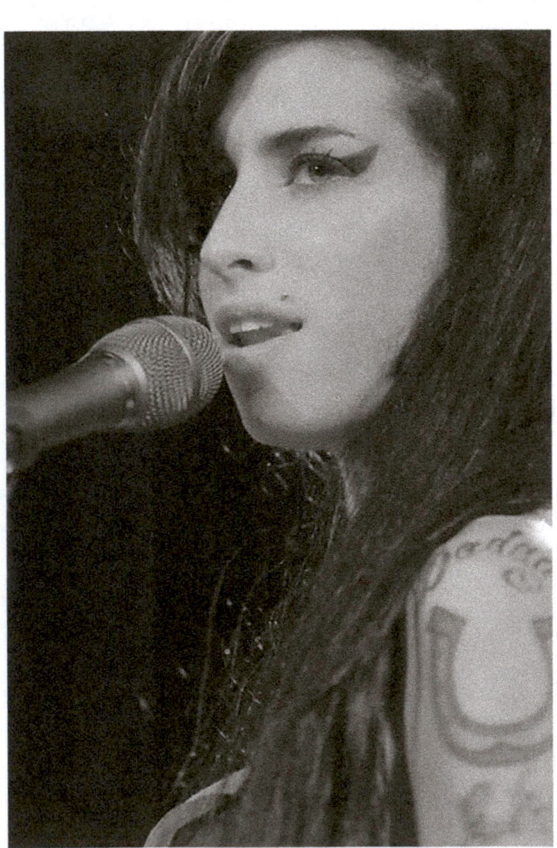

British singer-songwriter Amy Winehouse (1983–2011) captured tabloid headlines for her struggle with drug and alcohol abuse. (Shutterstock)

The influence on audiences of the death messages within artistic performances has its own research tradition. Congressional hearings have been conducted on the impact of television and popular music upon the homicidal and suicidal behaviors of children. In the late 1980s, the heavy metal group Judas Priest was sued for supposedly inspiring a suicide pact between two teenage boys. The unsuccessful suit, brought by the boys' parents, claimed subliminal messages within the *Stained Class* album facilitated self-destructive urges. Violent movies and television shows have inspired copycat behaviors, often with lethal consequences. After watching the movie *Natural Born Killers,* a 17-year-old shaved his head and began wearing tinted spectacles like the movie character Mickey, before driving to Salt Lake City and killing his stepmother and half sister.

In recent decades, a greater number of more gruesome deaths have resulted in a higher score on the Nielsen ratings of television shows and movie ticket revenues. In the world of fashion, the "skull fad" or "skull-chic" occurred concurrently with the "corpsification" of popular culture, by which symbolic images of death are rendered in vogue. Death has become increasingly graphic and intimate in television, as evidenced in programs like the highly rated *CSI: Crime Scene Investigation, Six Feet Under, Bones,* and *Dexter.* Touring the United States during the first decade of the new millennium was Gunther von Hagens's "Body Worlds" and its imitators (see **Body Worlds Exhibition**). The exhibition featured plastinated cadavers, often split or in other ways dissected, engaged in such life activities as playing chess, dancing, and riding on horses and bicycles. The living and the dead were also literally put together, hand to hand, by Tim Burton's animated movie *Corpse Bride* (2005).

It is often assumed in the social sciences that the inception of, and public reception given to, various themes in popular culture are products of their time. Consider, for example, death genres in cinema. It was in the decade following the detonation of the first thermonuclear weapons, in the midst of the 1950s postwar "Red Scare," that movies featuring massive mutants feasting on humanity appeared: *Godzilla, Them!* and *Rodan, the Flying Monster.* Following Rachel Carson's *Silent Spring,* scores of 1970s movies appeared concerning nature's revenge against man, such as *The Birds, The Swarm, Night of the Lepus, Day of the Animals,* and the *Planet of the Apes* series. The Vietnam War and Watergate produced a collective sense of breakdown of the moral order. A 1974 national survey conducted by the Center for Policy Research revealed that between 1964 and 1974, the percentage of the American public certain of God's existence dropped 8 percent to 69 percent, while during the same period, the percentage "definitely believing" in the existence of the devil increased by 11 percent to 48 percent, with another 20 percent considering his existence probable. From this milieu appeared the movies *Rosemary's Baby, The Exorcist,* and *The Omen.*

Public anxieties fueled by the 1970s publicity given to serial killers of young people such as Ted Bundy, David "Son of Sam" Berkowitz, and John Wayne Gacy, contributed to the appearance of such "slasher movies" as *Halloween* (1978), *Friday the 13th* (1980), *Eyes of a Stranger* (1981), *Madman* (1982), and *The House on Sorority Row* (1983). During the 1990s, popular culture was invaded by vampires, embodiments of collective fears of AIDS, with its associations between blood and romance. Capturing the apocalyptic fears surrounding the arrival of a new millennium, the deaths of but a handful of people would not do. The cinematic focus shifted to the earth-killing or mass-extinction scenarios of *Independence Day* (1996), *Deep Impact* (1998), *Armageddon* (1998), and *The Day After Tomorrow* (2004).

Over the past two decades, not only are there more roles for the dead in mainstream productions, but their roles in the plotline have also shifted from not only instilling terror but also serving as guardians for the living: *Field of Dreams* (1989), *Ghost* (1990), *Ghost Dad* (1990), *Casper* (1995), *City of Angels* (1998), *What Dreams May Come* (1998), *Meet Joe Black* (1998), *Jack Frost* (1999), *Sixth Sense* (1999), *The Gift* (2000), *What Lies Beneath* (2000), and *Dragonfly* (2002).

With science's blurring of the boundaries between life and death (i.e., the ability to keep the brain dead "alive" and to transplant deceased's organs into the living), new technologies now also allow the dead to perform with the living in popular culture. Thus, Natalie Cole sings with her long-deceased father Nat, and the surviving Beatles are reunited with John Lennon to perform "Free As a Bird" and "Real Love." In 2010, George Lucas announced a new movie project involving stars both living and dead, building upon such works as *Forrest Gump* (1994), wherein John Kennedy, George Wallace, Lyndon Johnson, John Lennon, and Elvis Presley were put to work from the grave to act with a very much alive Tom Hanks. Religion, with its conceptions of reincarnation, heaven and hell, no longer has a monopoly on the afterlife. In popular culture, one remains "alive" as long as one continues to make money.

Michael C. Kearl

See also: Public Dying; Public Mourning; Video Games.

Further Reading

Elliott, A. *The Mourning of John Lennon.* Berkeley, CA: University of California Press, 1999.

Kearl, M. *Endings: A Sociology of Death and Dying.* Oxford and New York: Oxford University Press, 1989.

Kearl, M. "The Proliferation of Postselves in American Civic and Popular Cultures." *Mortality,* 15(1) (2010): 47–63.

McIlwain, C. *When Death Goes Pop: Death, Media and the Remaking of Community.* New York: Peter Lang Publishing, 2004.

PROTESTANTISM

This is the name given to the religious movement that began with the Reformation in 16th-century Europe. It was an attempt to reform the Roman Catholic Church, which led to the splintering of Western Christianity into two major branches, a situation that still stands today. Further splintering among the Protestant branch created numerous and varied individual churches, sects and denominations. The term Protestant covers groups as varied as the Society of Friends (Quakers), Baptists, Presbyterians, Anglicans (Episcopalians), Assemblies of God, and Seventh-Day Adventists. What all these have in common are: reliance on the Bible as the primary, if not sole norm for Christian belief and practice; stress on "faith" in individual believers, and a rejection of the Papacy—the unified hierarchy of the Catholic Church. Protestantism, born as a protest movement, has always had as its hope the desire to purify the Church, and therefore historically has been suspicious of "tradition" as an independent source of authority. But Protestant groups vary greatly in how they interpret the Bible, in their understanding of the basic rites or sacraments or ordinances of the Church, and in their blueprints for the polity or proper organizational structure for the Church.

The major 16th-century reformers, Martin Luther and John Calvin, established different traditions, which today are represented by Lutheranism and the Reformed churches such as Presbyterians in the United States. Both founders continued the European model of "state churches," while other groups broke with this and wanted a Christianity separated from the world and more sect like. This "radical reformation" of the Anabaptists is today continued by Mennonites and the Amish. Later developments led to the reform movement led by John Wesley in Great Britain. This produced the Methodist Society, which became an independent denomination by the end of the 18th century. Most modern Evangelical Christians could trace their roots back to this era, when personal conversion experiences became the ideal for all Christians. By the end of the 19th century, these groups also reformed, producing both the Holiness movement, and early in the 20th century, the Pentecostal churches. Today, Pentecostalism is the most successful worldwide branch of Protestantism, especially in traditionally non-Protestant areas such as Latin America and Africa. Pentecostals are deeply committed to spiritual healing, although not necessarily opposed to conventional scientific medicine. In the United States, Protestants make up approximately 52 percent of the total population.

The significance of Protestantism for death and dying is two-fold. Because the Bible alone was considered authoritative, traditional teachings about Purgatory were rejected (see **Purgatory**). Protestants accepted an afterlife with the possibilities of Heaven and Hell for the dead, and a Last Judgment for everyone at the end of time. But without Purgatory, there was no religious connection to the dead, nothing that the living could do for or with them. The second major effect of Protestants' teaching was the de-emphasis on sacraments, in favor of personal faith. Thus, Christian dying was no longer accompanied by "last rites," the sacrament of Extreme Unction (now, Anointing of the Sick). However, this is somewhat misleading. Protestant dying through the 19th century at least was a sacred situation, in which the individual confessed sins, expressed faith in Christ, and hoped for a blessed existence in Heaven (see also **Ars Moriendi**).

Sociologists of religion believe that there is an additional effect of Protestantism as a social and religious outlook. According to Max Weber, "the Protestant ethic" led to a disenchantment of the world, an innerworldly asceticism, the rise of capitalism, and the rationalization of work and daily life. Protestantism was therefore one of the forces that led into modernity, with its focus on rationality, technology, and bureaucracy. Even as Protestant religious groups founded hospitals and schools, the ideological underpinnings of the modern secular order subtly undermined the religious basis of such institutions. The movement that began as an effort to reform Christianity from within, may thus have contributed, eventually, to its withdrawal from major areas of modern life. Health care and education today, even when under religious auspices, are examples of Weber's thesis regarding Protestantism's relation to modernity.

Lucy Bregman

Further Reading

Brown, R. *The Spirit of Protestantism.* New York: Oxford University Press, 1965.
Weber, Max. *The Protestant Ethic and the Spirit of Capitalism.* New York: Charles Scribner's Sons, 1958/1920.

PSYCHOLOGY

Psychology is the study of the mind and human behavior. Because of the pervasiveness of death in human experience, psychology has attempted to explore the ways that death affects human behavior. While human beings have traits in common with other living organisms, such as the instinct to survive, humans are seen to be unique in their capacity for abstract thought. This abstracting ability means that an individual can think of events from the past, and is able to project possible events that may occur in the future, including the death of one's self and others. This awareness of mortality, and the death anxiety that occurs as a result of this awareness (see **Death Anxiety**), is a key component of many important psychological theories.

The following are the specific psychological approaches to death:

Freud

When psychology was in its infancy as a distinct area of study, Sigmund Freud postulated that human beings have an innate death drive, which countered the drive of life energy, or the libido. Freud stated that the death drive, or the instinct of destruction, could be directed outwardly and expressed as a desire for mastery, control, or power. In his essay, "Mourning and Melancholia," Freud attempted to theorize the emotional reaction to loss, describing the similarities between individuals who experience profound grief over the loss of a loved one, and the condition of melancholia, which is akin to how depression is currently described. Freud stated that an individual's grief would come to an abrupt end once the bereaved individual detached emotional energy from the deceased loved one and reattached this energy to a new object (a process termed "decathexis").

Bowlby and Attachment Theory

In the 1940s, John Bowlby, a British psychologist and psychiatrist, drew from his knowledge of biology, psychology, and ethology (the study of animal behavior) in his observations of children who had been separated from their parents during World War II. His work and observations led to his development of attachment theory, which postulates that separation distress (and later grief) is an instinctually modulated response that occurs when the attachment system of an individual is threatened. Bowlby stated that individuals seek out secure attachments with others in order to feel safe in the world; the death or loss of an attachment figure triggers a grief response, which is seen as an adaptive response that serves the purpose of ensuring the safety and security of the one who is left behind.

Attachment Style and Grief

Recent work in the area of bereavement research by Margaret Stoebe, Henk Schut, and Wolfgang Stroebe at the University of Utrecht in the Netherlands, has built upon Bowlby's theory of attachment, providing insights into how attachment style moderates the grief response and predicts bereavement outcomes in specific individuals. Their model of bereavement, the Dual Process Model, is based upon attachment theory.

Terror Management Theory

Social psychologists Sheldon Solomon, Thomas Pyszczynski, and Jeff Greenberg were highly influenced by the work of Ernest Becker, an anthropologist and philosopher who argued that humans live with an innate fear of death that motivates them to behave in specific ways when confronted with reminders of their mortality. These psychologists have explored the relationship between death awareness and human behavior by observing the impact of death awareness upon human behavior, both individually and in social groups. They proposed the Terror Management Theory (TMT) which states that human behavior is chiefly motivated by the fear of mortality (see **Terror Management Theory**). Proponents of TMT state that the terror of absolute annihilation creates a profound (yet subconscious) anxiety in people, and that human beings spend their lives attempting to make sense of, avoid, or somehow overcome death through symbolic means, such as artistic works, monuments, or legacies that will be recognized after their death. These psychologists devised research experiments to demonstrate proof that *mortality salience,* or the awareness of one's own death, profoundly affects the decision-making of individuals and groups of people.

Existential Psychology

Existential psychologists focus upon issues related to purpose and meaning in life. Irvin Yalom, a well-known psychiatrist who trained in humanistic/existential psychology, has explored how individuals approach their fear of death and the ending of their physical existence. Yalom states that the fear of death is the one thing that unites all human beings. He also emphasizes that confrontation with one's fear of death allows an individual to appreciate life more and to live more fully.

Constructivist Psychology

More recently, constructivist psychology has focused upon the ways that human beings create systems for meaningfully understanding their world and their experiences, including death, dying, and grief. In this view, individuals are considered to be fundamentally engaged in making sense of the events that occur to them, and in verifying how much of that sense is useful for living. According to constructivist psychological theory, one's own death, the death of a loved one, or life after a loved one has died are all events that require an individual to rebuild previously held assumptions about how the world works and how others now occupy that world. The process of rebuilding, or adapting one's previously held assumptions about the world (in order to accommodate the presence of death and loss in life) involves making meaning of these events, resulting in a change in one's worldview that can accommodate and make sense of death and loss in everyday life. Robert Neimeyer is one of the leading researchers in this area.

Current Issues

Recent controversies taking place at the intersection of psychology and death pertain to the distinction of grief as a separate entity from depression, whether or not to include various types of disordered grieving into the upcoming fifth edition of the *Diagnostic and Statistical Manual of Mental Disorders* (*DSM-5*), and the appropriate psychological approaches and treatment of complicated grief.

Darcy Harris

Further Reading

Bowlby, John. *Secure Base: Clinical Applications of Attachment Theory.* London: Routledge, 1998.

Brennan, Michael. *Mourning and Disaster: Finding Meaning in the Mourning for Hillsborough and Diana* (especially chapter 2). Newcastle-Upon-Tyne: Cambridge Scholars Publishing, 2008.

Greenberg, Jeff, Sander L. Koole, and Tom Pyszczynski. *Handbook of Experimental Existential Psychology.* New York: Guilford Press, 2004.

Kastenbaum, Robert J. *The Psychology of Death,* 3rd edition. New York: Springer. 2006.

Neimeyer, Robert A. *Meaning Reconstruction and the Experience of Loss.* New York: Routledge, 2001.

Stroebe, Margaret S., Robert O. Hansson, Henk Schut, and Wolfgang Stroebe. *Handbook of Bereavement Research and Practice: Advances in Theory and Intervention.* Washington, DC: APA, 2008.

Yalom, Irwin D. *Staring at the Sun: Overcoming the Fear of Death.* New York: Jossey Bass, 2008.

PUBLIC DYING

The term public dying refers to the ways in which the process and experience of dying are made visible and accessible in the public domain. In the emerging field of death studies during the 1980s and 1990s, one of the forerunners examining the phenomena of public dying was A. H. Hawkins, who coined the term "pathographies" to refer to accounts of illness and dying published in books. Over the years, the appetite among the general public for these types of published accounts of dying has grown, with more recent examples, both firsthand and in recollections from close relatives, including Jim Beaver's *Life's That Way* and John Diamond's *C: Because Cowards Get Cancer Too.*

Historical Overview

Debates about the visibility and accessibility of dying have been central to the development and evolution of death studies, seen most clearly in the influential historical analysis of the status of death in Western Europe by Philippe Ariès (1974) (see **Ariès, Philippe**). Much of the discussions that have evolved since the publication of Ariès's work have been framed by argument about whether or not death is taboo, denied or sequestered in modern society.

There are two sides to this discussion. The first is that through the development of modern medicine, the institutionalization of health care, and the decline of organized religion, dying has become increasingly concealed from public view. The opposing argument is that through death registration and documentation, and the publication of accounts and imagery of death and dying in the media, death and dying are now more visible than ever.

A contrasting perspective is that many of the accounts and images of dying accessible in the media are of violent and sensational deaths, the result of war or famine rather than more "everyday" mundane deaths, such as those from heart disease and old age. This is a view first postulated by Geoffrey Gorer in his hugely influential essay "The Pornography of Death," published in 1955. In it Gorer claimed that media representation of death had become a source of titillation that bore little resemblance to the reality of death itself. This avoidance of engagement with the actual realities of death during much of the 20th century can itself be seen as a strategy by which death was denied and held at arm's length (see **Death Denial**).

The Influence of Technology

In the 21st century, one of the most significant contributors to the changing profile of dying in public has been the evolution of communication technology and the globalization of news media. Through 24/7 rolling news channels and the Internet, the almost minute-by-minute decline of an individual can be charted in detail. Celebrities and well-known individuals are the particular focus of such attention, as could be seen in 2005 during the last days of Pope John Paul II.

The Internet has also opened up opportunities for both disseminating and consuming news of an individual's health and subsequent dying. Via social networking sites (SNS) such as Facebook (see also **Cyberspace; Facebook**), discussion and hypothesizing about death and dying are rife. After Michael Jackson died in 2009, Twitter—the instantaneous microblogging community where people can post 140 character-long messages—was full of speculation about the contributory factors that led to his death. There was also much hypothesizing about the health of Apple cofounder and chief executive Steve Jobs in 2011, as his pancreatic cancer resulted in extreme weight loss, with much rumor that he was dying. This echoed comparable speculation a few years ago in 2008–2009 when photographs of an emaciated Patrick Swayze, the actor who also had pancreatic cancer, were published via celebrity magazines and became a subject of much speculation on the Internet.

This "citizen journalism," whereby anyone can produce hypotheses, has irrevocably redrawn the boundaries in both the provision of detail of someone's dying, and its consumption. New opportunities have been derived from this, specifically the way in which the news and details thereof can be woven into a biographical narrative and commodified.

Commodifying Dying

In the early 2000s, a particularly pertinent example of public dying—especially the way in which it was presented and consumed—was exemplified by the case of Jade Goody in the United Kingdom. Goody was a young woman who became a well-known "reality TV" personality as a result of being in the television show, *Big Brother.* Following her time in the *Big Brother* house, Goody demonstrated a readiness and enthusiasm to expose many facets of her private life in the tabloid press and celebrity magazines. This included her diagnosis of cervical cancer and subsequent experience of dying.

Goody died in March 2009, leaving behind a well-documented account of dying in print media on both sides of the Atlantic, several television shows that included recordings of her treatment, and a diary published shortly after her death. Throughout this, Goody was explicit in her desire to publicize her experience to raise sufficient income so that her two young sons could attend a fee-paying school. In other words, Goody deliberately and overtly chose to "sell" her experience of dying.

Much like the death of Diana, Princess of Wales, in 1997, being heralded as a benchmark for the phenomenon of public mourning (see **Public Mourning**), the commercializing of dying by Goody may well become a yardstick by which public dying will be measured.

Kate Woodthorpe

Further Reading

Ariès, Philippe. *Western Attitudes towards Death: From the Middle Ages to the Present.* Translated by P. M. Ranum. London: Baltimore, 1974.

Beaver, Jim. *Life's that Way: A Memoir*. New York: G.P. Putnam's Sons, 2009.

Diamond, John. *C: Because Cowards Get Cancer Too.* London: Vermilion, 1999.

Gorer, Geoffrey. "The Pornography of Death." *Encounter,* October, 1955. (This is available in the appendix of Geoffrey Gorer's *Death, Grief and Mourning.* Garden City, NY: Doubleday, 1965).

Woodthorpe, Kate. "Public Dying: Death in the Media and Jade Goody." *Sociology Compass,* 4(5) (2010): 283–94.

PUBLIC MOURNING

Public mourning refers to the widespread expression of grief following the death of celebrities, public figures, and victims of disasters or wars. It typically involves mourning for people who are not known to us in a personal capacity or through face-to-face relationships. The most spectacular and widely reported episode of public mourning in recent years followed the death of Diana, Princess of Wales, in 1997. This has since provided a benchmark, especially for those in the media, with which to compare other examples of public mourning, such as that following

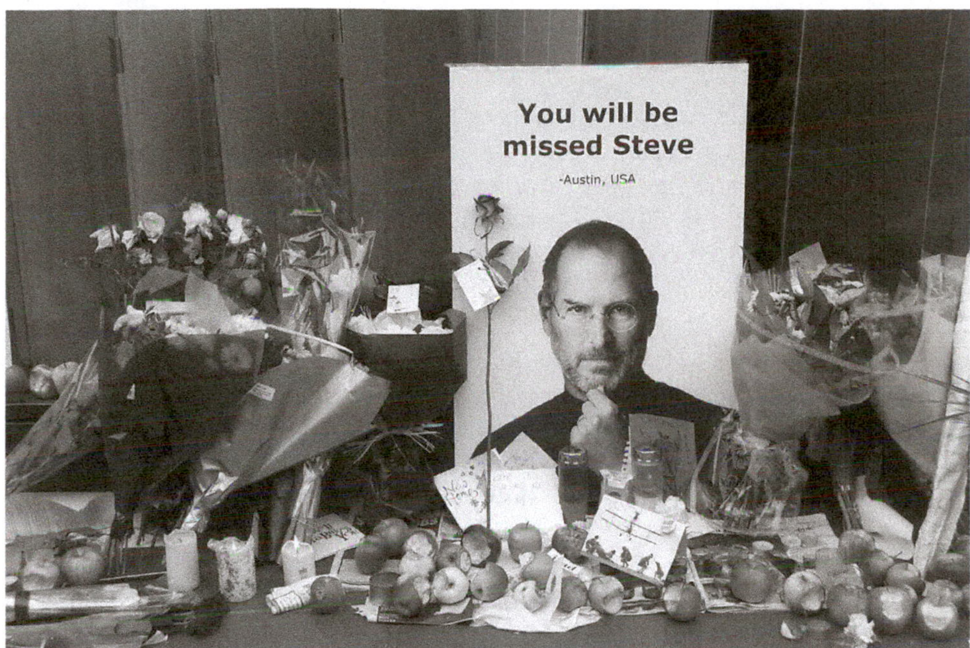

Memorial to Steve Jobs at the Apple store on Regent Street in London, 2011. After Jobs's death on October 5, 2011, public memorials began appearing all over the world, from China to Europe and North America. (Jenny Matthews/In Pictures/Corbis)

the terrorist attacks of September 11, 2001, the Columbia Space Shuttle disaster in 2003, and the death of pop star Michael Jackson in 2009.

New and Old Public Mourning

Old public mourning includes the public display of grief following the death of a person occupying a position of power or prestige within society. An example would be following the death of a king or chief in a traditional tribal society. It may also include the compulsory attendance at a leader's funeral in societies that are undemocratic, such as following the death of Kim Il Sung in North Korea in 1994. A further example would be the dutiful obligation to attend a ceremony of public mourning, such as the thousands of people that visited the Tomb of the Unknown Warrior at the end of World War I; or the peasants in early modern England who were paid with a loaf of bread to attend the funeral of the lord of the manor so as to swell the numbers and reinforce his importance within the community.

New public mourning, in contrast, is less orchestrated, more spontaneous, and characterizes the type of grieving following the death of celebrities and disasters in which the mourner has invested part of his or her identity. In recent years, such displays of public mourning have typically included one or more of the following features:

- Widespread media coverage
- The opening and signing of books of condolence (both paper and electronic)

- The creation of makeshift shrines using various elements of popular culture, including flowers, cards, candles, balloons, and soft toys

In the Challenger and Columbia Space Shuttle disasters of 1986 and 2003, as well as in the events of September 11, 2001, not only did the public mourning that followed receive widespread television coverage, but events themselves were captured on live television. This added to the sense of trauma and the intensity of mourning experienced by the wider public that witnessed these events. In the public mourning following the death of Princess Diana, large crowds of people gathered together in London, England, outside Buckingham and Kensington Palace, where they left an estimated 10,000 tons of flowers. The media coverage that accompanied the mourning for Diana was equally large in scale, with a record estimated television audience of 2.5 billion people worldwide tuning in to watch a funeral attended by world leaders, heads of state, and celebrities.

Criticism and Controversy

New forms of public mourning, such as that following the death of Princess Diana, have, however, generated criticism and controversy. Many in the media have questioned the authenticity of the public's grief for a distant celebrity or public figure whom they have never met. There is evidence to suggest that public mourning differs from the mourning following the loss of a face-to-face relationship in two key ways: (1) it is shorter in duration and (2) does not demand the psychosocial transition required following the loss of a close personal companion. There is, at the same time, evidence to suggest that the grief experienced following the deaths of celebrities, public figures, and public disasters extends well beyond simple empathy for people killed and bereaved and is instead experienced *as if* it were for the loss of a close personal relationship. This profound grief-like response may also serve as a trigger for personal losses that could not, for various different reasons, be properly grieved. The rituals of grief characteristic of public mourning can thus be seen as helping to validate the personal grief that has been disenfranchised by society's refusal to recognize it (see **Grief**).

Understanding Public Mourning

Public mourning for those not known to us personally can be better understood by placing it within a wider social and historical context. It was not uncommon, for example, in early periods of history within Western societies for a whole community, including people who did not know or even like the deceased, to demonstrate their support to the bereaved by attending a funeral as an act of duty or social support. Even today, in societies like Japan, it is customary—and a reflection of the respect for social hierarchy in that society—for a worker to attend the funeral of a boss' parent, even though the worker may never have met the deceased. When placed in this wider social context—and against a backdrop within Western societies in which death and grief were confined to the private family sphere during much of the 20th century—the public display of grief for people we have never met appears far less unusual or strange (see **Death Denial**).

Explanations

A number of different explanations have been put forward to account for the growth and spread of new public mourning. Five in particular stand out as worthy of attention:

1. ***Media amplification***
   The media play a pivotal role in facilitating new forms of public mourning by helping to stimulate more public interest than would otherwise be the case. Not only do people learn the behavior characteristic of these events from watching others on television, but the media also help to amplify and spread the phenomenon of public mourning by giving the illusion that it is more widespread than is actually the case.
2. ***Identification with celebrities***
   Social-psychologists have suggested that the grief-like response generated by the death of celebrities and public disasters can be understood in terms of the close personal identifications we make with celebrities and victims of disasters. In the case of celebrities, it is not uncommon for people to have maintained an ongoing "imagined relationship" with them through the media in ways that fill gaps that may exist in our personal or family lives. When a particular celebrity dies, we may seek comfort in public mourning as a way of making sense of, and coming to terms with, the shock of their sudden and unexpected departure. The public grieving for Kurt Cobain following his death in 1994 symbolized the close identification made by his fans with a genre of music and lifestyle that spoke to their sense of disaffection. Similarly, when Steve Jobs died in 2011, fans and users of Apple computers and electronic devices from around the world gathered outside Apple stores, leaving personal tributes, including half-eaten apples (the logo of Apple computers). Their actions reflected their identification with, and affection for, the products the cofounder of Apple computers helped design that so revolutionized their lives.
3. ***Expressivism***
   New public mourning can be linked to the growth of emotional expressivism among a generation of "baby boomers" who are much more comfortable with talking about their feelings. The public mourning in Britain following the death of Princess Diana can thus be seen to reflect a generational shift that contrasts sharply with earlier wartime generations whose daily existence was governed by the basic need for ensuring their physical survival rather than the expression of feelings.
4. ***Globalization***
   Globalization plays a role in the spread of new public mourning by diffusing ideas and practices from one particular part of the world to others. Travel, television, and the worldwide web all provide the opportunity to adopt a mourning practice seen in another culture by assimilating it within their own. Visitors to Mexico, for example, may have witnessed and been influenced by the colorfully decorated alters—including photos of the deceased—used to celebrate the Day of the Dead (see **Day of the Dead**). This might help to explain why some cultures, which have traditionally observed somewhat austere mourning practices, have recently come to adopt more celebratory ones, such as a minute's applause to celebrate the life of the deceased instead of a minute's silence.

5. ***Individualism***
   The growth of individualism and personal choice today allows us to pick and choose the individuals and events we mourn rather than to feel obligated to mourn during official memorial days sanctioned by the state (see **Memorial Day**).

Public mourning, both old and new, includes a wide variety of disparate events. While there are common elements linking all of them, the specific mourning witnessed in each is related to the unique set of circumstances surrounding the event or persons being grieved.

Michael Brennan

See also: Cyberspace; Facebook; Popular Culture; Public Dying.

Further Reading

Brennan, Michael. *Mourning and Disaster: Finding Meaning in the Mourning for Hillsborough and Diana.* Newcastle upon Tyne, UK: Cambridge Scholars Publishing, 2008.

Kear, Adrian and Deborah Lynn Steinberg (eds.). *Mourning Diana: Nation and the Performance of Grief.* London and New York: Routledge, 1999.

Walter, Tony (ed.). *The Mourning for Diana.* Oxford, UK: Berg, 1999.

Walter, Tony. "The New Public Mourning." In *Handbook of Bereavement Research and Practice: Advances in Theory and Practice,* edited by Margaret S. Stroebe, Robert O. Hansson, Henk Schut, and Wolfgang Stroebe (pp. 241–62). Washington, DC: American Psychological Association, 2008.

PURGATORY

This is the destination for those dead whose sins, although forgiven, have not been fully expiated, according to Roman Catholic Christianity. Purgatory becomes an "intermediate state," inhabited by the souls who need "purgation" or cleansing, between the time of their deaths and such time as they are truly ready to enter Heaven. This belief, although controversial in Christian history, allows the living to offer prayers to improve the condition of their beloved dead, and resolves some dilemmas about the sinful, imperfect lives of Christians whose faith was real, but whose deeds were not fully meritorious.

The origins of Purgatory as a realm for the dead are found in the verse in II Maccabees where Judas the hero makes a sacrifice on behalf of some dead comrades who wore idolatrous amulets. "Thus he made atonement for the dead that they might be freed from this sin" (II Maccabees, 12:46). But this idea of how the living might help the dead became a part of ancient Christianity. Particularly in the text of Gregory the Great, the saying of Masses for the dead was recommended as a means to hasten their cleansing. Nevertheless, until the high middle ages in the Western, Latin Church, this belief was not a major theological force. It became such in the 12th and 13th centuries. In contrast, the Eastern Orthodox Churches never accepted the entire doctrine, nor did they literalize it as Western Christians came to do. At its height, when affirmed at the First Lateran Council of 1215, the doctrine taught that although Christ made atonement for sin, the sinner's confession and absolution must be completed by his/her working out the effects of sin. For those who were "late repentant," for example, a last-minute change of heart, even with sacramental absolution, was not enough. They needed to pay the penalty. Or, as we might say, they needed rehabilitation in order to become persons for whom Heaven was a fitting destination. This view, found so eloquently in Dante's *Divine Comedy* that it stuck as the official teaching, makes Purgatory a gateway into Heaven. All those in Purgatory, eventually, will ascend to the Beatific Vision. Earlier beliefs had made Purgatory much more "hellish," and various locations for it—as in "St. Patrick's Purgatory" in western Ireland, focused on its sinister and underworldly character. The Dante version made it a place of hope. Although there is suffering there, it is suffering with a purpose and the souls know it to be only temporary.

Why was this belief important? The practice of praying for the dead, and offering Masses for their purgation, was enormously important in how medieval Christians saw the roles of the dead and the living. While saints in Heaven could help the living, the dead in Purgatory needed our help. Since Masses for the dead required priests, the practice of saying Masses with no congregation became normal. A "chantry priest" was one whose main task was to dutifully perform this function for the dead, especially for dead patrons who endowed chapels specifically for this purpose. A major function of Wills was not just to distribute property to the living, but to guarantee the soul's speedy transit through Purgatory by such endowments.

At the time of the Reformation, this was one of the practices targeted by the Reformers. They saw the whole system of Purgatory prayers as the use of the dead to make money for the church; priests were those who fed off the dead ("Totenfresser"). Moreover, Purgatory was not in the Bible, and II Maccabees was declared "Apocrypha" and out of the Christian canon probably for this reason, as well as because it was not included in the official Jewish canon either. The views of Martin Luther and John Calvin focused on God's election of those whom God wished to save, and not on what humans could do to influence the status of the dead, nor on speculation about their destinations. Thus an important link between the living and the dead was severed. Although Protestants kept the two ultimate destinations, Heaven and Hell, and saw these as clearly taught in the New Testament, they rejected Purgatory as a human add-on, and rejected as well all the financial transactions that had grown up as part of the theology.

Lucy Bregman

See also: Catholicism; Heaven; Hell.

Further Reading

Alighieri, Dante. *The Purgatorio,* Volume 2 of *The Divine Comedy.* Translated by John Ciardi. New York: New American Library, 1957/c.1320

LeGoff, J. *The Birth of Purgatory.* Chicago: University of Chicago Press, 1984.

R

REINCARNATION

Reincarnation refers to some mental, emotional, and/or spiritual aspect of a deceased person becoming associated with a new physical body. Acceptance of reincarnation is very widespread, and although specifics vary from culture to culture, beliefs about reincarnation typically incorporate some of the deepest structures of a people's worldview.

One important shared cultural concern around reincarnation is what component of a person gets reborn; what is so essential that it persists from one lifetime to the next. Hindus generally believe that each living being has a soul (*ātman*) which survives the death of one body and enters the new mother's womb at the time of conception. The peoples of sub-Saharan Africa also generally believe in a nonphysical soul which survives the death of the old body and comes to animate that of an infant. Buddhists, by contrast, hold that there is no eternal, unchanging soul animating a body but that each moment of a person's mind creates the next moment. In this way, people's experiences seem continuous, and after a person's death, the disembodied mind continues to experience one moment after another until it becomes associated with a new body (which can be either physical or immaterial).

Ian Stevenson, a University of Virginia psychiatrist who researched children who claimed to remember previous lives, concluded that for many cases reincarnation is the most probable explanation. However, despite researching thousands of case studies over several decades, he was unable to posit any mechanism for transmitting a person's identity from one lifetime to the next. These examples demonstrate the way that beliefs in *what* is reincarnated tend to mirror cultures' formulations of the core identity of a person, whether they theorize that as a discrete soul, as a mental continuum, or as the intangible, but vivid, memories and tendencies that constitute a self.

Reincarnation also reflects a culture's understanding of the relationship between humans and nonhuman animals. Hindu and Buddhist cultures generally accept that a person can be reborn as an animal (or in various nonphysical realms). Hindu, Buddhist, and ancient Greek cultures, among others, praised a vegetarian lifestyle for that reason. Many New Age groups that accept the doctrine of reincarnation, however, tend to reject the idea that humans could be reborn as nonhuman animals. Following the modern, Euro-American trust in progress, they hold that souls can only progress, not regress, from one lifetime to another until, ultimately, they attain full awakening (however a given group conceptualizes that).

Stevenson's research relied on talking with children and their families for verifiable or falsifiable information regarding previous lives, so investigating alleged previous lives as animals was not possible. However, he did have a few reported cases in which a child claimed to remember a life as a nonhuman animal. Many Amerindian societies, even those which may not believe in human reincarnation, hold that animals return to the spirit world following a successful hunt, and the proper rituals must be performed in order for that animal to return to the physical world and provide the human community with food again. Some also consider human-to-animal and animal-to-human reincarnations possible.

An important reincarnation-related question for many African and Asian societies is whether a deceased ancestor can simultaneously be reborn into the family and remain as an ally in the spirit world. Ancestors, and their correct propitiation (appeasement), are very important in Indian societies to this day, and while most Hindus accept the official doctrine of reincarnation, many families also maintain their ritual duties toward their ancestors. In African and East Asian societies, these two afterlife narratives also seem less to compete than to *complement* each other, with the spirit realm in which the ancestors operate seen as intimately connected with the physical realm peopled with the current incarnations of lineage ancestors.

In some cultures, the process of reincarnation is held to end at some point, while in others it renews society generation after generation. Hindus and Buddhists believe that reincarnation occurs because the being who dies is enmeshed in the illusion that the visible world is real as it appears, and on the basis of that misconception, it longs for continued bodily life and pleasures. Both traditions claim that this cycle of mistaken reincarnations will end with the person's final apprehension of reality (*moksha* or *nirvāna*), though they disagree about the final nature of reality. Arctic Amerindian people who believe in reincarnation, by contrast, do not conceive of rebirth as a failure to recognize one's true nature but as the natural way of the world. Their system does not look outside the continuity of the social and natural worlds to explain why humans and/or animals should be reborn. Much of Stevenson's research was conducted in Asian societies familiar with the idea that rebirth might end with liberation, but of course a social scientist would have no empirical way to investigate whether people can attain *moksha* or *nirvāna* and cease to reincarnate.

Finally, what is the relationship between death and reincarnation? Many societies that believe in reincarnation hold that the manner of someone's death can significantly influence the next incarnation of that person. Amerindians believe that an animal for whom proper rites are not preformed will not return to offer itself as food again. Buddhists, with their emphasis on the power and continuity of mind, hold that a life that ends in extreme anger or fear (such as a death by murder or in battle) is more likely to trigger the negative karmic imprints of the dying person and lead to a negative rebirth. Stevenson found that children were much more likely to remember traumatic or early deaths than peaceful ones, and many of the children who claimed to have memories of lives that ended in murder or a fatal accident seemed to have posttraumatic symptoms related to the previous personality's mode of death.

Claire Villarreal

See also: Buddhism; Hinduism.

Further Reading

Mills, Antonia and Richard Slobodin (eds.). *Amerindian Rebirth: Reincarnation Belief among North American Indians and Inuit.* Toronto: University of Toronto Press, 1993.

Stevenson, Ian. *Children Who Remember Previous Lives: A Question of Reincarnation.* Jefferson, NC: McFarland, 2001.

RELIGION

Death and destiny have long been associated with ritual behavior, beliefs, places, leaders, and often with supernatural figures, which have all, at one time or another, and in different social contexts, been described as "religion." This notion of religion solidified during the 19th century as part of what became known as the "comparative study of religion." Some scholars see this term as the outcome of Western societies that differentiate religion from much else in a society's economic, political, or kinship life; others argue that religion is absent from some cultures and should not, therefore, be imposed upon them. Smith (1963), for example, demonstrated how the word "religion," and its Latin and European derivatives, developed from classical times to the present; he concluded that the term "religion" should be replaced by the terms "cumulative tradition," covering various *cultural* phenomena, and "faith," encompassing *personal-emotional* factors.

Historically, religion became increasingly evident in large-scale, urban-focused societies where aspects of life had become differentiated from each other, such as work from home, public from private. Just as hospitals, doctors, and funeral directors professionalized sickness, death, and corpses, so churches, temples, and priests professionalized ideas of supernatural forces, human thriving, destiny, and death rites. Cities and nation states often witnessed religious phenomena complementing political institutions. Sometimes, the head of state was also the head of its religious institutions, as with the Dalai Lama in traditional Tibet, or the Queen and the Church of England. The Pope remains in a similar, albeit much reduced, status today.

Many see secularization, especially from the later 20th century in Western Europe, as a process in which religious institutions lose their wider influence and social significance, with matters of faith becoming a personal and private concern. At the same time, there has been a purported growth in diverse ritual and ideological routes to self-understanding, whereby religion becomes "de-differentiated" and synonymous with the term "spirituality," which was once restricted to descriptions of personal-emotional engagement within formal religious traditions, but which has now come to be used for this diverse search for self-discovery, whether religious or secular. By the 21st century, spirituality has become a serious matter within medical domains, such as palliative care, that engage with the ethical-emotional dimensions of the meaning people attach to their lives, especially in terms of end-of-life care and death. In some healthcare contexts, spiritual care workers have either replaced, or work alongside traditional clergy in providing pastoral support to the sick and dying.

Early anthropology (see **Anthropology**) approached religion as something that had evolved, and some anthropologists asked how it related to magic and science. In his classic book, *The Elementary Forms of the Religious Life,* Emile Durkheim (1912) developed the ideas of W. R. Smith on ancient sacrifice, arguing that communal rites integrated individuals within a unified community, including ancestors and deities, conferring a strength that elevated individuals above themselves. What people saw as God was, in Durkheim's view, a sense of society itself, and hence, religion, for Durkheim, was understood as the ritual worship of society and the values and institutions it cherished. Smith also influenced Sigmund Freud, who saw religion as an illusion in which the desire for security reached beyond that derived from human fathers into a belief in a supernatural divine father god.

Karl Marx had also seen religion as a device compensating for life in a heartlessly cold world; famously, as the "opium of the people," in which the poorest and most downtrodden in society were duped into accepting the injustices of capitalist society by the promise of a glorious and heavenly afterlife. Bronislaw Malinowski took funeral rites to be at the core of religion as a means of fostering hope amidst death and despair. Indeed, Malinowski believed the existential fear generated by the thought of death was the basis and origin for the emergence of religious belief itself. This emphasizes the fact that religions frequently provide the major means of dealing philosophically with death, and ritually with corpses, framing all with beliefs about the meaning of life and afterlife identity. Clifford Geertz produced a well-known cultural definition of religion as just such a system of symbols energizing emotional moods and motivations for living and creating both an explanation of the reality of life and a sense of its utter uniqueness. Not dissimilarly, American sociologist of religion, Milton Yinger (1970, 7), has provided a functional and inclusive definition of religion, as "a system of beliefs and practices by means of which a group of people struggles with the ultimate problems of human life," in which we can include death and serious illness. However, the religion that makes identity and destiny so real to some believers that it constitutes salvation can, correspondingly, make them devalue other religions as not "as real'" or true (Davies, 1984). This is certainly the case with Scientology, which is often derided in its attempt to be defined as a "religion."

Since death, funeral rites, and afterlife destiny have been so central to many religious traditions, it is interesting that, today, some funeral rites and ideological explanations of life are provided by secular, humanist, or nonreligious agencies. The same could be said for the era of the Soviet Union or The People's Republic of China. This highlights the profound difficulties in attempting to define "religion," for if "religion" majors on conducting funeral rites and the articulation of core values around them, we may well ask if this makes secular rites count as "religious"?

Many would object to this, arguing that some reference to supernatural agents is necessary for inclusion in the "religious" category.

Explanations as to the power of belief in supernatural agents have recently come from cognitive science and evolutionary biology, focusing on the human propensity to see reasons for events, and to read intention and active agency in the environment, even where none exists (Boyer, 2001). Another view—based on the psychology of trauma—defines "two modes" of religion (Whitehouse, 2004): the "doctrinal" mode of explicit ideas learned in formal ways and spread through missionary teaching to many peoples, and the "imagistic" mode arising amongst a small group, whose deep emotional and painful initiation ceremonies become embedded in a person's memory. As with traumatic events of war or catastrophe, such times are experienced as what psychologists call "flashbulb memories": they are vividly experienced yet seldom discussed and have no doctrinal scheme but possess great power to bind followers together. Restricted to small groups, this "imagistic" mode is not suited for widespread missionary "teaching."

What is obvious is that religious traditions, and their secular counterparts, influence and manage people's emotional lives and group identity, seeking to bring meaning and hope amidst potential confusion and despair, most especially surrounding death and human destiny (Davies, 2011).

Douglas J. Davies

See also: Afterlife Beliefs; Buddhism; Catholicism; Christianity; Cults; Heaven; Hell; Hinduism; Islam; Judaism; Protestantism; Purgatory; Spirituality; Totemism.

Further Reading

Boyer, P. *Religion Explained.* London: W. Heinemann, 2001.
Brennan, M. "Explaining Religion." *Sociology Review,* 20(3) (2011): 30–3.
Davies, D.J. *Emotion, Identity, and Religion: Hope, Reciprocity and Otherness.* Oxford: Oxford University Press, 2011.
Davies, D.J. *Meaning and Salvation in Religious Studies.* Leiden: Brill, 1984.
Durkheim, E. *The Elementary Forms of the Religious Life.* London: Nesbitt, 1912.
Geertz, C. "Religion as a Cultural System." In *Anthropological Approaches to the Study of Religion,* edited by M. Banton (pp. 1–46). London: Tavistock Press, 1973/1966.
Malinowski, B. *Magic, Science, and Religion.* London: Souvenir Press, 1974/1948.
McCutcheon, R.T. *The Discipline of Religion: Structure, Meaning, Rhetoric.* London: Routledge, 2003.
Smith. W.C. *The Meaning and End of Religion.* New York: Macmillan, 1963.
Tylor, E.B. *Primitive Culture.* Cambridge: Cambridge University Press, 2010/1871.
Whitehouse, H. *Modes of Religiosity.* New York: Altamira Press, 2004.
Yinger, J.M. *The Scientific Study of Religion.* New York: Macmillan, 1970.

RIGHT-TO-DIE MOVEMENT

The right-to-die movement is made up of number of individuals, organizations, and groups who have advocated in favor of the legalization of voluntary euthanasia and the individual's right to refuse life-sustaining medical treatment, especially in circumstances in which a person's quality of life is so radically diminished, that preservation of that life is considered as merely prolonging suffering. Sometimes also referred to as the dignity-in-death movement, campaigners have asserted the individual's right to die in a dignified, peaceful, and pain-free manner as a fundamental human right underscored by choice, freedom, and autonomy in ways that are uniquely modern. The assertion of these rights can be understood in both a "positive" sense, as the entitlement *to* something (in this instance, the right to self-determination and to choose to end one's own life); as well as in a "negative" sense, as the right to noninterference in the realm of personal activities by some external agency such as the state (in this case, the right *not* to have one's life maintained artificially and against one's wishes).

While the end of 20th and the beginning of the 21st century has seen an upsurge in activities and publicity surrounding the right-to-die movement, its origin can be traced to the early part of the 20th century and the establishment, first, of the Voluntary Euthanasia Society (VES) in Great Britain in 1935, followed in 1938 by the founding of the Euthanasia Society of America. Eclipsed by the events of World War II and its aftermath, the activities of right-to-die campaigners waned until the 1950s and 1960s, when the development of new life-sustaining medical technology raised ethical questions about the desirability of artificially preserving human life in circumstances where cognitive and neurological activities had betrayed it.

It was, however, the landmark legal ruling and controversy surrounding the case of Karen Ann Quinlan in 1975 that served to energize and provide a focus for the right-to-die movement. Quinlan, who at the age of 21, had been found in her bed not breathing after a night at a local bar, was admitted to a New Jersey hospital, where she remained in a coma and unresponsive for several months, her breathing and nutrition sustained artificially, until her parents requested that hospital authorities withdraw her life support. Hospital officials, however, refused this request and the case reached the New Jersey Supreme Court, who set a legal precedent by ruling that artificial respiration could be withdrawn. In the years that followed, other high-profile legal cases such as that of Nancy Beth Cruzan and Terri Schiavo, not only highlighted the need for advance directives (see **Advance Directives**)—indicating an individual's desire to refuse medical intervention should they be unable to communicate their wishes following permanent brain injury and impairment—but galvanized right-to-die campaigners in their pursuit of legal reform and drive to influence public opinion.

By the 1990s, there were an array of advocacy and lobby groups providing information and support to those who wished to terminate their own lives, notably The Hemlock Society, founded in 1980 by Derek Humphry, and Exit International, established in 1997 following repeal of the first law in the world legalizing voluntary euthanasia (the Rights of the Terminally Ill Act) in the Northern Territories of Australia by the Federal Parliament in Canberra. It was also in the 1990s that the right-to-die movement received widespread media attention through the activities of Dr. Jack Kevorkian, the Michigan pathologist who had famously helped terminally ill patients to die and was later imprisoned for second-degree murder (see **Kevorkian, Jack**).

Today, a range of activist groups providing legal counsel and expert advice on how to end one's own life, sponsoring opinion polls, and lobbying for legal reform exist throughout the United States, Great Britain, and Australia. The Hemlock Society, which became known as End of Life Choices in 2003, and later merged with Compassion in Dying in 2005 to form Compassion and Choices, claims some 60,000 supporters across the United States.

The right-to-die movement has not been without its detractors and critics, most notably the religious right, whose arguments stand in diametric opposition, and for whom the choice as to when and how we die can only be made by God alone.

The success of the right-to-die movement can be measured by the extent to which it has managed not only to raise voluntary euthanasia and assisted dying as issues of public debate, but also by the impact it has had on affecting legal reform in states like Oregon, Washington, and Montana, where physician-assisted suicide is permitted under certain circumstances. Its success can also be measured by the extent to which issues that were once somewhat marginal have fully entered the mainstream, as seen in widely aired television documentaries such as the 2006 film *The Suicide Tourist,* the 2010 PBS Frontline documentary *Facing Death,* and the 2011 BBC documentary *Choosing to Die,* featuring British author and advocate of the right-to-die, Terry Pratchett. In the decades to come, as the proportion of the aged population within Western societies grows and the number of individuals suffering from Alzheimer's disease increases, debates surrounding the right-to-die are certain to intensify.

Michael Brennan

See also: Alzheimer's Disease; Death Awareness Movement; Dignitas; Euthanasia; Good Death; Physician-Assisted Suicide.

Further Reading

Compassion and Choices: www.compassionandchoices.org

Dignity in Dying: www.dignityindying.org.uk

Exit International: www.exitinternational.net

Hillyard, Daniel and John Dombrink. *Dying Right: The Death with Dignity Movement.* London: Routledge, 2001.

Humphry, Derek and Mary Clement. *Freedom to Die: People, Politics and the Right to Die Movement.* New York: St. Martin's Press, 2000.

Woodman, Sue. *Last Rights: The Struggle over the Right to Die.* Cambridge, MA: Perseus Publishing, 2001.

RIGOR MORTIS

Rigor mortis is the postmortem contraction of skeletal muscles fixing the joints in place and making limbs stiff and difficult to move. This phenomenon is temporary and occurs anywhere from one to several hours after death, lasting up to 72 hours depending upon the person's age, sex, physical condition, and muscular build. This explains why rigor mortis is less pronounced in infants, children, and people who have been confined to bed for long periods of time, and who have smaller muscle mass. Rigor mortis is caused by hardening of the muscular tissues as a consequence of muscles being deprived of adenosine triphosphate (ATP). This condition is temporary and disappears gradually as muscle protein begins to decompose. Knowledge of the progression of rigor mortis can be very useful for pathologists and forensic investigators in attempting to determine the approximate time of death and amount of time that has lapsed since death. Rigor mortis usually follows a downward progression that usually begins in the involuntary muscles of the eye, then moves to the face, neck, upper extremities, trunk, and then lower extremities. This pattern of rigor is known as Nysten's law, after a French pediatrician named Pierre-Hubert Nysten, who recorded his observation that rigor mortis follows a particular pattern of progression. This principle likely reflects the fact that rigor mortis, while affecting all muscles in the same way at the same time, becomes noticeable first in small muscle groups, such as those around the eyes, mouth, and jaws, and becomes pronounced somewhat later in the larger muscles of the lower limbs.

Michael Matthews

Further Reading

Iserson, Kenneth V. *Death to Dust: What Happens to Dead Bodies?* Tucson, AZ: Galen Press, 2001.

Stedman's Medical Dictionary, 26th edition. Philadelphia: Lippincott Williams and Wilkins, 1995.

S

SCHOOL SHOOTINGS

School shootings occur on a small scale, where individuals either in school or on school property are killed by firearms, or on a larger scale, when shooter(s) enter school property and shoots multiple victims. School shootings have been recorded since the 1800s, but in the past three decades, the media has made these occurrences more widely known. The federal government defines school violence as that which occurs on school property, on the way to or from school, or on the way to or from a school sponsored event. Despite media attention, the Centers for Disease Control and Prevention (CDC) reports that violent deaths at school (including shootings) accounted for less than 1 percent of the homicides and suicides among children aged 5–18. According to a 2010 report by the National Center for Education Statistics, "The percentage of youth homicides occurring at school remained at less than 2 percent of the total number of youth homicides, and the percentage of youth suicides occurring at school remained at less than 1 percent of the total number of youth suicides over all available survey years" (Robers et al., 2010, 6).

The CDC reports that 5 percent of students surveyed in 2009 admitted to having carried a weapon to school in the previous 30 days, and 7.7 percent of students in the same survey reported being threatened with a weapon at school in the previous 12 months. Rates of school-associated student homicides decreased between 1992 and 2006. Of these homicides, 65 percent were due to gunshot wounds. Rates were significantly higher for males, students in secondary schools, and students in central cities.

Even if students, faculty, and staff escape the bullets of the shooter, they can be affected by the shooting for years to come. Some report that they are anxious and unduly affected by popping noises. Others need to be treated for post-traumatic stress disorder (PTSD). Those who witness violence are often called "silent victims," and though they may be physically unaffected, can be emotionally harmed. School shootings are not limited to the United States nor are they confined to the past three decades. However, some of the most deadly include the following:

1966 Charles Whitman, a student at The University of Texas at Austin, climbed the University's tower, killing 3 people on the way up and 16 people from the top of the tower; 32 other people were wounded.

1989 An adult male, Marc Lepine, entered the Ecole Polytechnique in Montreal, Canada. He separated the male and female students and shot only the

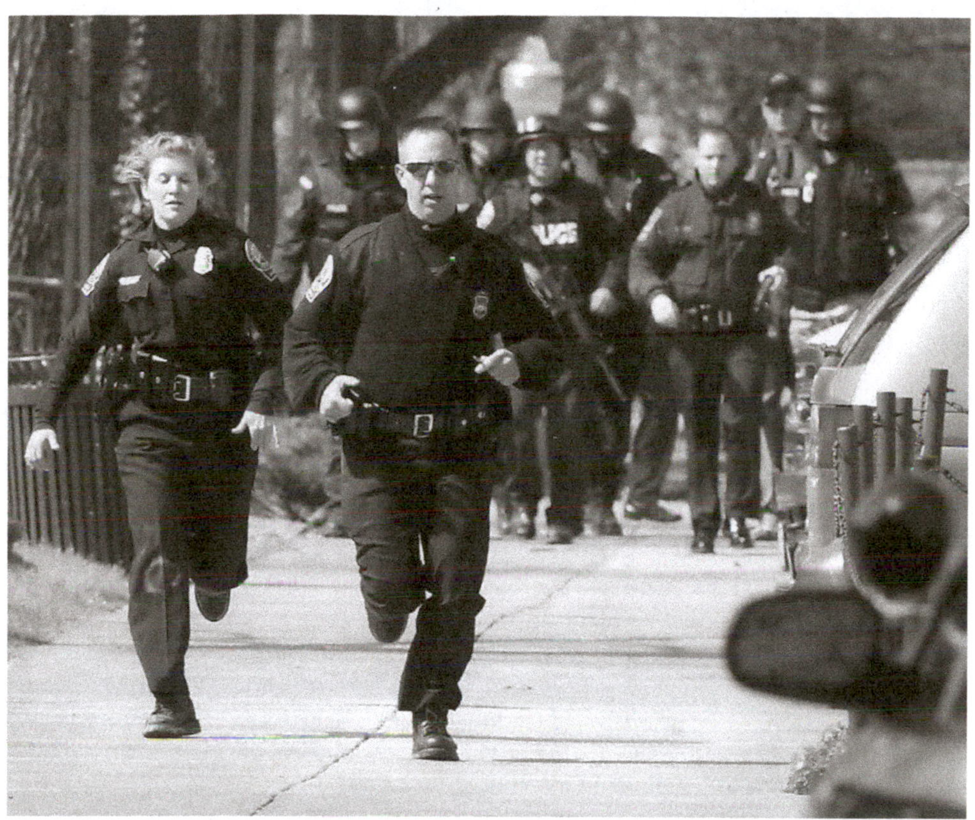

Police officers run from Norris Hall on the Virginia Tech campus to a classroom building across campus after learning that the shooter continued his rampage there in Blacksburg, Virginia, on April 16, 2007. (AP/Wide World Photos)

	women. He killed 14 women and injured 10 women before completing suicide.
1996	The Dunblane Primary School shooting in Scotland occurred during a first-year gym session. Sixteen children and a teacher were killed by an adult male, Thomas Hamilton, who later killed himself; 10 children were wounded in the attack.
1999	Columbine High School in Colorado was the site of a shooting spree by two students, Dylan Klebold and Eric Harris. By the end of the incident, both shooters, 12 other students, as well as 1 teacher had died. 23 students were wounded.
2002	Eighteen people died in Erfurt, Germany, when a student who had been expelled, Robert Steinhauser, fired upon students and teachers at the Gutenberg-Gymnasium Erfurt, a high school. 10 people were wounded.
2005	After killing his grandfather and his girlfriend, Jeff Weise, 16, drove to Red Lake Senior High School in Red Lake, Minnesota, and killed a teacher, an unarmed security guard, five students, and then himself, wounding five others.

2006 Charles Carl Roberts, an adult male, took students hostage in a one-room Amish schoolhouse and killed five female students and wounded five others before taking his own life.

2007 Seung-Ho Cho, a senior at Virginia Tech University, killed 32 people and wounded 25 others in two separate shooting sprees. He killed two students in a dormitory and then, two hours later, chained the entrance to Norris Hall shut and began shooting, killing 30 and wounding 15 people, before completing suicide.

2007 Pekka-Eric Auvinen, an 18-year-old student at Jokela High School in Tuusula, Finland, killed five boys, two girls, and the female principal of the school, wounding one other person. He shot himself and later died of his wounds in hospital.

2008 A student at the Kauhajoki School of Hospitality at Seinajoki University of Applied Sciences in Kauhajoki, Finland, fatally shot 10 people and then turned the gun on himself. One other student at the University was injured in the shooting.

2008 Stephen Kazmierczak, a former student at Northern Illinois University, opened fire in a University lecture hall, killing 5 students and then himself, wounding 17 others.

2009 A recent graduate of the Winnenden Secondary School in southwestern Germany, Tim Kretschemer, killed nine students and three teachers, as well as three other people after leaving the school. He then killed himself after police had wounded him.

2009 The Azerbaijan State Oil Academy, a university-level institution in Baku, Azerbaijan, was the scene of a shooting. Twelve students and staff members were killed by Farda Gadyrov, an adult male who killed himself as the police closed in. Several students were also wounded in the attack.

2011 In the first school shooting reported in Brazil, an armed adult male, Wellington Oliveira, shot 10 girls and 2 boys dead in an eighth-grade classroom at Tasso da Silveira Municipal School in Realengo, Brazil. Oliveira was a former student of the school. After police shot him, he completed suicide.

2012 On the morning of December 14, several days before Christmas break, 20-year-old Adam Lanza killed his mother at their family home, before driving some 5 miles to Sandy Hook Elementary School in Newtown, Connecticut, where, heavily armed with a semiautomatic rifle, he fatally wounded 20 children (some as young as 5 years old) and 6 adults, before eventually killing himself. This was the second deadliest mass shooting in American history, after the shooting at Virginia Tech University in 2007.

Preventing School Shootings

Though school shootings do receive a great deal of press, the United States Department of Education reports that school is one of the safest places for children and adolescents. The U.S. Secret Service's study, published in 2002, notes that the adults in students' lives (parents, teachers, school administrators, counselors, and coaches) can prevent violence on school grounds by monitoring and listening to what students are saying. The study found that students who planned to perpetrate a school shooting tell at least one person, often giving out specifics before the event takes place. The study also found that school shooters were rarely impulsive in their attacks.

Contrary to popular belief, there is not an accurate or useful profile for school shooters. In their study, the Secret Service determined that family situations, academic performance, mental disorder, or drug usage varied across perpetrators. Instead, they suggest that a student's behaviors are better indicators of possible violence. Most attackers had access to firearms. Bullying was often a factor in the decision to attack, though the report makes it clear that bullying is not a factor in every case, nor will every child who is bullied prove to be a risk.

School staff members were often those who stopped the attacker rather than law enforcement officers. The study calls for schools to work with law enforcement on both prevention and critical incident response plans. The report notes that warning signs are common—in more than half of the cases, at least one person was concerned about the shooter's behavior.

A significant problem in preventing targeted violence is determining how best to respond to students who are already known to be in trouble. This study indicates the importance of giving attention to students who are having difficulty coping with major losses or perceived failures, particularly when feelings of desperation and hopelessness are involved.

Explanations of School Shootings

School shootings affect communities for years after the actual event. A search on the Internet regarding any of the school shootings listed above usually results in recent commemorations of the event. Certainly, media outlets highlight the anniversaries of the most well-known events. School shootings cause both children and adults to pause—the latter feeling that they should protect their youngsters, and the former fearing that what should be a safe place no longer is.

After school shootings, the general public, as well as media organizations and professional groups, attempt to theorize about the cause of such violence. The availability of firearms, mental illness, bullying, video games, domestic abuse, "lax parenting," the media, and peer groups are all indicted. Others suggest that schools do not teach moral values and that this produces amoral people who are willing to sacrifice both their own lives and the lives of others. Yet, it is likely that a combination of some, or all of these factors, is responsible for each individual incident of school violence.

Jane Moore

Further Reading

Centers for Disease Control and Prevention. "School Associated Student Homicides, United States, 1992–2006." *MMWR*, 57(02) (2008): 33–36. http://www.cdc.gov/mmwr/preview/mmwrhtml/mm5702a1.htm

Centers for Disease Control and Prevention. "School-Associated Violent Death Study, 2010." http://www.cdc.gov/ViolencePrevention/youthviolence/schoolviolence/SAVD.html

Centers for Disease Control and Prevention. "Youth Risk Behavioral Surveillance, United States, 2011." *MMWR*, 61(4) (2012). http://www.cdc.gov/mmwr/pdf/ss/ss6104.pdf

Robers, S., J. Zhang, and J. Truman. "Indicators of School Crime and Safety, 2010." *National Center for Education Statistics, U.S. Department of Education, and Bureau of Justice of Statistics.* Office of Justice Programs, U.S. Department of Justice. Washington, DC, 2010. http://nces.ed.gov/pubs2011/2011002.pdf

U.S. Secret Service. "Preventing School Shootings: A Summary of a U.S. Secret Service School Initiative Report." *National Institute of Justice Journal*, 248 (2002): 11–15.

SEX AND DEATH

Although seemingly unlikely bedfellows, the links between sex and death are perhaps more common than first thought. As heavily taboo topics, Geoffrey Gorer's (1955) essay, "The Pornography of Death," drew attention to the way in which death in the 20th century had replaced sex in the 19th as a subject that was smothered in prudery, a source of fantasized and voyeuristic titillation that bore little resemblance to the real thing and had thus become "pornographic." Elsewhere, in "Beyond the Pleasure Principle," Sigmund Freud (1920) postulated the idea that the unconscious desire manifested in sexual activity for self-preservation (and that of the species as a whole) was undercut by a competing desire for self-destruction, a struggle represented in the poetic metaphor between Eros (the Greek God of life and love) and Thanatos (the Greek God of death).

Further examples of the link between sex and death can be found in the anecdotal evidence presented by some historians of sexual arousal among males engaged in face-to-face killing—a very literal form of "bloodlust." It can be found too in evidence of the desire for greater sexual intimacy in the face of destruction and annihilation provided by warfare and terrorism. Grounded in terror management theory (see **Terror Management Theory**), recent research in this area suggests that as awareness of death (mortality salience) increases, so too does the desire for sexual activity and the likelihood of sexual risk taking. In what has been termed by some as "terror sex," research has also indicated an increase in unprotected sex among gay and bisexual men in the aftermath of 9/11.

Further connections between sex and death can be found in research that suggests a link between extended life expectancy and those who not only remain sexually active in later life but who report greater frequency of orgasms. It can be found too in recent research by U.S. scientists, which suggests that children with older fathers and grandfathers appear "genetically programmed" to live longer. In the opposite direction, the link between sex and premature death is dramatically illustrated in sub-Saharan Africa, where sexually contracted HIV/AIDS is the leading cause of death among females aged 15–49.

Finally, the link between sex and death can also be found in recent bioethical debates surrounding posthumous pregnancies using the cryopreservation of spermatozoa.

Michael Brennan

Further Reading

Freud, Sigmund. "Beyond the Pleasure Principle." In *The Standard Edition of the Complete Psychological Works of Sigmund Freud,* edited by James Strachey, Vol. 18 (pp. 1–64). London: Hogarth Press, 1955/1920.

Gorer, Geoffrey. "The Pornography of Death." *Encounter,* October, 1955. (This is available in the appendix of Geoffrey Gorer's *Death, Grief and Mourning.* Garden City, NY: Doubleday, 1965).

SOCIAL CLASS

Death is often referred to as the "great leveler" in that one of the few facts of life is that we must all die. There are, however, many factors that will influence the nature and timing of death, and social class is one such factor in that it affects life experiences, health and access to medicine, and health care services. Social class refers to social divisions in society whereby people who share the same socioeconomic status, share the same social class position. Almost all societies have some form of social stratification that separates people according to hierarchies of status. For example, the caste system in India is a form of social stratification. In modern Western societies, despite a commitment to equality in the eyes of the law, there are clear social divisions that give people different access to goods and services that effectively result in disparities in lifestyle, for example, in terms of access to health care, hospice, and funeral services.

An understanding of social class is important as it provides insights into power and inequality in societies, as well as to cultural distinctions that affect behavior and people's life experiences. Despite the fact that there is no clearly agreed-upon definition of the concept, social class divisions are largely based on access to power in society and are influenced by education, occupation, and income. In the United Kingdom, for example, when referring to social class, sociologists tend to rely on the Registrar General's categorization that divides society into socioeconomic groups ranging from Social Class I—professional—to Social Class V—unskilled occupations. Social class affects life experiences of housing, choices of regional location, geographical and social mobility, the nature of schooling (private or public and well or poorly resourced schools), educational qualifications, and occupation. There are also cultural factors and traditions associated with different socioeconomic groups that may be significant in guiding behavior, with individuals from lower socioeconomic groups thought to be more likely to smoke and to be involved in high-risk behavior.

Studies that have focused on the impact of health and social inequality on mortality rates have shown that economic factors are central to the understanding of inequalities in mortality. People in the lower social classes have a reduced life expectancy compared to those in higher social classes. In the United Kingdom, for example, men in the professional classes can, on average, expect to live almost 10 years longer than those in the manual classes. Explanations for these differences can be found in the greater life chances and better quality of life for people in higher socioeconomic groups. For example, members of lower classes are more at risk of workplace accidents and related diseases such as asbestosis. A lower life expectancy rate for this group is also associated with poor living conditions, environmental hazards, and the greater likelihood of dying suddenly or in violent circumstances.

In singling out the importance of social class for mortality, it is worth remembering that the effects of social class, and those that are related to experiences of ethnicity, are sometimes difficult to separate. Both are factors commonly associated with low life expectancy and premature death. For minority ethnic groups in Western societies, socioeconomic conditions may be even more damaging to health than those experienced solely as a result of social class position. For example, Aboriginal peoples living in Australia have an average life expectancy that is much lower than that of their white Australian counterparts. In the U.S., Native Americans, rural African Americans, and the inner city poor have levels of health more commonly associated with those living in developing countries, and white women in the U.S. live, on average, five years longer than black women.

In the context of death and dying, cultural practices associated with social class distinction impact on experiences of dying, funeral, and memorial beliefs and practices, as well as on ways of grieving and remembering the dead. Historical research that has considered social class differences in death and dying traditions includes the work of David Vincent, who, in 1980, published an article entitled, "Love and death in the nineteenth-century working class." This was based on his research of autobiographical accounts that explored experiences of love and death among working-class people in England during the 19th century. His findings were that working-class people could scarcely afford the luxury of intense emotion occasioned by the loss of someone close to them, and he concluded that the loss of a family member was so bound up with the potential loss of his income or his work within the home, that it simply exacerbated and intensified the misery of their everyday existence. Research into working class experiences of death and bereavement in Britain in the 19th century was extended by Julie-Marie Strange in 2005 when she produced a detailed description of some of the experiences of the working class poor. She demonstrated that social and cultural influences structure people's experiences of grief and showed that working-class cultures in the United Kingdom differed substantially from more prosperous middle-class experiences. For example, funerals in the 19th century could be extremely elaborate affairs for the higher social classes, often involving mutes (professional mourners), feathermen (who would carry black, dyed ostrich feathers), and pages, as well as ornate hearses for transporting the coffin accompanied by black-clad mourners in the funeral procession. The cost and nature of the funeral demonstrated the social class of the deceased person and her family, and as such, were used as a means of displaying status and power in society. At the other extreme was the pauper funeral that entailed anonymous burial in a mass grave. As the concern over funeral extravagance increased, the middle classes began to criticize the poor for their "unreasonable" expenditure on funerals and developed a stereotype of a working class who would rather see their children starve than undergo a pauper burial.

The distinction in funeral and mourning practices during the 20th century was highlighted in 1950 by the sociologist W. M. Kephart, who published a paper entitled "Status after Death" that explored social class variations in funeral preferences in the city of Philadelphia, Pennsylvania. His survey demonstrated significant differences between the behavioral patterns of upper and lower social class groups, with the middle classes falling somewhere in between the two, having few distinctive patterns. Kephart found that cremation was more popular among the upper classes and was rarely used by those from the lower classes. He also found that people in the lower social classes spent a greater percentage of their income on funerals compared with those in other classes, but that they were more likely to have taken out life insurance to pay for the costs. He also found that the time from death to the funeral was shorter among the upper classes; that viewing of the deceased's body, and comments on its appearance, were more likely by lower class groups. The lower classes were also more likely to display their emotions openly and to purchase flowers, particularly set piece formations such as "bleeding hearts," "clocks" or "gates," and wreathes with phrases such as "beloved father."

More recently, the importance of working-class experiences of bereavement have been a focus of research by Chris Allen. As a sociologist of crime and deviance, Allen's research into heroin use in deprived urban areas highlighted the issue of how working-class people coped with the intense feelings of grief that might follow bereavement. Like many previous studies, he found what was described as a stoical approach to coping with grief that entailed trying to put the loss to one side because of the need to get on with the struggles of day-to-day life.

Other research into social class has tended to focus on upper and middle-class experiences of death and bereavement. These studies are important in furthering our understanding of the values, belief systems, and cultural mores surrounding the experiences of higher social groups. Regrettably, they are sometimes presented as a model or framework for understanding the meanings that people from all social classes construct around their engagement with death and they often, erroneously, suggest that the experiences and behaviors of people in the higher social classes "filter down the social ladder."

Glennys Howarth

Further Reading

Allen, Chris. "The Poverty of Death: Social Class, Urban Deprivation, and the Criminological Consequences of Sequestration of Death." *Mortality,* 12(1) (2007): 79–93.

SOCIAL DEATH

The term social death describes the process of marginalization and isolation experienced by the long-term sick and dying, whereby they are rendered *socially dead* even before actual physical death occurs. The concept is most closely associated with David Sudnow (1967), who, in his classic ethnographic study *Passing On*, analyzed the social relations between those who were dying, their loved ones, and health care providers within the institutional context of the modern hospital. The core idea, in which the dying are screened off from others, socially shunned, and treated as already dead by the rest of society, gave impetus to the newly emerging hospice movement in the 1960s and its powerful critique of modern health care, which, it argued, had effectively turned the natural process of dying into a medical event to which the dying were no longer privy. Key elements comprising the social death include the process by which the dying are excluded from communications; removed from public gaze by their transfer to terminal hospital wards; and treated with awkwardness, embarrassment, or as social lepers. Elaborations of the concept of social death can also be found in texts that have become classics within the field of death studies, such as Glaser and Strauss's (1965) famous study of "awareness contexts," Elisabeth Kübler-Ross's best-selling book *On Death and Dying* (1969), and Norbert Elias's *The Loneliness of the Dying* (1985).

Michael Brennan

See also: Awareness Contexts; Death Awareness Movement; Hospice Movement; Kübler-Ross, Elisabeth.

Further Reading

Glaser, Barney G. and Anselm L. Strauss. *Awareness of Dying*. Chicago: Aldine, 1965.
Sudnow, David. *Passing On: The Social Organization of Dying*. Englewood Cliffs, NJ: Prentice-Hall, 1967.

SOCIOLOGY

Sociology is defined as the scientific study of society. The term itself has been widely attributed to Auguste Comte (1798–1857), and combines the Latin word *socius* (meaning companion) with the Greek word *logos* (meaning the study of). Comte also referred to sociology as a "social physics," and it is this that gives some clue to sociology as the study of the dynamics underpinning *social relations*. Originating in France in the mid to late 1800s, it shares much in common with other social science disciplines such as psychology and anthropology, each underscored by the pursuit of evidence-based knowledge grounded in the scientific method. It is commonly taught at universities across the United States and throughout the world, and has spawned a number of specialty subdisciplines, including the sociology of death.

Structure/Agency

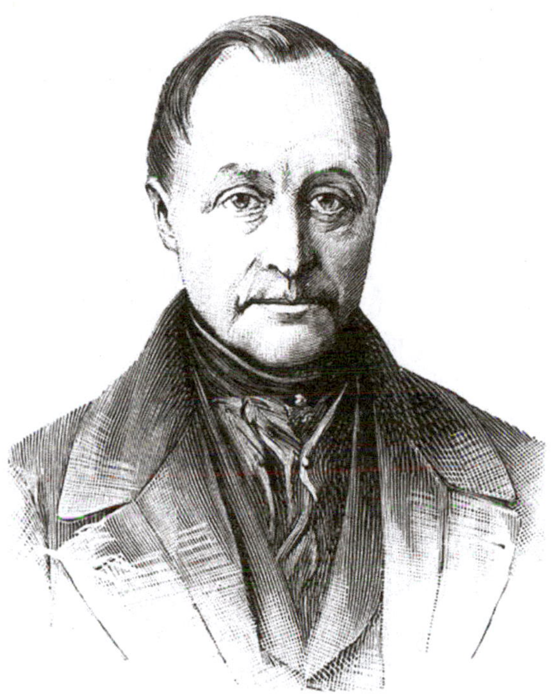

A brilliant polymath, Auguste Comte was a leader of the scientific intellectualism movement of the 19th century. He is best known for developing the philosophy of positivism and for coining the term sociology. (Library of Congress)

One of the key debates within sociology is the extent to which human behavior is shaped either by factors external to a person (social structure) or as a result of individual choice (human agency). This dualism, in which there are two competing ways of viewing the same phenomenon (in this case human behavior), has characterized sociology since its inception and is commonly known as the structure/agency debate. On the one hand, we could argue, for example, that society is made up of social structures that influence behavior, such as religion, education, politics, and the economy. Culture itself, with its commensurate set of unwritten social norms, can be seen as part of this social structure, whereby customs, traditions, and values help determine and shape the decisions we make as individuals. On the other hand, we could say that individuals have "agency" in that they can determine their own life, independent of socially sanctioned customs and traditions. When it comes to understanding death from a sociological perspective, one of the issues routinely explored is the extent to which cultural expectations and practices associated with dying and bereavement are shaped by society or come from individuals themselves. In terms of making sense of this disjuncture between control and free will, sociologists are often drawn to concerns about the exercise of power and distribution of resources in society.

Social Inequality

Sociologists are particularly interested in social inequality, also referred to as "social divisions" or social stratification. These divisions can be seen in terms of gender, age, race, ethnicity, class, education, religion, and sexuality. On the surface, it is apparent that these factors will influence peoples' experiences of death, dying, and bereavement. For example, older people are more likely to die and/or suffer bereavement through losing members of their peer group, while people with different religious beliefs will understand and mark someone's death differently.

Issues related to socioeconomic status, such as income, social deprivation, and the impact these may have on experiences of death, dying, and bereavement, have however been largely overlooked by many sociologists specializing in this area. There is recent evidence that this trend is now beginning to turn, with a growing awareness of the disparity in mortality rates among people from different socioeconomic backgrounds (see also **Mortality Rates**). Data released by the Congressional Budget Office in 2008 suggests that individuals from the highest socioeconomic group can expect to live 4.5 years longer than people from the lowest socioeconomic group. Similar inequalities in life expectancy are repeated in terms of gender and race. Here, data from the Center for Health Statistics indicate that in 2007 whites in the United States could expect to live 4.8 years longer than blacks (78.4 to 73.6 years), and that women could expect to live 5 years longer than men (80.4 to 75.4 years). Sociologists have explained these differences in mortality by pointing to the *social determinants of health:* factors, including poverty, education, occupation, income, and lifestyle choices, which determine our health as well as how long we can expect to live.

The Sociology of Death

Until fairly recently, sociology has typically been overlooked as making a significant contribution to debates about death, dying, and bereavement, with psychology and anthropology regarded as being the dominant contributory disciplines to this field (see **Anthropology; Psychology**). This, however, neglects the very substantial contribution that sociologists have made to the study of death and dying. For example, sociologists have been closely engaged in debates involving the removal of death from public life in modern Western societies (referred to as "sequestration"); the extent to which death is—if at all—still a taboo within contemporary society (see **Taboo**); and the social dynamics surrounding public mourning, public dying, and a host of other socially relevant issues connected with death, grief, and bereavement. Additionally, death has been central to the development of sociology as an academic discipline.

Durkheim and Suicide

One of the founders of sociology was Emile Durkheim (1858–1917), whose systematic study of suicide rates in different European countries at the turn of the 19th century became a classic and seminal piece of sociological theory and research. This study was important in demonstrating that there were *social* and not just psychological factors influencing a person's decision to take his own life. By comparing statistics on suicide from across a variety of European countries, Durkheim was able to demonstrate particular patterns underlying aspects of human behavior. One such pattern was that Protestants had consistently higher rates of suicide than Catholics. Durkheim inferred from this that lower levels of social integration among Protestants than Catholics (whose life revolved around the community of the Church) may well have been a contributory factor in their higher rates of suicide. In this study, Durkheim was effectively establishing the comparative method as a cornerstone of sociological theory and practice.

Research Methods

The study of death by sociologists has also made a significant contribution to the development of contemporary research methods within the social sciences more generally. In the 1960s, Barney Glaser and Anselm Strauss developed the idea of "awareness contexts" (see **Awareness Contexts**). As a contribution to qualitative research (the in-depth investigation of small-group behavior), Glaser and Strauss's work demonstrated the productive relationship between theory and methods through their development of "grounded theory," whereby theory is developed not in abstraction but on the basis of empirical research.

Recent Sociological Work

Since the 1990s, there has been a growth in sociological work on death and dying. Some of the innovative research to emerge has looked at near-death experiences and the afterlife; other research has examined the ethics associated with life and death from a social perspective, such as brain death and organ transplantation. Sociologists have also been working with specialists in public health to explore the delivery of palliative care to communities. As the study of society, and everything it comprises, the scope and focus of sociology is very wide ranging.

Interconnectedness

Overall, it is important to recognize that these discipline-specific contributions to the study of death are not mutually exclusive, and that sociology and sociological insight should not be regarded in isolation from the rest of the social sciences. Rather, the growth of the academic study of death is interdisciplinary and has come from scholars working in a wide range of disciplines who have integrated and developed theoretical insights from their own respective fields.

Kate Woodthorpe and Michael Brennan

See also: Anthropology; Psychology; Thanatology.

Further Reading

Allen, Chris. "The Poverty of Death: Social Class, Urban Deprivation and the Criminological Consequences of Sequestration of Death." *Mortality,* 12(1) (2007): 79–93.

Brennan, Mike. "Death and Dying." *Sociology Review,* 14(3) (2005): 26–28.

Congressional Budget Office. Economic and Budget Issue Brief: Growing Disparities in Life Expectancy, April 17, 2008. http://www.cbo.gov/sites/default/files/cbofiles/ftpdocs/91xx/doc9104/04–17-lifeexpectancy_brief.pdf

Howarth, Glennys. *Death and Dying: A Sociological Introduction.* Cambridge: Polity Press, 2007.

Kellehear, Allan. "Dying as a Social Relationship: A Sociological Review of Debates on the Determination of Death." *Social Science & Medicine,* 66(7) (2008): 1533–44.

National Center for Health Statistics. Health, United States, 2010: with Special Feature on Death and Dying, 2011. http://www.cdc.gov/nchs/data/hus/hus10.pdf#specialfeature

Walter, Tony. "The Sociology of Death." *Sociology Compass,* 2(1) (2008): 317–36.

SPIRITUALITY

At the end of the 18th century, Christian theologians began to think about religion as an innate human capacity that was separate from doctrines and religious institutions. It seemed to them that religious doctrines and institutions had been the cause of the wars that had ravaged the continent for hundreds of years. These theologians wanted an individual faith without the problematic superstructure of organized religion. In 1799, Friedrich Schleiermacher defined religion as a "feeling" of surrender to the "Whole," of absolute dependence, or "sense and taste for the Infinite."

At the turn of the 20th century, William James, one of the founders of American psychology, defined religion as the feelings, acts, and experiences of individuals "in their solitude, so far as they apprehend themselves to stand in relation to whatever they may consider the divine."

Both definitions leave open the question of what God, or the gods do *for,* or want *from,* humans. Religion is what humans *do,* not what clergy or religious institutions *say* it is. Indeed, God or gods were not necessary for religion in these definitions. The problem, of course, was that religion already had a definition. Existing religions, such as Christianity, Islam, Judaism, Buddhism, Hinduism, and so on, had traditions, institutions, teachings, and rules that did not depend upon an individual's feelings or actions to be what they were.

Europeans and Americans thus searched for a term that would refer *only* to the innate capacity, not to institutions or doctrine. For the first two-thirds of the 20th century, Evelyn Underhill's use of the term *mysticism* was used by scholars and philosophers to refer to the journey full of ecstasy and agony that individuals take to find direct experience of what Underhill called "the Absolute." Mysticism could be like music: in each generation there are virtuosos who can create and express the full depth of the art, but the rest of us, some more than others, can appreciate as we listen, and perhaps in our limited way, make music ourselves.

By the closing decades of the 20th century, the use of the term mysticism waned. Contemporary people have little taste for agony in the quest for meaning, and ecstasy was associated with the secular pursuit of extreme experiences, often using psychedelic and hallucinatory drugs. Still, more and more people did not feel connected to institutions in the culture (Putnam, 2000). Further, mysticism seemed to demand withdrawal from everyday life and years of disciplined dedication. A new word was needed and *spirituality* appeared to be it.

The new definition of spirituality was rapidly taken into the emergent interest in death and dying in the last decades of the 20th century. Because spirituality was not necessarily about God or the objects of faith, the concept could be used in the new hospice movement (see also **Hospice Movement; Palliative Care**) to cover the spiritual needs of any dying patient, no matter their cultural or religious heritage. The term could be associated with early concepts in the study of death and dying. For example, Elisabeth Kübler-Ross described "acceptance," the last of her five stages of dying, as a spiritual state. She contrasted "acceptance" to "resignation," which she did not consider to be spiritual.

Just as in the early theories of religion, which treated it as an innate human capacity, the actual content of spirituality is not so important or easy to define. Indeed, there is no agreement on what thoughts, feelings, or behaviors comprise spirituality. When Unruh, Versnel, and Kerr (2002) surveyed as many empirical and clinical studies as they could find which focused on "spirituality," they discovered 92 definitions that could, with some difficulty, be assigned to seven general categories.

Nevertheless, as Lucy Bregman notes, the term spirituality fills an important niche in the contemporary Western worldview, which she describes as "a glowing and useful term in search of a meaning." As participation in civic and political organizations has declined, and individuals come to define themselves increasingly through, or in relation to, mass market products or entertainment, spirituality is a good way to describe our sense and taste for the "Infinite" in those moments that connect us with whatever we may consider the divine.

Dennis Klass

See also: Kübler-Ross, Elisabeth; Religion.

Further Reading

Bregman, L. *Death and Dying, Spirituality and Religions.* New York: Peter Lang Publishing, 2003.

Bregman, L. *The Ecology of Spirituality.* Waco, TX: Baylor University Press, forthcoming 2014.

Bregman, L. "Spirituality: A Glowing and Useful Term in Search of a Meaning." *Omega, Journal of Death and Dying,* 53(1/2) (2006): 5–26.

James, W. *The Varieties of Religious Experience: A Study in Human Nature.* New York: Random House, 1994/1902.

Putnam, R. D. *Bowling Alone: The Collapse and Revival of American Community.* New York: Simon & Schuster, 2000.

Schleiermacher, F. *On Religion: Speeches to Its Cultured Despisers.* New York: Harper and Row, 1958/1799.

Underhill, E. *Mysticism: A Study of the Nature and Development of Man's Spiritual Consciousness.* New York: Dutton, 1930.

Unruh, A., J. Versnel, and N. Kerr. "Spirituality Unplugged: A Review of Commonalities and Contentions, and a Resolution." *Canadian Journal of Occupational Therapy,* 69(1) Feb. (2002): 5–19.

SPONTANEOUS SHRINES/ ROADSIDE MEMORIALS

The placing of flowers, cards, and mementos as a response to fatal crashes, disasters, or tragedies is a familiar sight. These are recognizable communal responses to tragedy and are often referred to as spontaneous shrines. These shrines express attempts to make a catastrophe, on either a large or small scale, more manageable. This form of public mourning was evident for Diana, Princess of Wales in 1997, and following the terrorist attacks of September 11, 2001, as well as other tragedies (see also **Public Mourning**). They facilitate a broader response from a larger public audience, beyond family and friends, as anyone can add a token if they wish. Creating these shrines can help give people a sense of purpose and they often emerge swiftly, sometimes within hours of the event, and may only remain in place for a short period of time.

Roadside memorials, in the form of flowers, cards, mementos, or crosses, are a form of a spontaneous shrine in response to a sudden death on the road, but are generally placed by people connected to the person who has died rather than the public at large. These memorials make grief very visible and can be of great importance to bereaved families and friends, marking the place where their loved ones lost their life, and serving as powerful reminders of tragic intimate experiences, even though they are in public places. While they generally mark motor vehicle accidents, some also mark suicides, deaths by drowning, and other tragic deaths.

Unlike the form of spontaneous shrine that emerges as a form of public mourning, and which remain for just a short period of time, some roadside memorials become a more permanent fixture. These memorials have been documented throughout Europe, Canada, Australia, and North and South America. In some countries, they seem to be a relatively new phenomenon, particularly so in Australia, where they do not appear to have been present prior to the 1980s. Elsewhere, they seem to be part of a continuing tradition, and probably a Roman Catholic tradition, of remembering the dead and marking death in open places.

Roadside memorials can be deeply personal sites of remembrance and may provide a continuing connection with the deceased (see also **Continuing Bonds**). For some family members and friends, the place of death and the site of the memorial have become the locations where the living may feel closest to the deceased and may become a type of sacred place and a site of pilgrimage, being visited and maintained for months or years. There is evidence that many roadside memorials are revisited on holidays, the birthday of the deceased, and the anniversary of the death—for example, during Christmas, memorials may be draped with tinsel or hung with seasonal decorations.

Roadside memorials and spontaneous shrines also serve as an effective warning for road users of the dangers of the road. A U.K. charity, RoadPeace, dedicated to supporting bereaved and injured crash victims, developed a program of providing standardized memorials to be placed by friends or family of someone killed on the road. This program—"Remember Me"—has erected over 2,000 markers since its launch on August 31, 2003. These markers are black A4 size (approximately 11 inches × 8 inches) signs depicting a red anemone flower and are intended to be noticeable, nondenominational reminders of the dangers on the roads. In the United States, Mothers Against Drunk Driving (MADD) have erected roadside memorials to those who have died, especially as a result of drunk driving. Families involved in the erection of roadside memorials saw part of their purpose as that of educating the public about the dangers of a particular road, with the memorial serving as a warning to other road users.

Newer forms of roadside memorials are now emerging, for example, a Ghost Bike campaign began in St. Louis, MO, in 2003 to mark a place where a cyclist was struck by a car. Ghost Bikes are small and somber memorials for bicyclists who are killed or hit on the street. A bicycle is painted all white and locked to a street sign near the crash site, accompanied by a small plaque. They serve as reminders of the tragedy that took place on an otherwise anonymous street corner, and as quiet statements in support of cyclists' right to safe travel.

Ghost Bikes have spread throughout the United States and are now appearing in cities worldwide. Since 2006, they have also been erected in many places in the United Kingdom, many by cycling groups that want not only to remember the dead but also to draw attention to the vulnerability of cyclists. These bikes incorporate the dual purpose of other memorials—acting both as a shrine and as a warning.

Roadside memorials may be used as a warning about the dangers of the road but responses to these memorials, both public and private, are varied, and rarely neutral. Concerns have been expressed that the memorials serve as a distraction on the road, thus becoming a further danger to road users. Frequently, they can meet with strong opposition. Differing attitudes across the United States have meant that they are banned in some states yet may be facilitated in others, such as Alaska and West Virginia—where they may be permitted if particular procedures, including guidelines about size and position, are adhered to. In Canada, there has been a variety of official and unofficial responses to these memorials with state and local authorities demonstrating awareness of the sensitive nature of these memorials, while trying to balance issues of driver and road safety.

Una MacConville

Further Reading

Everett, H. *Roadside Crosses in Contemporary Memorial Culture.* Austin, TX: Texas University Press, 2002.

Grider, S. "Spontaneous Shrines: A Modern Response to Tragedy and Disaster." *New Directions in Folklore,* 5 (2001). https://scholarworks.iu.edu/dspace/handle/2022/7196?show=full

MacConville, Una. "Roadside Memorials—Making Grief Visible." *Bereavement Care,* 20 (3) (2010): 34–36.

Santino, Jack. *Signs of War and Peace.* London: Palgrave Macmillan, 2001.

SUDDEN INFANT DEATH SYNDROME

Sudden infant death syndrome (SIDS) is the sudden and unexpected death of a seemingly healthy infant less than one year of age. For a case to be considered that of SIDS, the death must be unexplained, even following a full investigation. SIDS usually occurs while the baby is asleep with no outward signs of distress or struggle; the infant may simply stop breathing. Most SIDS deaths occur among infants under six months of age, with the majority occurring under four months of age. The syndrome is more common in male babies than in female babies.

Prevalence/Incidence

Despite a decline in rates of SIDS of more than 50 percent in Canada, the United States, and many other developed countries since the early 1990s, SIDS continues to be a leading cause of death among infants, accounting for approximately 25 percent of all deaths between one month and one year of age. SIDS rates in Canada and the United States in 1990 were 0.8 and 1.3 per 1,000 live births respectively, dropping to 0.3 and 0.8 per 1,000 live births in 2002. The declines in rates have been attributed mostly to public education advocating that infants be placed on their backs to sleep and that specific modifications to the baby's environment be made.

Causes

Factors that are thought to be relevant to SIDS include those that can be associated with the mother, the infant, and the environment:

- ***Maternal factors***
  There has been a higher incidence of SIDS associated with mothers who are very young, who smoke or use illicit drugs, who have other health issues, or where there were complications during the pregnancy.
- ***Infant factors***
  SIDS has been more commonly associated with infants who are preterm or who have a sibling that previously died from SIDS. In addition, male babies seem to be more prone to SIDS. Some infants may have poor temperature control. Despite the fact that SIDS babies may appear to be in perfectly good health, they may have an abnormality of the central nervous system (brain, nerves, or spinal cord) that has yet to be identified. Some infants, for example, may have underdeveloped parts of their central nervous systems that are not yet mature. Babies affected by SIDS may have some flaw in their breathing control or ability.
- ***Environmental or care factors***
  These factors may relate to infants who are not placed on their backs to sleep, whose sleeping area is overly soft or has loose bedding, being exposed to smoke, living in environments that are too warm, or living in poverty. It used to be that the majority of SIDS deaths occurred in winter, possibly due to babies being overwrapped in clothes and therefore at risk of becoming overheated. Now, there is evidence showing no difference in the number of SIDS deaths associated with different seasons. Overheating, however, is still considered a risk for SIDS. These factors are all seen as contributory; however, there is no evidence for a specific cause-and-effect relationship between any of these factors individually and death from SIDS.

Social Aspects

Parents who have lost a baby as a result of SIDS are often overcome with grief and guilt, feeling responsible for the death of their child. Not only must these parents struggle with the loss of their baby, but they frequently must also endure a police investigation of the death, and there is often a prolonged wait for the cause of death to be determined. The loss of the baby comes as a profound shock to the parents, and the traumatic nature of the death and the inability to find a concrete cause of death can further complicate their grief (see **Grief**). Although there is greater public awareness regarding SIDS, a SIDS death can carry stigma for the parents due to erroneous assumptions about causation and perceived parental deficiency or inadequacy of some type. It is important for these parents to have access to information, support, and counseling to help them get through this difficult time. Organizations dedicated to helping families after a SIDS loss, such as First Candle, may provide much-needed information as well as support.

Darcy Harris

See also: Children; Infant Mortality; Perinatal Death.

Further Reading

American Academy of Pediatrics Task Force on Sudden Infant Death Syndrome. "The Changing Concept of Sudden Infant Death Syndrome: Diagnostic Coding Shifts, Controversies Regarding the Sleeping Environment, and New Variables to Consider in Reducing Risk." *Pediatrics,* 116(2005): 1245–55. http://www.firstcandle.org

Hunt, Carl E. and Fern R. Hauck. "Sudden Infant Death Syndrome." *Canadian Medical Association Journal,* 174(13) (2006): 1861–69.

Moon, Rachel Y. and Linda Y. Fu. "Sudden Infant Death Syndrome." *Pediatrics in Review,* 28(6) (2007): 209–14.

SUICIDE

Suicide—the act of killing oneself—has been present in some form or another in almost all cultures, countries, and civilizations as long as written history has existed, and probably before. Sometimes, people have given additional names to the act to differentiate one "kind" of suicide from another. In Japan, the royal samurai in centuries past called it *harikari,* and it was an honorable act. In recent decades in the United States, the term "rational suicide" has been given to those deaths where people had a "good reason" to kill themselves, for instance, a terminal disease. The "suicide bombers" of the Middle East are differentiated from those who kill themselves because of mental distress, by their goal, which is not to destroy themselves, but to destroy others and to achieve martyrdom (see **Martyrs**). However, the most common reason people die by suicide is due to the desire to end seemingly intractable mental pain.

How Much Suicide Is There?

According to the World Health Organization, approximately 1 million people in the world die by suicide every year. Worldwide, the annual number of suicides is greater than the number of deaths from war and homicide combined. Suicide is a serious public health problem in many countries, and is a leading cause of death among teenagers and young adults. Despite these numbers, it is a statistically rare event and one which is very hard to predict on a case-to-case basis, with 16 deaths by suicide occurring for every 100,000 people.

In the United States, approximately 36,000 people die by suicide every year, making it the 10th leading cause of death. A suicide attempt occurs every minute in the United States; while someone dies by suicide every 16 minutes. Suicide rates vary depending on gender, age, marital status, race, geography, and social class. For instance, four times as many men die by suicide compared to women. However, three times as many women *attempt* suicide compared to men. One reason for this may be that men tend to choose more lethal means such as firearms. In terms of age, those 65 and older are the most likely cohort to end their lives. Though teenagers and young adults are less likely to take their lives than the elderly, in 2010, suicide was the third leading cause of death for young people between the ages of 15 to 24.

Those widowed and divorced are more likely to die by suicide than those who are married, most likely because of the lack of a strong social support network. Those who live in more rural or remote regions compared to those in urban areas are also more likely to die by suicide, due to social isolation. Finally, there is also evidence that people with less money are more at risk of death by suicide. While poverty may not be a direct cause of suicide, it may indirectly affect access to health care, likelihood of trauma, and other factors associated with a high suicide risk.

The true number of suicides has always been difficult to pin down. For many years, it was well known that coroners, other medical personnel, and the police listed other causes of death—such as accident or heart attack—on official reports, rather than subject families and others left behind to the shame and public shunning that often resulted from knowing that a person had killed himself. Thus, it may be that the numbers listed above are smaller than the actual numbers of annual suicides.

The rate of suicide in some countries is historically higher than others, though that can vary, too. For years, it was assumed that the Scandinavian countries had higher rates than other countries, because of the dark winters and other factors. In fact, Hungary was, for many years, the site of the highest number of suicides. After the fall of the Soviet Union in 1991, some of the former republics climbed to the top of the suicide list. In 2010, it was estimated that South Korea has the highest number of suicides worldwide.

Attitudes toward Suicide

Different cultures and religions have often taken different attitudes toward suicide. In ancient Rome, it was considered an act not only of courage, but of honor, to kill oneself after failing in a battle. For a great deal of Judea-Christian cultures, however, it has been considered an immoral, if not illegal act, with those who had died by suicide refused burial in sanctified ground, their families shunned, and, attempted suicide considered a crime, actually punishable by jail time. More recently, a variety of religions have changed their stance, understanding suicide to be an outcome of illness rather than an immoral act.

Though overall attitudes toward suicide have often been negative, there is some evidence that very public suicides may draw others to take their lives as well. It has been thought that the rate of suicide can spike following the death of celebrities by suicide. Data suggest this may have been the case when Marilyn Monroe died. However, when the celebrated musician Kurt Cobain died, his wife, Courtney Love, displayed public anger at him for his act. Experts believe that her public reaction to his death helped prevent future suicides from occurring among vulnerable and impressionable people. In the United States, there was fear in the last part of the 20th century that teenagers would emulate the suicide of other teens in a "copy-cat" fashion because of the adulation of those who had died; in fact, there is evidence to suggest that the way in which the media and communities portray a death by suicide can influence the likelihood of other suicides.

Suicide among the terminally ill, or those suffering from painful, distressing, or otherwise incurable diseases, has acquired some notoriety over the past 40 years, in large part because of the concept of "assisted suicide." This term became publicly well known in large part because of Dr. Jack Kevorkian, who offered his services to those who wished to die, but could not do it by themselves. The controversy over assisted suicide continues (see **Kevorkian, Jack; Physician-Assisted Suicide; Right-to-Die Movement**). As of 2012, three states in the United States (Montana, Oregon, and Washington) now legally permit assisted suicide for residents of those states under specific circumstances. Since legislation was first passed in Oregon in 1997 under the Death with Dignity Act (DWDA), a total of 401 patients have died in Oregon with the assistance of their physicians (DeSpleder and Strickland, 2011: 224). In all other states, however, it is still a crime to help someone kill him- or herself.

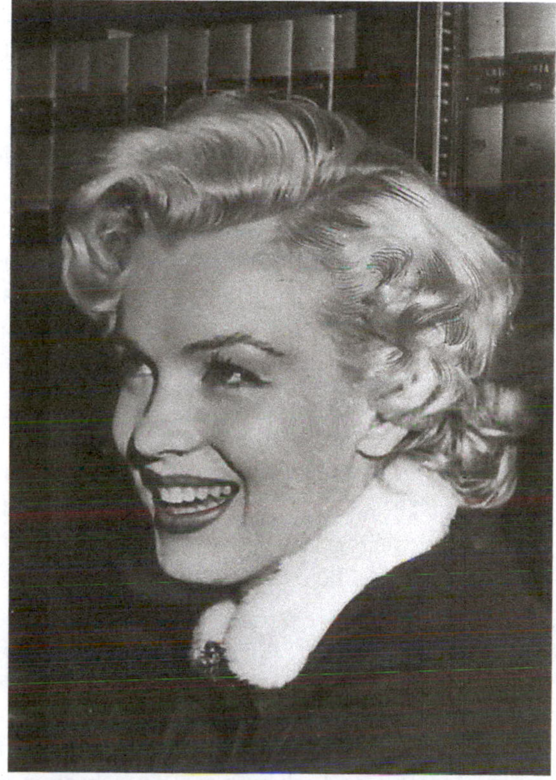

Marilyn Monroe rose to fame as a film star, but her glamorous looks, breathy voice, and personal mystique caused her fame to soar far beyond her talents as an actress. (The Illustrated London News Picture Library)

While current attitudes toward suicide have changed radically in the United States, including much public dialogue about suicide, anyone associated with public health is aware that stigma still surrounds suicide. Religious leaders do not now consider suicide a sin, but many still report some negative reaction to such a death, partly because in some religions only God has the right to give or take away life.

Nevertheless, the days of burying a person who killed him- or herself on the crossroads of a highway, or whispering the word "suicide" behind one's hand, or crossing the street to avoid talking to the relative of a dead person is, for the most part, behind us. But, there is still a great deal of negative feeling about people who attempt or complete a suicide, as well as toward their families and physicians. And for those left behind, suicide can be a powerfully damaging force.

Causes of Suicide

Many factors may contribute to a death by suicide. The presence of a mental illness, the presence of drugs and alcohol, access to means (i.e., guns, bridges, etc.) and a history of a recent loss can all contribute to the likelihood of a suicide. Most often, there is no single factor that causes a suicide to occur, though the media often portrays these deaths in a simplistic and sensational way. Some special cases of suicide are often reported in the media and acquire considerable notoriety. Harassment or bullying in schools, "outing" a gay person, and other events that capture public attention are not the single causes of most suicides. Instead, there is usually a combination of underlying risk factors and circumstances that together create a "perfect storm."

The question of whether suicide "runs" in families, or has some genetic basis, is still being debated. It may be said that the tendency toward suicide can run in families, to the extent that depression, bipolar disorder, or addictive tendencies can be hereditary. There is also some evidence that the instance of a suicide in a family "as a way of solving problems" has some effect upon other family members.

Biology also contributes to the risk of suicide. Depression affects a large number of people, in America perhaps as many as 38,000,000. Clinical depression, as well as other illnesses, cause physiological changes and can render people at their wit's end. "I can't go on"; "I'm at the end of my rope"; and "There is nothing hopeful in my future" are the kinds of thoughts that severely depressed people may have. Winston Churchill called his depression his "black dog" and there are plenty of books and diaries that spell out the debilitating force of clinical depression. However, it is important to remember that people who complete suicide as a way out of depression are a small percentage of those who are depressed.

Another important factor associated with suicide is perceived isolation, a lack of interpersonal connectedness, or a sense of burdensomeness (Joiner, 2005). Finally, access to means is another important factor that can increase the likelihood that a suicide will occur. This may be why some professions such as policemen and physicians have higher rates of suicide than other professions, precisely because they have easy access to guns and lethal medications. It has also been found that when states or countries change their access to lethal means, such as making guns less available and creating barriers to bridges, suicide rates drop.

The American Association for Suicidology (AAS) has produced a helpful mnemonic device, known as, IS PATH WARM in order to help people remember the warning signs of suicide. Though not all items are present in every suicide, most tend to be quite common:

I deation (thoughts about suicide)
S ubstance Abuse
P urposelessness
A nxiety
T rapped
H opelessness
W ithrawing
A nger
R ecklessness
M ood changes

Myths about Suicide

Because suicide is often such a taboo topic, there are many ideas relating to it that are, in fact, untrue. These myths are unfortunate because they often perpetuate the stigma surrounding suicide and sometimes serve as a barrier for those who are scared to communicate their suicidal thoughts, or for those who do communicate them, but are not taken seriously. Here are some of the common myths:

1. If people talk about suicide they will not act on it.
   False: Many people who take their life have told others in the days or weeks preceding their death.
2. If someone wants to die, there is nothing that can be done to prevent it.
   False: Many suicidal people are in fact quite ambivalent and can resolve their suicidal crisis unharmed.
3. Talking to someone about suicide might put the idea of suicide in their head.
   False: Asking someone if they are suicidal can be a relief to someone who is, and will not create suicidal ideas in someone who is not.

Vanessa McGann

See also: Suicide Prevention and Postvention.

Further Reading

DeSpelder, Lynne Ann and Albert Lee Strickland. *The Last Dance: Encountering Death and Dying,* 9th edition. Boston: McGraw-Hill, 2011.
Hendin, Herbert. *Suicide in America.* New York: W. W. Norton, 1995.
Jamison, Kay Redfield. *Night Falls Fast: Understanding Suicide.* New York: Vintage Books, 1997.
Joiner, Thomas. *Why People Die by Suicide.* Cambridge: Harvard University Press, 2005.
Maltsberger, John T. and Mark Goldblatt (eds.). *Essential Papers on Suicide.* New York: New York University Press, 1996.
Shneidman, Edwin. *Definition of Suicide.* Northvale, NJ: Jason Aronson, 1985.

SUICIDE PREVENTION AND POSTVENTION

The term "suicide prevention" refers to efforts of governments, organizations, and individuals to reduce the incidence of suicide. The term "suicide postvention" is a fairly recent concept. It refers to efforts to intervene in a person or a community's psychological life after a death by suicide, in order to restore well-being to those affected.

Prevention

In recent years, there has been an increasing awareness that suicide is a public health issue and thus interventions should not be made exclusively with individuals but with society as a whole. As part of this effort, in 2001, the U.S. Department of Health and Human Services created a National Strategy for Suicide Prevention in order to reduce the number of annual suicides. Suicide prevention can occur on many different levels, and various strategies have been implemented to achieve this goal. These involve: public awareness campaigns, gatekeeper training, screenings, means restrictions, and treatment.

Public awareness campaigns: Since there is much stigma about suicide and many myths about suicide continue to exist, one strategy to prevent suicide has been to educate the general public as to the prevalence, risk factors, and warning signs of suicide. Organizations such as the American Association for Suicidology, the American Foundation for Suicide Prevention, and the Suicide Prevention Resource Center, all have materials to educate the general public about the prevention of suicide. In addition, the American Foundation for Suicide Prevention and other organizations have sponsored walks and other public events to raise funds for, and awareness about, suicide prevention.

Gatekeeper training: Another strategy to prevent suicide has been to train those in key positions who come into contact with people at high risk of suicide. Teachers, parole officers, doctors, and nursing home staff are all examples of professionals who have begun to receive training on how to recognize and respond to suicidal signs in individuals.

Screening: Screening refers to the testing or questioning of large groups of people who are potentially at risk in order to determine who is in danger, so that interventions can be made. Some schools, clinics, and colleges have begun to utilize routine screening. One difficulty with this approach is that there can be many false positives and quality follow-up needs to be in place for those who are flagged. Many feel that physicians ought to routinely screen for thoughts of suicide, as it has been found that of those people who die by suicide, approximately 75 percent have visited their physician in the year before their death.

Means restriction: Reducing the likelihood that someone considering suicide will have access to the means to kill him- or herself has been found to be a powerful way to prevent suicide. Means restriction was shown to work in a dramatic way when the United Kingdom changed to a nonlethal form of natural gas and suicide rates decreased as a direct result. Many in the suicide prevention community feel that stronger gun control laws will help to reduce the number of suicides; stronger gun control has reduced the number of suicides in many communities. Other examples of means restriction that are being pursued include the use of barriers on bridges, rooftops, and other high places, and individually packaged "blister packs" of medication so as to make it difficult to take drugs by the handful.

Suicide hotlines: Suicide telephone hotlines have been around in the United States since the 1970s. The goal of hotlines is to get help to people who are considering suicide as quickly as possible. Because suicidal individuals often do not feel like they can talk to those around them, and because suicide is often a very impulsive act, access to free, universal 24-hour help is one strategy for suicide prevention.

Treatment: Research shows that up to 90 percent of individuals who die by suicide have a diagnosable mental disorder, such as bipolar illness, depression, or schizophrenia, as well as posttraumatic stress disorder (PTSD) and substance abuse. Thus, another focus of prevention has been on the treatment of psychiatric illnesses. Finding the right kind of preventive techniques for potentially suicidal people has not always been easy, nor has any particular treatment proven 100 percent successful. Clinicians and researchers are always looking toward developing new and better ways to provide relief to chronic and acutely suicidal individuals. Doing so can obviously save lives. Psychotherapy and medication both reduce suicidal thoughts and behaviors.

For the severely depressed adult or young person, various kinds of "talking therapy" have been used for many years. Among the most successful of such techniques is cognitive therapy, in which a therapist helps a patient change his or her way of *thinking* about events in life, and thus changing the way he or she *behaves.* Dialectical behavioral therapy has also shown to be effective in decreasing suicidal thoughts and behaviors.

With the development of antidepressant and antipsychotic medications, as well as mood stabilizers during the last half of the 20th century, many people can become psychiatrically stable and thus less suicidal. While some medications may increase suicidal thoughts in a small subset of people, many have been found to reduce them.

Postvention

There is no doubt that those left behind after the suicide of a friend, colleague, or family member suffer considerable grief. Whether that grief is greater than, or simply equal to, the bereavement people feel after any sudden death is of some debate within the field of suicidology. Whatever the case, suicide leaves in its wake a number of questions and feelings that create waves of pain in the survivors, (the term "survivor" is used for those left behind, not for those who have tried to kill themselves and not succeeded.)

These feelings include shock, anger, denial, physical illness, depression, anxiety, and accusations and self-questioning. "What could we have done?" "What *didn't* we do?" "Who is to blame?" The underlying or expressed sense that a survivor has somehow failed because of the death of a loved one, friend, or colleague can surpass any reasonable expectation by others, yet the feelings can remain.

While focused attention to survivors did not surface in clinical or written work until the mid-1980s, there is strong evidence that this kind of grief interferes with the quality of life of those left behind. This can be seen in communities such as schools or colleges, as well as within families. The feelings can go on for years, and there is some evidence that survivors are more likely to kill themselves than the general population if not attended to. As Edwin Shneidman, the founder of "suicidology" has claimed, good postvention is prevention for the next generation.

Moreover, estimates of the number of survivors have escalated in the past two decades. Originally, a number of five to seven survivors for every suicide was used as a guide. In the United States, for instance, that would imply that every year up to a quarter of a million new survivors are added. Lately, however, a different kind of estimation has been used, with some experts judging that up to 60 percent of the U.S. population will experience the death by suicide of someone they know. Thus, there has been an increased effort to develop effective postvention strategies. These postvention strategies can be broken down into three areas: (1) the individual, (2) the community, and (3) the culture at large.

1. ***Individual postvention***

On an individual level, postvention may include counseling, support groups, and psychotherapy. In the last few decades, peer-led "survivor" support groups have grown and can now be found in almost every state. One of the benefits of this postvention is that it shows the survivor that he or she is not alone in experiencing the terrible feelings that follow a suicide. Kept to oneself, it is possible to assume that one is going crazy or is alone in these kinds of experiences. With inclusion at a conference, in a discussion group, or with an experienced counselor, the feelings are brought to the surface and the survivor can recognize that their feelings may be unpleasant and painful, but not abnormal. In addition, by meeting people who have gone through the same experience over time, a recent survivor can see that there is light at the end of the tunnel.

There has also been a huge growth of organizations designed to help survivors directly. In some countries or areas these are called SOS—Survivors of Suicide groups. Australia now has a telephone helpline dedicated exclusively to those who have lost a loved one to suicide. Likewise, the Internet has provided a large number of sites where survivors can seek solace or advice. In addition, organizations whose purpose it is to study suicide, have added survivor activities to their research activities. Memorial quilts, seasonal commemorative events such as walks, conferences, and education have become a regular part of their work.

2. ***Community postvention***

Many organizations, including schools, hospitals, and workplaces, are unprepared and confused, if not traumatized, in the wake of a death by suicide. Because of this, articles, guidelines, and protocols have recently been developed with the common goals of restoring equilibrium, offering comfort, and reducing suicide risk to those left behind. While differing in details, they all stress the importance of having a place to share one's feelings while maintaining a sense of everyday routine (thereby decreasing the chances of rumor and chaos), meeting in small groups, and honoring—not glorifying—the death of the deceased. In addition, they stress the importance of actively looking for signs of distress or imbalance in any of the remaining community members, so as to get them the help they might need. Community postvention also often offers guidelines for memorials and funerals, as it has been shown that certain types of memorializations might run the risk of "contagion," or further suicides, especially among teens and other vulnerable populations.

3. ***Postvention for the culture at large***

On an even larger scale, there has been some focus on how to help society at large to better understand and mourn when a public figure takes his or her life. The focus of this type of postvention is often aimed at the media and their portrayal of suicide. There is some evidence to suggest that the way in which a story is reported can increase the likelihood of other suicides. Refraining from using the word "suicide" in a headline, depicting the act of suicide as resulting from multiple causes rather than pointing the finger at someone to blame, as well as offering information on how to get help if one is feeling suicidal, are all examples of ways the media can cover the story of a suicide while proactively trying to help the broader community understand and heal.

Vanessa McGann

Further Reading

http://www.suicidology.org
http://www.afsp.org
http://www.sprc.org
Jamison, Kay Redfield. *Night Falls Fast: Understanding Suicide.* New York: Vintage Books, 1997.
Jordan, John R. and John L. McIntosh (eds.). *Grief after Suicide: Understanding the Consequences and Caring for the Survivors.* New York: Routledge, 2011.
Marcus, Eric. *Why Suicide? Questions and Answers about Suicide, Suicide Prevention, and Coping with the Suicide of Someone You Know.* New York: Harper Collins Publishing, 2010.
Myers, Michael F. and Carla Fine. *Touched by Suicide. Hope and Healing after Loss.* New York: Gotham Books, 2006.
Shneidman, Edwin. Foreword to *Survivors of Suicide,* by Albert. C. Cain, ix–xi. Springfield IL: Charles C. Thomas, 1972.

SUPERSTITIONS

There are countless superstitions surrounding the study of death and dying. The majority of these superstitions stem from ancient beliefs and rituals. For example, people would perform different rites and rituals to keep the ghosts away from the living as they believed that they could "catch" death from a dead person. Due to that particular superstition, people began shutting the eyes of the dead, as it was believed that the eyes would be a window into the spirit world. Today, people throughout the world still shut the eyes of the dead almost immediately after death occurs. Many cultures have also believed in burning a dead person's house down or moving far away so that the spirit of the dead would not have a place to haunt and come back. Similarly, the Early English Saxons cut the feet off of the dead to prevent them from walking away. Some Aborigine tribes cut off the heads of the dead to prevent the spirits from coming back, believing they would be too confused to return without their head. Many cultures believe that one must cover the mirrors immediately after someone dies so that they are not used as a "portal" for the dead. Several superstitions relate to birds flying in or near a home, or clocks suddenly chiming, signaling a familial death being near. Finding a hat on a bed, or dropping an umbrella on the floor, are superstitions that have been connected with the message that someone in the house would die or be murdered. There are also a number of superstitions surrounding the cemetery, such as holding one's breath while passing a cemetery so not to breath in the spirits of the dead. Another superstition is that nothing new should be worn to a funeral, especially shoes, or if there is water in a grave, the deceased will have a restless spirit.

Andrea Malkin Brenner

Further Reading

Opie, Iona and Moira Tatem. *A Dictionary of Superstitions.* Oxford and New York: Oxford University Press, 2005.

T

TABOO

The word "taboo" is derived from the Polynesian term *tapu*, meaning marked off. It has long since become used to describe an activity or practice (and often discussion thereof) that is socially forbidden, beyond the acceptable parameters and socially approved etiquette of a community, culture, or society. Within many societies, powerful social mores govern the customs surrounding death and dying. In the Indian caste system, for example, and because it is considered taboo to touch a dead body, the only people permitted to handle dead bodies (in mortuaries and in preparation for funeral pyres) are the dalits or "untouchables," the lowest rank within the caste system, the oldest existing system of social stratification.

In some Asian cultures, discussion of death is largely taboo, and therefore heavily quarantined, because it is believed that talking about death will hasten its occurrence. Death taboos can also be found in certain tribes within American Indian culture, especially among Navajos, who favor bringing the sick into hospitals to die so that death does not pollute the family home. Another manifestation of the death taboo can be found in the name avoidance practiced in some cultures, whereby the deceased are never again mentioned by name so as to prevent disturbing them in the afterlife.

In contemporary Western societies, there has been much discussion among scholars in recent years as to whether, and to what extent, death and dying can any longer be considered taboo topics. Geoffrey Gorer first identified death as *the* taboo topic dominating the first half of the 20th century, eclipsing sex as the taboo that had preoccupied the Victorians a century earlier. However, by the end of 20th and beginning of the 21st century, the huge proliferation of media interest in death and dying (from newspaper and magazine articles, through movies, television series, and documentaries, to social media sites, blogs, and Internet websites) has meant that for some the suggestion that death is any longer a taboo is difficult to sustain.

In what now has become a seminal work within the field of death studies, Tony Walter in his paper "Modern Death: Taboo or Not Taboo?" has offered a nuanced approach to discussion, suggesting that while death may once have been a taboo, any such prohibitions have since melted away. Instead, Walter suggests that death is "sequestered" or hidden away within particular domains (especially health care) rather than forbidden; that it may be limited to certain social groups and classes within modern society (rather than apply equally across all social groups); and that we may well still have "conversational unease" about death and dying because of the lack of appropriate language for discussing it, but this is not to the same as it being taboo. Walter also suggests that, to a certain extent, death must be accepted and at the same time denied by all societies, for modern society would be hampered in its ability to function if it were continually preoccupied by death.

Even if we acknowledge that death in modern Western societies is no longer the forbidden topic it once was (as evidenced by the willingness to engage, second hand, in public news stories and events about the deaths of distant others), certain types of death continue to attract social stigma in ways suggestive of a taboo, none less so than death by suicide. Such a death complicates the grieving process for survivors in ways that make it very difficult to communicate their feelings (of anger, guilt, sorrow, etc.) with others; and also for friends and coworkers of suicide survivors who are reluctant to reach out and offer support for the fear of saying the wrong thing and of breaching the taboo. In short, and as Edwin S. Shneidman, one of America's most eminent suicidologists has pointed out, taboos include things you should not *do,* words you must not *say,* and ideas you must not even *think about.* Suicide transgresses all three of these: prohibitions against murder (or suicide as self-homicide), interdictions on speech about it (in ways that increase the sense of social isolation of survivors), and in the taboos surrounding explicit acknowledgement of suicidal ideation as the first step toward getting help.

Laurel Hilliker and Michael Brennan

See also: Death Denial; Euphemisms; Humor; Media and Death; Sex and Death; Suicide.

Further Reading

Kellehear, A. "Are We a Death-Denying Society? A Sociological Review." *Social Science & Medicine,* 18 (1984): 17–23.

Lee, R. "Modernity, Mortality and Re-Enchantment: The Death Taboo Revisited." *Sociology,* 42(4) (2008): 745–59.

Shneidman, Edwin S. "Suicide." In *Taboo Topics,* edited by Norman L. Farberow (pp. 33–43). New York: Atherton Press, 1963.

Walter, T. "Modern Death: Taboo or Not Taboo?" *Sociology,* 25(2) (1991): 293–310.

Walter, T. "The Sociology of Death." *Sociology Compass,* 2(1) (2008): 317–36.

TAXIDERMY

Taxidermy is the art of preparing, stuffing, and mounting the skins of animals, especially vertebrates. In recent years, freeze drying (the removal of moisture and preservation of the animal's natural body form) has become an increasingly popular process used by taxidermists. Animals "preserved" using these processes can be found in natural history museums or sometimes at the zoo, if a beloved resident is preserved after death. Some pet owners seek the services of a taxidermist to create a pet memorial to cope with the death of a beloved pet (see also **Pets**). Pets have been described as "honorary humans" and have been preserved throughout history. Ancient Egyptians believed in the immortality of cats and the wealthy would embalm their pet cats after death to preserve the body of the cat for the return of the soul. Nowadays, some veterinarians offer preservation as an option to bereaved pet owners and refer them to taxidermists.

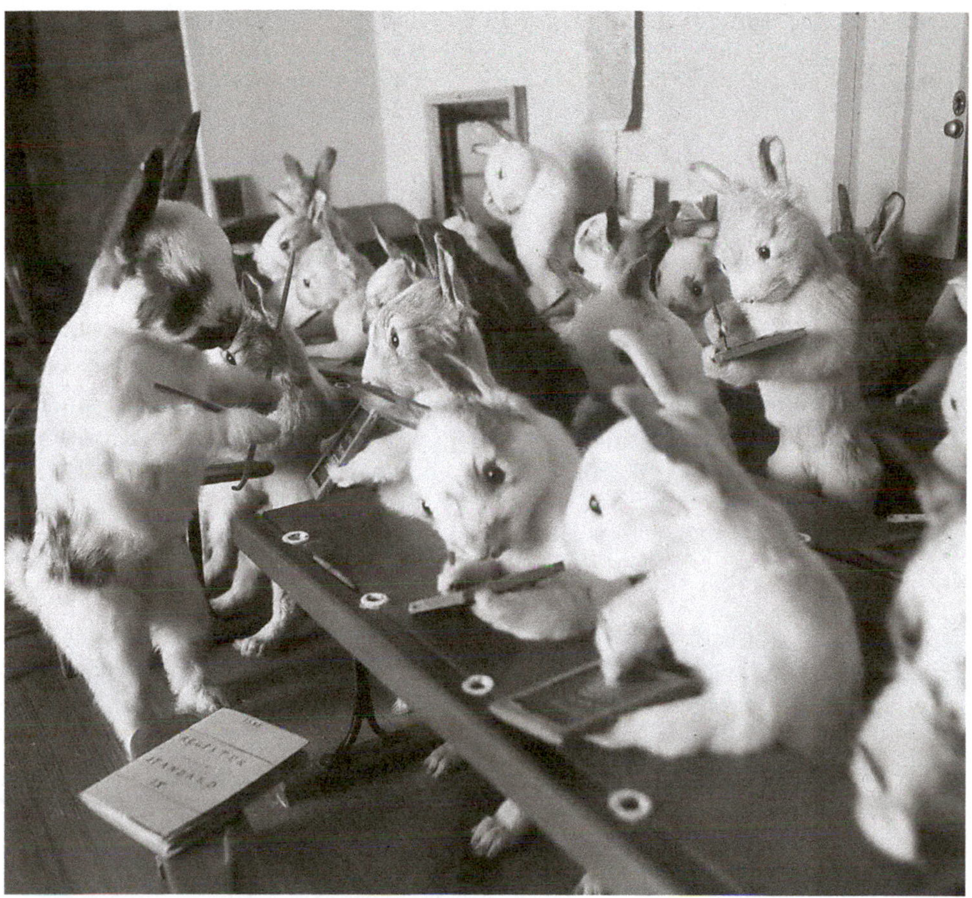

Victorian stuffed animals created by taxidermist Walter Potter at Potter's Museum of Curiosity in Bolventor, Cornwall, England. Potter created anthropomorphic tableaus based on nursery rhymes. (Graham French/BIPs/Getty Images)

Another style of taxidermy—anthropomorphic taxidermy—involves stuffed animals dressed as people or displayed as if engaged in human activities. This style, popular in Victorian and Edwardian times, has been revived by a group of artists (Loved to Death™) who "take the time to honor the living soul that has passed by making mementos out of their precious remains," a style referred to as "taxidermy *memento mori*" (see also **Memento Mori**). These creations provide a unique way for humans to memorialize deceased animals.

Carla Sofka

Further Reading

Benbow, S.M.P. "Death and Dying at the Zoo." *The Journal of Popular Culture*, 37(3) (2004): 379–98.

Grossman, Anna Jane. "Preserving Memories of Pets, and Then Some." October 11, 2011. http://cityroom.blogs.nytimes.com/2011/10/11/preserving-memories-of-pets-and-then-some/?hpw.

Madden, D. *The Authentic Animal: Inside the Odd and Obsessive World of Taxidermy.* New York: St. Martin's Press, 2011.
Morris, P. A. *Walter Potter's Curious World of Taxidermy*. London: Constable and Robinson, 2013.

TERMINAL ILLNESS AND CARE

A terminal illness is one that leads to death. An illness is usually described as "terminal" when the person who is dying is expected to die within hours, days, or weeks. Specialized care for terminally ill or dying people is available throughout the world in the form of hospice and palliative care services (see **Hospice Movement; Palliative Care**). These services are designed to meet the complex physical, emotional, spiritual, and social needs of the dying and their families. Terminal care is provided at the very end stage of palliative care in purpose- built hospices, selected hospitals, and residential care facilities, as well as in the dying person's home.

Terminal Illness and Death

Death may be caused by organ failure resulting from illnesses such as cancer and HIV/AIDS, neurological disease or chronic heart failure, a series of strokes, end-stage renal disease, or respiratory failure. The terminal stage of illness may be the result of one major condition or a combination of illnesses. It is sometimes difficult to pinpoint the actual beginning of a terminal phase. Elderly people who have been chronically ill for a number of years, and suffer from various medical conditions, sometimes die without being identified as "terminally ill." In these circumstances, dying could be said to be "ambiguous." Since most dying today occurs within the context of chronic illness and old age, the process of dying is becoming more uncertain and ambiguous than ever (see **Disease**).

Communication about Dying

While there may be cultural differences in how dying people are approached, open and supportive communication about death and dying is now generally preferred to denial, avoidance, and a "conspiracy of silence" that existed in the past. A high level of fear and anxiety about the subject of death puts the person who is terminally ill at risk of being avoided and neglected. In some situations, a person with a terminal or irreversible condition such as dementia may be treated by family, friends, and caregivers as "already dead" or "as good as dead." The withdrawal of compassionate care and full engagement with the ill, disabled, and dying person can lead to what has been termed by sociologists as a form of "social death" that actually precedes biological death (see **Social Death**).

Care of the Dying

The systems of care that have been developed for the terminally ill over the past 40 years in various parts of the world are commonly described as hospice care, palliative care, and end-of-life care. All of these terms are used interchangeably with "terminal care" although "terminal care" is usually reserved for the very end of life. Given the more predictable illness trajectory and distressing symptoms often associated with terminal cancer, the initial focus of hospice care was on cancer patients (see also **Dying Trajectory**). Hospice and palliative care for people with HIV/AIDS and severe neurological conditions was developed in subsequent years.

Pioneers in Terminal Care

The care of dying people was revolutionized in the 1960s through the pioneering efforts of two remarkable women, both doctors. With a background in nursing, social work, and medicine, Dame Cicely Saunders (1918–2005) established St. Christopher's Hospice in London, England, in 1967. Saunders and her colleagues aimed to meet the physical, emotional, and spiritual needs of dying patients in a more enlightened and holistic way than had been previously offered. Saunders developed a highly effective use of narcotics and opiates in relieving terminal cancer pain, as part of what she described as a "high person, low technology" system of health care for relieving distressing symptoms and providing end-of-life care. Recognizing the patient and family as the unit of care led to the provision of grief counseling (see **Grief Counseling**) and support for key survivors before and after the patient's death.

It was also in the late 1960s that Swiss American psychiatrist, Elisabeth Kübler-Ross (1926–2004) began her worldwide pioneering work on death and dying, by raising public awareness of the special needs of dying people. In her famous book, *On Death and Dying*, published in 1969, Kübler-Ross challenged people to overcome their fear and denial about death in order to provide better care for the dying. Kübler-Ross suggested that dying people moved through five stages of dying: denial, anger, bargaining, depression, and acceptance (see **Kübler-Ross, Elisabeth**). For many years, this was the preferred model for understanding the grief of a terminally ill person and indeed, all people experiencing significant loss and bereavement. However, subsequent research has shown that each dying person's experience is unique, and far more complex than was first thought. Stage models are no longer considered to be helpful as they tend to categorize and oversimplify the experience of dying and grieving.

Over the past 50 years, the hospice and palliative care movement has spread to many parts of the world and continues to progress in developing countries. The word "hospice" dates back to medieval times when hospices were established by religious orders to care for sick and dying pilgrims traveling to holy places. However, the more secular term "palliative," which means to relieve or soothe symptoms, was first introduced by Balfour Mount, who established the first hospital-based palliative care unit in the world at Royal Victoria Hospital, Montreal, Canada, in 1974.

Irene Renzenbrink

Further Reading

Bern-Klug, M. "The Ambiguous Dying Syndrome." *Health and Social Work,* 29(1) (2004): 55–65.
Elias, N. *The Loneliness of the Dying.* Oxford: Basil Blackwell, 1985.
Holden, C. "Hospices for the Dying, Relief from Pain and Fear." In *A Hospice Handbook: A New Way to Care for the Dying,* edited by Michael Hamilton and Helen Reid (pp. 57–63). Grand Rapids, MI: William B. Eerdmans Publishing Company, 1980.
Kübler-Ross, E. *Death: The Final Stage of Growth.* New York: Simon and Schuster/Touchstone, 1974.
Stoddard, S. *The Hospice Movement: A Better Way of Caring for the Dying.* New York: Vintage Books, 1992.
Sudnow, D. *Passing On: The Social Organizing of Dying.* Englewood Cliffs, NJ: Prentice Hall, 1967.

TERROR MANAGEMENT THEORY

Terror management theory (TMT) is rooted within the field of social psychology, and is derived from the Freudian-inspired ideas of cultural anthropologist Ernest Becker. Developed in the 1980s by researchers Jeff Greenberg, Tom Pyszczynski, and Sheldon Solomon, the essence of the theory lies in the assumption that anxiety about our own mortality is a motivating factor in human behavior. This key assumption revolves around the idea that an unconscious awareness of death leads us, as human beings, to develop psychological defense mechanisms (of denial and displacement) aimed at warding off the fear of death through the establishment of immortality ideologies designed to ensure that our lives are experienced as meaningful and secure. These ideologies are wide ranging and include cultural and religious beliefs about the afterlife and immortality of the soul; scientific assertions about the projected mastery and defeat of human mortality (including cryogenics and some aspects of medical science); as well as attempts at political and economic domination witnessed during colonialism, and more recently, the Cold War.

Crucially, according to Terror Management theorists, while an awareness of our own mortality may inspire us to produce positive enduring accomplishments that may serve to guarantee our own immortality (be it by writing a book, inventing a product, or producing a work of art), it more often triggers a negative response to others (whether at the everyday interpersonal level or at the level of geopolitical decision making) that is manifested in outbursts of violence and aggression.

In order to establish the empirical basis of TMT, researchers established a series of experiments (which, since the theory was first developed, have now exceeded well over 250) in order to test what they described as the "mortality salience hypothesis." This hypothesis is underscored by two key components: (1) that individuals within all societies have a felt need to be able to maintain faith in a meaningful worldview supportive and reflective of their beliefs; and (2) that individuals have a need to experience themselves as objects of significance—as valued and protected members of society in ways that provide a sense of self-esteem. By reminding people of their own mortality, an assumption underpinning the hypothesis is that not only will we see a temporary increase in the need for death-denying aspects of culture supportive of a particular worldview, but that a reminder of the salience of our own mortality will be reflected in our attitudes and behaviors toward others. In essence, what this amounts to is an increased identification with others who we perceive as similar (in terms of race, religion, politics, nationality, etc.) and a commensurate disidentification with, and hostility toward, others whom we perceive as different.

The assertions of terror management theorists have been confirmed by a series of experiments. One such example included a study conducted with municipal judges in Tucson, Arizona, in which half were given a questionnaire containing reminders of their own mortality and half were not. When asked to examine a hypothetical court case involving solicitation for prostitution, the half who had been given mortality reminders were much more punitive in their judgments (suggesting that their worldview of themselves as judges, operating fairly and as upholders of the law, had been violated), recommending a bond for the prostitute at $450 compared to $50 by judges who had not been given reminders of their own death.

In another such study, participants were again divided equally between a control group exposed to a questionnaire containing questions about their own mortality, and the rest of the group, who were not. In a separate, and what participants were led to believe was an unrelated study, they were then asked to administer a portion of hot chili sauce to a participant of differing political views for them to taste and rate. As anticipated, and consistent with TMT, those participants exposed to reminders of their own mortality administered portions twice as large as those who did not, thereby confirming an intention to harm or act maliciously toward others dissimilar from themselves when given reminders of their own mortality.

All of this can help us to understand the spiral of violence and aggression toward others, whether in the microaggressions of the workplace or the internecine conflict between nations and extraterritorial opponents of nations. The attacks of 9/11, for example, can be understood as a case study of TMT writ large, whereby an attack on the people and cultural symbols of the United States provided an existential threat and reminder for other Americans on their own vulnerability in ways that help precipitate an aggressive reaction not only toward the perpetrators (Al Qaeda and other rogue states perceived as harbingers of terrorism), but also toward innocent others because of their perceived difference. In the days and weeks following the 9/11 attacks, hostilities toward American Muslims (and other racialized minorities, including Hindus and Sikhs) were reported across the United States. Understood using TMT, such tribal and racist responses can be interpreted as brutal behaviors borne of our unconscious desire to escape death by inflicting it on others.

Michael Brennan

See also: Death Anxiety; Death Denial; Immortality.

Further Reading

Becker, E. *The Denial of Death.* New York: Free Press, 1973.

Flight from Death: The Quest for Immortality. DVD-Video. Directed by Patrick Shen. Los Angeles, CA: Transcendental Media, 2005. http://www.flightfromdeath.com/

Goldenberg, Jamie, Tom Pyszczynski, Jeff Greenberg, and Sheldon Solomon. "Fleeing the Body: A Terror Management Perspective on the Problem of Human Corporeality." *Personality & Social Psychology Review,* 4 (2000): 215–18.

Pyszczynski, Tom, Sheldon Solomon, and Jeff Greenberg. *In the Wake of 9/11: The Psychology of Terror.* Washington, DC: American Psychological Association, 2003.

Solomon, Sheldon., Jeff Greenberg, and Tom Pyszczynski. "The Cultural Animal: Twenty Years of Terror Management Theory and Research." In *Handbook of Experimental Existential Psychology,* edited by Jeff Greenberg, S. Koole, and Tom Pyszczynski (pp. 13–34). New York: Guilford Press, 2004.

TERRORISM

Terrorism is a practice that involves violent activities, intended to cause the death of people within a certain population in order to terrorize it for certain purposes. Long before September 11, 2001, and the ensuing War on Terrorism, definitions of terrorism had abounded. More than 100 such definitions were enumerated in Schmid and Jongman's *Political Terrorism,* published in 1988. The current number of definitions is higher still.

One reason for the present abundance of definitions of terrorism is the practical fragmentation of counterterrorism. A simple example would be the nature of international conventions on counterterrorism. The first one is the 1963 *United Nations Convention on Offences and Certain Other Acts Committed On Board Aircrafts.* A more recent one is the 1997 United Nations *Convention for the Suppression of Terrorist Bombings,* which bans use of explosives and other lethal devices in public places. The most recent one among the 14 United Nations Conventions against terrorism is a 2010 *United Nations Convention on the Suppression of Unlawful Acts Relating to International Civil Aviation,* which criminalizes various uses of a civil aircraft as a weapon, to discharge biological, chemical, or nuclear (BCN) weapons, among other related acts. Such fragmentation seemingly avoids the problem of establishing a uniform working definition of terrorism.

This, however, is not at the root of the abundance of definitions of terrorism. At the root is not a practical aspect of explicit counterterrorism, but rather, to put it plainly, a political aspect of implicit support of terrorism. Whenever a general definition of terrorism is put forward, attempts are made to exclude or excuse parties, actions, and conditions from being related to terrorism. The most famous line of argument invokes the apparent observation (ascribed to the British writer Gerald Seymour, in his 1975 novel *Harry's Game,* which is about an IRA terrorist act) that one person's terrorist is another person's freedom fighter. It would, however, be wrong to exempt a person from the blame of committing terrorist acts on grounds of his cause being "freedom." The end does not justify the means: fighting for freedom does not, as such, justify resorting to terrorist means of killing people.

A universal definition of terrorist acts is perhaps beyond present political reach, but it is not beyond conceptual characterization. Here are conceptual elements of terrorism that are shared by many definitions:

1. It is a practice of violence.
2. The practice involves acts or threats to perform acts of killing and injuring people who do not jeopardize the life or health of the agents of the practice; Notice that condition (2) is couched in terms of "people" and not in terms of noncombatant victims. Acts of terrorism can be directed against people in military uniform, when they are not engaged in fighting agents of the practice or anybody else.
3. The practice is used against members of a certain clearly identifiable population.
4. The practice is used repeatedly.
5. The practice is used in order to terrorize that population.
6. The practice is used in order to change the political situation by means of terrorizing the population.
7. The practice is used on political, ideological, or religious grounds that justify it in the eyes of its agents.

Justification

No act of terrorism is morally justifiable. If it is an act of terrorism, it includes the intention to kill people, or otherwise injure them, in order to terrorize the population in which they are members so as to gain some political benefit. Such an intention is utterly different from the intention of self-defense. The people intended to be killed, often children, are not attacking the terrorist. By killing them, the terrorist does not foil an attempt on their part on the terrorist's life or liberty. The terrorist intends to kill in order to use death to terrorize the population and thereby exert on it pressure, of a kind that the terrorist hopes would lead to a change of the political situation. However, using the life or well-being of a person as a mere means in pursuit of an end of any kind is morally wrong. It treats human beings as if they are tools, thus breaching the duty to respect the life of every person, including the people who are to become the victims of the intended act of terrorism.

Distinctions

Several distinctions ought to be made in order to facilitate further discussion of justifiability and counterterrorism. First, terrorism should not be confused with guerilla warfare, though often the same organization resorts to both modes of operation. The gist of the difference is that unlike terrorism, as discussed above, guerilla activity is directed solely against combatants and is carried out in a military way.

Second, terrorism can be domestic or international. The difference is in the nature of the population the terrorist intends to terrorize. The moral significance of the distinction is manifest in the practice of employing police against domestic terrorism and military forces against international terrorism. Police ethics are indeed much more restrictive than military ethics.

Third, terrorism can be carried out by a state, by a nonstate organization, or by unorganized groups or individuals. When a state is involved in acts of terrorism directed at people outside its borders, the ensuing armed conflict ought to be governed by international law. When the agents of terrorism are not state agents, doctrines are required for morally governing the armed conflict. Individual terrorism is a novelty of Osama bin Laden, who declared with his associates in their 1998 *World Islamic Front Statement* that the "holy struggle" (*Jihad*) is an individual duty of Muslims.

Counterterrorism

A democratic state ought to defend its citizens against terrorism. The moral problem it faces is how to provide its citizens with effective defense against terrorism, while paying due respect to the human rights of every person, whether a citizen or not.

The most conspicuous difficulty in defending citizens against terrorist lethal violence is the seeming necessity to cause collateral damage. When there is no way to capture a terrorist, whose activities jeopardize the life of citizens, it may be necessary to attack terrorists in order to kill them. However, quite often, terrorists reside, plan their activities, and carry them out in the vicinity of people who are not involved in terrorism, but whose life is jeopardized when the terrorists' are attacked. Thus, a state defends its citizens against terrorists intending to cause their death, by attacking the terrorists and thereby causing the death of some of their neighbors.

This common practice allows the state to cause collateral damage for self-defense, if certain conditions obtain. This practice has been defended by philosophers on grounds of a classical doctrine of double effect and forms part of international law of armed conflict. The doctrine of double effect rests on the distinction between evil that is intended and pursued and evil that is not intended, considered undesirable, and minimized under the circumstances. Among the conditions that have to be met for an act of self-defense that causes collateral damage to be morally and legally justified, most important is the condition of proportionality. The essence of this condition is that the benefit a state wishes to gain by an act of self-defense that causes collateral damage justifies the evil of causing that collateral damage. Comparisons of benefits and damages are often not easy to make.

International law aptly leaves the duty of making these comparisons to military commanders (whose own acts are under the consideration of international law). It is a tragic element of fighting terrorism that in order to save life from death by terrorism, one sometimes has no choice but to kill not only the aggressive terrorist, but also some people who are not involved in terrorism at all.

Asa Kasher

See also: Jihad; Martyrs; Megadeath; War.

Further Reading

Fotion, N., B. Kashnikov, and J. K. Lekea. *Terrorism: The New World Disorder.* London and New York: Continuum, 2007.

Kasher, A. and A. Yadlin. "Military Ethics of Fighting Terror: An Israeli Perspective." *Journal of Military Ethics,* 4(1) (2005): 3–32.

Nesi, G. (ed.). *Counter-Terrorism: The United Nations and Regional Organizations in the Fight against Terrorism.* Aldershot, England and Burlington, VT: Ashgate, 2006.
Primoratz, I. "The Morality of Terrorism." *Journal of Applied Philosophy,* 143 (1997): 221–33.
Schmid, A. P. and A. J. Jongman. *Political Terrorism: A New Guide, to Actors, Authors, Concepts, Data Bases, Theories, and Literature.* New Brunswick, NJ: Transaction Books, 1988.
Thackrah, J. R. *Dictionary of Terrorism,* 2nd edition. London and New York: Routledge, 2004.
Walzer, M. "Terrorism and Just War." *Philosophia,* 34(1) (2006): 3–12.

THANATOLOGY

Derived from a combination of the Greek words thanatos (*death*) and *logos* (the study of), thanatology is the interdisciplinary study of death, grief, and bereavement. Drawing from a wide variety of academic disciplines, including psychology, sociology, anthropology, philosophy, history, theology, medicine, and law, thanatology has witnessed tremendous growth since the 1950s. This was a period of profound death denial in American society, when death was regarded as something of an obscenity and early pioneers of the study of death and dying encountered a widespread culture of resistance in their attempts to establish it as a topic of academic inquiry. Since then, thanatology has grown into a full-fledged academic subdiscipline, with its own professional organization, ADEC (whose subtitle is "The Thanatology Association"), conferences, and academic journals (*Death Studies, Mortality,* and *Omega: The Journal of Death and Dying,* which takes its name from the last letter of the Greek alphabet). Thanatology is today a part of the academic curriculum in universities and colleges across the United States, and at graduate and professional levels, it provides a focus for those whose work brings them into contact with the dead, dying, and bereaved, from social workers and clergy, to funeral directors, educators, and counselors. Thanatology covers a wide array of areas—from all types of death and the emotional response to loss across the life span, to beliefs and practices about bodily disposal and life after death—reflective of human life in all its diversity and richness. This emphasis, on death as an integral part of life, is a reminder of an overriding thanatological concern to integrate all facets of the human experience within the study of death and dying.

Michael Brennan

See also: ADEC; Death Awareness Movement; Death Education.

TOBACCO

Tobacco is a leaf of various plants that belong to the genus *Nicotiana.* The leaves are dried and then used in various methods for the desired effect on the human body.

How Is Tobacco Used?

After tobacco is processed, it can be used in a variety of ways. A popular method to introduce tobacco into the body is by smoking the substance in cigarette form.

Other popular methods to smoke tobacco include through cigars, homemade blunts, and pipes.

Loose leaf chew, chewing tobacco, and snuff are typically used by placing a pinch of the substance between your bottom lip and gums. The nicotine is then absorbed through the lip and the desired effect on the body is initiated.

Diversity of Tobacco

Tobacco can come in many forms, sizes, and shapes. Depending upon what country you are in, certain methods of tobacco use are more popular than others. In the United States, for example, the most popular way to use tobacco is through smokeless tobacco like snuff. It is popular in parts of India to use qiwam, which is tobacco in paste form used by placing the paste in your mouth and chewing on it.

Age Range

Nine out of 10 smokers begin smoking before the age of 18. This has been a major issue, as much of the marketing for tobacco use has often been designed to appeal to children and adolescents. Joe Camel was the mascot/representative for Camel cigarettes from 1987 until 1997. His hip, popular, and colorful image helped to make Camel cigarettes one of the highest grossing cigarette companies in the 1990s. In 1991, the *Journal of the American Medical Association* published a study which found that by age six, nearly as many kids could identify that "Joe Camel" was associated with cigarettes as could identify that the Disney Channel logo was associated with Mickey Mouse. It was this type of study and pressure from Congress that ended Joe Camel's run as the mascot for Camel Cigarettes in 1997.

Tobacco-Related Deaths

Tobacco use is the leading preventable cause of death in the United States. On average, adults who smoke cigarettes die 14 years earlier than nonsmokers. There is no doubt that tobacco use causes death and disease. Lung cancer is the number one disease that kills tobacco users. Ischemic heart disease is the second highest killer of tobacco users.

The World Lung Federation (WLF) reported in 2012 that smoking rates in the developed world continue to decline, but the numbers are growing quickly in poorer regions of the world. Tobacco is the number one killer in China, causing over 1 million deaths per year, with a projection of 3.5 million people dying per year in 2030.

Withdrawal

Tobacco is an addictive drug and causes withdrawal symptoms if the user attempts to quit using it. When a user stops using tobacco, the reduced nicotine intake will disrupt the balance of the central nervous system, causing withdrawal symptoms. The most common withdrawal symptoms include craving for tobacco, anger, increased appetite, irritability, and anxiety. Tobacco withdrawal symptoms tend to last for a few weeks, but some people may experience a few of these symptoms for a longer period of time.

Additional Impact

Not only is tobacco proven to cause death and disease, but it also contributes to the diminished quality of life in tobacco users, as well as those affected not only directly from their tobacco use, but by second-hand smoke. There are two types of second-hand smoke: sidestream smoke and mainstream smoke. Sidestream smoke is the smoke from a lighted end of a cigarette, cigar, etc. Mainstream smoke is the smoke exhaled by the smoker. Sidestream smoke is the more dangerous of the two types of second-hand smoke because it contains more carcinogens with smaller particles, which make their way into the lungs more easily. Second-hand smoke kills over 50,000 people a year through disease such as heart disease, lung cancer, and sudden infant death syndrome (SIDS).

Public Health Policy

There are proactive measures being taken through the implementation of policy to fight the high number of deaths from users of tobacco and second-hand smoke. A few of the most successful public health policy changes include increased tax for tobacco products, smoke-free air laws, and allowing health insurance to cover tobacco cessation programs.

Jason Bertrand

See also: Alcohol; Drugs.

Further Reading

Farrington, K. *This Is Nicotine (Addiction)*. Houston, TX: Sanctuary Publishing, 2002.

McGinnis, J. "Actual Causes of Death in the United States." *Journal of American Medical Association,* 18 (1993): 2207–12.

Schroeder, S. "Confronting a Neglected Epidemic: Tobacco Cessation for Persons with Mental Illnesses and Substance Abuse Problems." *Annual Review of Public Health,* 31 (2010): 297–314.

Sidai, J. "Practices and Perceptions of Mental Health Counselors in Addressing Smoking Cessation." *Journal of Mental Health Counseling,* 33 (2011): 264–82.

TOMBS/MAUSOLEUMS

Tomb is a general term referring to a place of burial, often more elaborate than a simple earth burial. Complexity of construction varies greatly over time, space, culture, and available resources. Rock-cut tombs developed from a tradition of

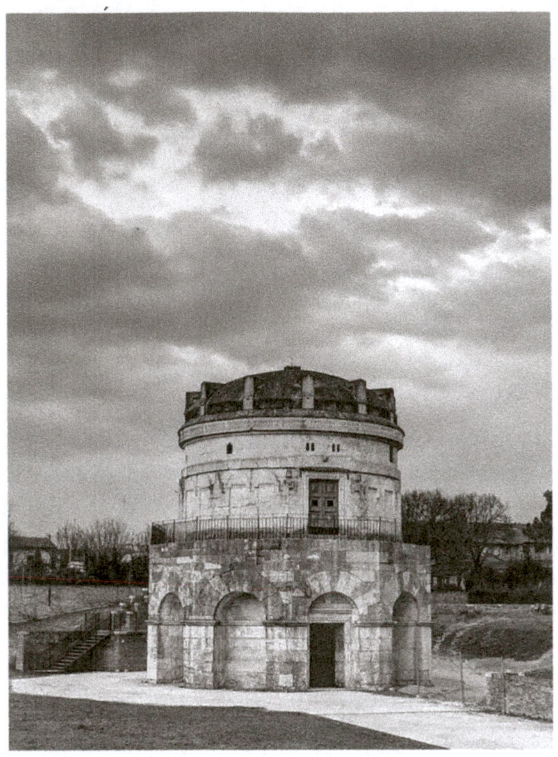
Theodoric's mausoleum, Ravenna, Italy. (Daderot)

cave burials in many areas; Christ was buried in a rock-cut tomb. Most tombs have a visible above-ground component, and elaborate free-standing examples can be called mausoleums.

Prehistoric communities often constructed communal tombs in which some or all of the population would be placed. Some, such as the megalithic monuments of Europe, were major features in the landscape and were centers for many forms of ritual activity. Famous examples include Newgrange and Knowth in the Boyne valley in Ireland, and West Kennett long barrow near Silbury Hill, England. These tombs required considerable effort from the population to construct and maintain them.

The pyramids of Egypt are tombs, as are many smaller structures for burial of members of the royal families and court officials that are set around them, still decorated with elaborate wall paintings, even if most of the contents have been removed. The Valley of the Kings contains many elaborate rock-cut tombs, often with many passages and rooms, though most failed to avoid robbing. The tomb of Tutenkhamun was a rare example that survived intact to be discovered by Howard Carter in 1922.

The most famous mausoleum of all was at Halicarnassus in what is now Turkey, built for Mausolus, king of that area in the fourth century BC. It is from this tomb that the term mausoleum derives; it was so impressive that it was one of the seven wonders of the ancient world. Tombs were often placed along the roads that led into Roman towns and could be based on buildings such as temples, as seen on the Via Appia in Rome and the Street of Tombs, Pompeii. Emperors such as Augustus and Hadrian had huge mausoleums constructed in Rome, where there is also the famous pyramid-shaped tomb of Caestius. Many wealthy families had much smaller tombs, and these were found throughout the Roman Empire. By the late Roman period, some revered Christians were placed in tombs that then became the focus for pilgrimage, and were later the sites of major churches and cathedrals.

Medieval tombs for important figures were usually placed within religious buildings, and some had their own chapels added to churches to house them. Many tombs included effigies, carved life-sized representations of the deceased.

In all cases, the bodies of the deceased are buried in the ground, in a wooden or stone coffin. They were often depicted as dressed in clothing of their rank such as priests, soldiers in armor, or high-status women in fashionable dress. In the 15th and 16th centuries, cadaver tombs were erected, with a carved version of the decaying body, usually with a more typical depiction above this of the person as if asleep.

Across the world, major rulers and some religious figures had mausoleums constructed for them. Some of the most famous include the 7th-century Qianling mausoleum, China, for the Li family, rulers in the Tang dynasty, and the 17th-century Taj Mahal, India, built by the Mughal emperor Shah Jahan for one of his wives.

Early modern European tombs often continue the effigy tradition, with the deceased in modern fashions or sometimes classical dress. Associated with these monuments are burial vaults of brick or stone, set under the church floor into which the coffins were placed. These vaults have often been used for generations. From the 18th century onward, tombs were more often outside, and also began to be placed in the countryside, away from churchyards. Early examples of mausoleums set on country estates are those at Castle Howard and Rockingham, England. Family mausoleums became extremely popular in European and North American cemeteries in the 19th and early 20th centuries. They occur in a range of revival styles, including Classical, Gothic, and Egyptian, and many are in use to this day, especially by communities with Mediterranean origins.

Harold Mytum

See also: Burial; Cemeteries.

Further Reading

Colvin, H. *Architecture and the After-Life*. New Haven, CT: Yale University Press, 1991.

Curl, J. S. *A Celebration of Death: An Introduction to Some of the Buildings, Monuments and Settings of Funerary Architecture in the Western European Tradition*. New York: Sterling, 1980.

McDowell, P. and R. E. Meyer. *The Revival Styles in American Memorial Art*. Bowling Green, OH: Bowling Green State University Popular Press, 1994.

TOTEMISM

Totemism was identified in ethnographic literature at the end of the 18th century as a most basic form of religion in Australian and North American tribes. As tribes divided into phratries (groups of clans), the phratry's totem, usually identified with some plant or animal, became a part of the tribe's totem, such as a wolf's eye. The clans among phratries each identified their own totem which was connected to, but not necessarily part of, the totem of the tribe. No two clans had the same totem. A person could adopt a totem from either the maternal or paternal line, or have their totem assigned by a mythic ancestor; this naming of the totem varied by tribe. Apart from the general totem of the clan, each person could, but did not have to, hold an individual totem. These were acquired through deliberate acts, or assigned by a more sacred person of the clan such as the oldest man or a shaman (religious leader). There continue to be many rituals surroundings totems. Tribe members are prohibited from both killing and eating any animal or plant that is represented in their totems. It is believed that such an act may result in the death of the individual. There are exceptions for certain ceremonies in which, for example, the blood of the animal is required. Because the totem is a sacred object, when a totem animal or plant is accidentally killed or found dead, it is cared and grieved for as if it were a member of the clan. This illustrates the way in which the totem comes to symbolically represent the group identity of the clan, thereby reflecting the link between culture and nature. Old men are often exempt because they are seen as holding a higher religious status in their particular communities. Tribe members are expected to bear an emblem of their totem on their being and to mark it on all personal belongings. Although the initial process differs from clan to clan, women and uninitiated men are traditionally forbidden from many rituals. Many of the rituals of totemism can still be found in Australian and North American tribes today.

Andrea Malkin Brenner

Further Reading

Durkheim, Emile. *The Elementary Forms of the Religious Life*. Translated by Karen E. Fields. New York: The Free Press, 1995/1912.

V

VALHALLA

In Norse mythology, Valhalla is the "Hall of the Slain" of the god Odin. Situated in Asgard (one of the nine realms of Norse cosmology and capital city of the Norse gods), Valhalla is a gigantic hall where courageous warriors slain in battle dwell, feasting by night and preparing by day in mock battles for the Ragnarök, a looming series of future events including a final battle of cosmic and cataclysmic proportion.

Each of Valhalla's 540 doors is large enough to permit 800 warriors to march through, shoulder to shoulder. Its roof is made of shields, the rafters of spears, and benches are covered with coats of mail (armor fashioned from small metal rings interlinked to form a mesh).

Entrance to Valhalla is barred by the river *Thund* and the gate *Valgrind.* Worthy warriors—the *einherjar* (adopted sons of Odin)—reach Valhalla only after being chosen and escorted by the Valkyries, blond, blue-eyed demigoddesses. Food and drink are served by the white-robed Valkyries, having set aside their scarlet corselets and swords and shields that call up the northern lights (a display of natural light visible in regions located at high latitude, such as Scandanavia). The *eiherjar's* mead (an alcoholic beverage also known as "honey wine") runs daily from the udders of the goat Heiðrun, while boiled flesh of the boar Saehrimni supplies meat for the nightly feasts.

A variant of the mythology of Valhalla states that one half of the worthy warriors dwell in Valhalla, while Folkvangr, the heavenly palace of the goddess Freyja, welcomes the rest. Another version stresses that unworthy warriors are consigned to an underworld of the dead, sometimes termed Hel, and viewed as a goddess cast into Niflheim, an abode of blood and hunger.

Some evidence suggests that the term *Valhalla* originally referred to a grave mound. A variation of Valhalla and the mythology surrounding it provides the basis of *Der Ring des Nibil,* Wagner's four-cycle opera.

Regina A. Boisclair

Further Reading

O'Donoghue, Heather. *From Asgard to Valhalla: The Remarkable History of the Norse Myths.* London: I. B. Tauris, 2007.

VAMPIRES

Vampires, as they are conceived of today, are reanimated corpses that differ from other reanimated corpses, such as zombies, in two essential respects: they must consume blood to survive, and their corpses do not decay. They are a subset of the undead—creatures that formerly were alive, but are not presently dead. The modern conception of the vampire is based largely on 18th-century Eastern European (primarily Slavic) folklore, although subsequent works of fiction and film have added to and altered that conception. Earlier conceptions of creatures with vampiric features include creatures called "shades" in Homer's *Odyssey* and the Hebrew legend Lilith in the *Babylonian Talmud.*

Common Attributes of Vampires

There are a number of traits commonly attributed to vampires. These traits can be mutually exclusive, depending on the particular details of the legend, so no vampire is required to possess each. Thus, what it means to be a vampire is to be in possession of *some* combination of the following set of attributes:

1. **Vampires drink blood**
   The drinking of blood is necessary for the survival of vampires. This is an essential feature of vampires. Thus, any creature that does not require blood for survival is not a vampire. This is the feature most commonly associated with vampires.
2. **Vampires are shape shifters**
   Vampires can change into other creatures at will. Most notably, vampires change into bats and wolves.
3. **Vampires are cursed or damned**
   A common thread running through tales about vampires is that upon becoming a vampire they become damned or cursed. In many cases, the vampire becomes one of Satan's legion.
4. **Vampires do not have a soul**
   Vampires are considered to be soulless. This attribute may be at odds with the previous one, as what it often means to be cursed or damned is for one's soul to be cursed or damned, although, according to some legends, vampires are damned to exist without a soul.
5. **Vampires do not have a reflection**
   It is often thought that in virtue of not having a soul, vampires do not cast a reflection.
6. **Vampires have fangs**
   A vampire's fangs are used for the extraction of blood. Fangs are also used to turn humans into vampires. Accounts of this phenomenon vary. According to some legends, being bitten by a vampire is sufficient to turn one into a vampire. Others hold that the vampire must ritualistically "turn" the human. This often involves the comingling of vampire and human blood.
7. **Vampires are harmed by sunlight**
   Direct exposure to sunlight will result in a vampire's death, typically via burning up. The sun, in many legends, represents God's goodness. As damned creatures,

exposure to Godly things causes burning. Similarly, crosses and holy water will burn vampires. On some accounts, garlic and silver are also thought to be harmful to vampires, though the religious basis for this is controversial and unclear. Consequently, one can protect oneself from vampires by being in possession of a cross, garlic, holy water, or silver.

8. **Vampires are immortal**
   Unless killed, vampires will live forever. Thus, unlike humans, vampires will not die of nonmurderous causes (with the exception of prolonged exposure to sunlight). Though there is much variation in the vampire legends about how to kill a vampire, it is most often held that in order to kill a vampire one must either drive a stake through its heart or cut off its head.
9. **Vampires sleep in a grave**
   Vampires are thought to rise nightly from their graves. In some cases, vampires sleep in coffins. In other cases, they sleep in mausoleums.
10. **Vampires have the ability to charm**
    Charming is akin to hypnotizing. Vampires charm their victims in order to effortlessly suck the victim's blood. Charming is also used to get humans to do the vampire's will.

Richard Greene

Further Reading

Cavendish, Richard (ed.). *Man, Myth and Magic: An Illustrated Encyclopedia of the Supernatural.* New York: BPC Publishing Ltd., 1970.
Greene, R. and K. Silem Mohammad (eds.). *Zombies, Vampires, and Philosophy.* Chicago, IL: Open Court Publishing Company, 2010.
Ramsland, Katherine. *The Science of Vampires.* New York: Berkley, 2002.

VIDEO GAMES

Video games are interactive games played electronically by a user(s) who manipulates images and/or information displayed on a computer screen or other electronic device. In the past few years, video game releases, particularly from the *Call of Duty* series have often surpassed the sales of blockbuster movies. Although video games span numerous genres, violent games are among the most popular. Games which feature war, violence, and death are financially lucrative, perhaps reflecting long-standing human interest in these aspects of human life stretching back as far as we have recorded literature. However, concerns about the potentially addictive quality and violent nature of some video games have provoked controversy and concern among some policy makers, advocates, and scholars. Such concerns have been heightened and highlighted by recent media stories reporting the deaths of young gamers during "marathon" sessions (sometimes spanning several days), in which gamers play without stopping for breaks, sleep, or food. Others claim that public fears about video games (and gaming itself), including those with violent and controversial content, are exaggerated and out of proportion with the actual threat they pose, reflecting instead a moral panic that is itself often generated by more traditional media, such as television and newspapers.

Death in Video Games

Video games emerged as a popular source of entertainment in the 1970s, even though most early games were simplistic and devoid of storyline or characterization. Although some of these early games such as *Pong* were nonviolent, most of the video games, which were popular in the 1970s, involved some form of cartoon-quality violence and death. Noteworthy examples of games involving machine-on-machine violence include *Asteroids* and *Space Invaders,* as well as *Pac Man* and *Centipede,* the main objective of which is to destroy insect pests and scorpion mushrooms in order to avoid being eaten by a descending centipede. Other games of this era, such as *Raiders of the Lost Arc,* began to allow primitive versions of human-against-human violence.

A game called *Death Race* is probably the first videogame known for the controversy generated by its portrayal of death. Released in 1976, *Death Race* involved the player driving a car whose aim was to score points by running over screaming gremlins. Reactions to this game were so heated that it was sometimes physically removed from arcades by irate activists. Death-related themes were also found in nonviolent games. Even relatively nonviolent games such as *Frogger,* in which players attempt to guide a frog across a river or street, culminate in the death of the player's main character.

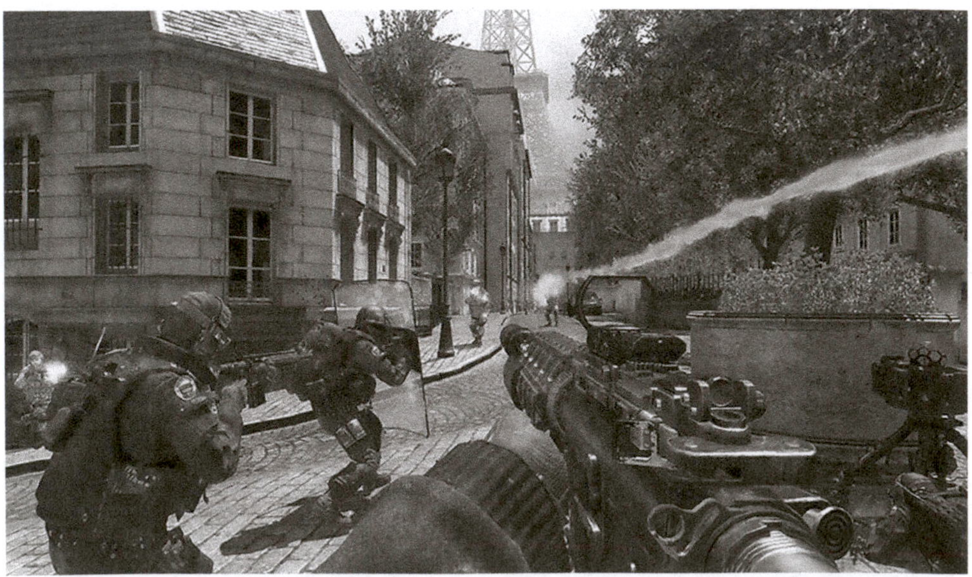

In this file video game image released by Activision, special forces try to repel a Russian invasion of Paris in *Call of Duty: Modern Warfare 3.* **(AP Photo/Activision, File)**

In many early games, players were rewarded with higher scores for violent acts. This has led to the common assumption that gamers "earn points" for violence despite the fact that, by the 1990s, most games phased out awarding scores. Themes related to violence and death continued to expand in computer and video games in the 1980s and 1990s. As graphics slowly improved and game play began to feature more human-on-human violence, controversy about violence in videogames continued. The interactive nature of video games emerged as a common focal point for concern, although no conclusive or definitive evidence emerged that video games had more effect than other media in generating real or actual violence in their users. Storylines also became more complex and artistic, allowing designers greater opportunity to explore themes that could, at times, be quite morbid.

From the early 1990s, games such as *Mortal Kombat, Streetfighter,* and *Doom* depicted the grizzly consequences of violence, attracting public criticism for doing so. During the period in which video games containing themes of violence and death grew in popularity, youth violence declined to lows seen only previously in the 1960s. The data, along with lack of scholarly research support, have led to a decline in the assumption that video games are "harmful." By the time of the *Brown v EMA* Supreme Court decision in 2011, in which the United States Supreme Court struck down a California law regulating violent video game sales to minors (referring to the available research evidence as unconvincing and inconsistent), increasing numbers of scholars have acknowledged that the research evidence does not support the supposed claims of harm caused by violent video games.

Depictions of Death in Video Games

As with certain aspects of television, such as children's action-adventure series' and war films, an early criticism of video games was that death was not portrayed in a realistic fashion. In early games, death was effectively trivialized, and was all part of the game; one could, after all, always overcome death by starting another game, thereby reviving the life of a game's key protagonist.

Even in more modern "action" games, death has tended to be treated in a transient way. In order to keep the action flowing, individual deaths quickly come and go, with players moving on to the next target. Relatively little emotional attachment is formed between the player and the majority of characters in the game. Increasingly, however, there are exceptions to this. Modern games such as *Bioshock 2* and the *Call of Duty* series often use "cut scenes" between periods of action to portray the death of important game characters as emotionally laden events. Typically, these cut scenes come as "chapter breaks" in the game and serve to move the story forward. Players may even see their characters die, permanently, as part of the game's storyline, such as in recent series of *Modern Warfare* releases.

Christopher J. Ferguson

Further Reading

Ferguson, C.J. "Violent Video Games and the Supreme Court: Lessons for the Scientific Community in the Wake of Brown *v.* EMA." *American Psychologist,* 68(2) (2013): 57–74.

Ferguson, C.J. and J.D. Ivory. "A Futile Game: On the Prevalence and Causes of Misguided Speculation about the Role of Violent Video Games in Mass School Shootings." In *School Shootings: Mediated Violence in a Global Age,* edited by Muschert, G.W. and J. Sumiala (pp. 47–67). Bingley, UK: Emerald Group Publishing Limited, 2012.

Hall, R., T. Day, and R. Hall. "A Plea for Caution: Violent Video Games, The Supreme Court, and the Role of Science." *Mayo Clinic Proceedings,* 86(4) (2011): 315–21.

Kent, S. *The Ultimate History of Video Games: From Pong to Pokemon.* New York: Three Rivers Press, 2001.

Olson, C. "Media Violence Research and Youth Violence Data: Why Do They Conflict?" *Academic Psychiatry,* 28 (2004): 144–50.

"When Killing Becomes a Game." *Al Jazeera,* November 26, 2012. http://stream.aljazeera.com/story/game-kill-0022412

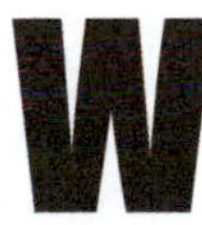

WAKES/VISITATIONS

A wake takes place between the time of death and the disposal of the deceased's body. This ritual may also be known as "visitation," "visiting" or "calling hours," "laying in state/honor/repose," or "waking the dead," depending upon a range of social and historical factors, including the social class, ethnic/cultural background, and religious/spiritual beliefs of the deceased and their family, as well as the geographical location and period in history in which the death occurred.

"Waking the Dead"

Prior to the widespread practice of embalming (see **Embalming**) and the emergence of modern medicine, with its ability to confirm physical and brain death (see **Definitions of Death**), a "wake" provided an interim period before burial that accomplished several purposes. Some religious belief systems and cultures practiced "watching" or "waking" the dead to confirm the death, a custom that might consist of a solemn vigil or the playing of practical jokes ("rousing the ghost") to frighten superstitious relatives. In addition, prayers might be offered for the deceased (see also **Purgatory**), and the bereaved were provided with the opportunity to begin the psychological process of adjusting to their loved one's death.

In earlier periods of history, when people typically died at home, and before the advent of modern funeral homes, the deceased were often laid out in the sitting room or "parlor" of their own home, and friends and family would come to "pay their respects" prior to the burial. In some cultures, wakes were solemn affairs. In other cultures, food and drink, wailing and keening (a vocal lament accompanying mourning), and participation in bawdy games were customary. "Sin eaters" agreed to take on the sins of the deceased by consuming ritual foods, and although the "price" of this action included becoming a social outcast, the poor and hungry welcomed an opportunity to eat.

Modern "Visitation"/"Lying in State"

Although wakes in the deceased's home sometimes occur in conjunction with hospice care, "visitation" or "calling hours" frequently take place in a funeral home. Friends and those who knew the deceased through work or other affiliations gather to say their goodbyes, and to provide support to the bereaved. "Viewing" of the deceased may occur if the casket is open. Families often compile photo collages to illustrate the deceased's life, and guests may share stories about the deceased.

Following the death of a government official (e.g., the president or person occupying some other high-level office), the wake may be held in the principal government building of a country and is described as "lying in state." In the United States, this term is used when the body is displayed in the Rotunda of the U.S. Capitol. On rare occasions, a person of great historical significance who is not a government official will "lie in honor" in the Rotunda, as for example, did Rosa Parks. Public display of a prominent individual's body in a non-government building is referred to as "lying in repose." Lying in state, honor, or repose commonly occurs in conjunction with other public displays of grief (see also **Public Mourning**).

Recent variations in traditional wakes and visitations have occurred due to the availability of technology as well as the "convenience culture" in which we live. For example, drive-thru visitation services are available at several funeral homes, and "cyber funerals" allow individuals who are unable to physically attend to participate in funeral rituals (see **Cyberspace**).

Carla Sofka

See also: Funerals.

Further Reading

Habenstein, Robert W. and William M. Lamers. *The History of American Funeral Directing*, 7th edition. Brookfield, WI: National Funeral Directors Association, 2010.

Jones, Constance. *R.I.P.: The Complete Book of Death and Dying*. New York: HarperCollins, 1997.

Puckle, Bertram S. *Funeral Customs: Their Origin and Development*. London: T. Werner Laurie Ltd., 2008/1926. Available on Google Books http://books.google.com/books?id=KgvdSnaSYpYC&pg=PA6&dq=Puckle,+Bertram+S.+Funeral+Customs:+Their+Origin+and+Development.&hl=en&sa=X&ei=AIzaT_q8O8qe2gXpsMGRBg&ved=0CDkQ6AEwAA#v=onepage&q&f=false

Seeman, Erik R. *Death in the New World: Cross-Cultural Encounters, 1492–1800*. Philadelphia: University of Pennsylvania Press, 2010.

WAR

War is the conflict between two or more opposing forces. These forces represent political communities, which may be nations, governments, or other entities, such as an organized terrorist group or an internal political faction within a particular country. The conflict typically involves the use of armed forces. However, it can also be primarily political in nature, with arms held in reserve and used only as a threat. The Cold War that spanned much of the second half of the 20th century between the Soviet Union and the United States would be an example of such a war.

War is characterized by intentional violence carried out by groups of individuals trained specifically for that purpose. Wars can be fought internally between political groups with opposing beliefs and goals (a civil war) or against an external enemy. An external enemy may be a nation state or an organized group that aspires to statehood or to gain influence in a state (such as modern terrorist groups). A war may even be waged against private groups with no ambitions of statehood, such as drug traffickers targeted in the U.S. war on drugs or a small dissident group of guerillas within a country. This last group carries out a type of war known as a guerilla war (a name that means, literally, "little war"). Guerilla wars were most common during the last third of the 20th century. The key element in a guerilla war is that the guerillas, although typically facing much larger and often better-armed forces, have widespread support from the people. They attack and harass government forces to try to undermine rule by that government in an area. An example would be the guerilla war waged by the Afghan Mujahideen against the occupying forces of the Soviet Union, following their invasion of Afghanistan in 1979.

The Goals of War

Wars vary in motivation and goals. They have been fought for land, resources, national independence, religion, self-defense, and because of irreconcilable political differences. The Prussian military soldier and strategist, Carl von Clausewitz (1780–1831), once claimed that "No one starts a war . . . without first being clear in his mind what he intends to achieve by that war and how he intends to conduct it." That point, the need to have a clear objective before starting a war, would seem to be obvious. However, some wars are started without a clear agreement on the goals of the war or how they are to be achieved. Those who study America's involvement in Vietnam, or that of the Soviet Union in Afghanistan, often find that there was widespread disagreement as to the objective of each of these wars, even among government officials.

In every war, each side wishes to defeat its enemy. However, there is also lack of agreement on what constitutes a "defeat." The defeat of an enemy's forces and its ability to wage war would seem to be a clear defeat of that enemy. That, however, may not always be the case. Von Clausewitz once said that it was not always necessary to conquer all of an enemy's territory, but there were times when, even if it were done, it might not be enough to defeat that enemy.

War is an extension of national policy. The policy of the nation waging a war will therefore play a major role in determining the "character" of the war that is waged. A similar idea has been advanced by Sir John Keegan, author of *A History of Warfare*. Keegan has suggested that war is a universal phenomenon whose form and scope is *defined by the society that wages it*. When that society holds the goals of a war to be of absolute importance, the ultimate result can be total or absolute war.

The Nature of War

Wars can be conventional or nonconventional in nature. Conventional war consists of the use, by opposing sides, of armed forces in battle. As the size of the forces grew and the type of arms used became more sophisticated, the numbers of people killed and wounded rose drastically. Unconventional war tries to defeat an enemy using methods other than traditional armaments and may result in high death tolls among combatants as well as civilian population.

In World War I, a new type of weapon emerged with the introduction of chemical agents to the battlefield. The chief of these was mustard gas, a poison that attacked the respiratory and nervous systems. Chemical warfare was thought to be so devastating that its use was banned by the Geneva Protocol of 1929. This followed a precedent set by the Hague Conventions of 1899 and 1907, which had established rules by which war was to be conducted and what weapons could be used to conduct such wars. The conventions were, in part, violated in World War II, but the ban against chemical agents on the battlefield was observed.

The age of nonconventional war can be said to have truly begun in 1945, when nuclear bombs were used to annihilate the Japanese cities of Hiroshima and Nagasaki. In the same year, the cities of Tokyo, Dresden, and Hamburg had most of their populations wiped out by fire bombs targeted against each city and all of its inhabitants. Technology had outpaced the ability of "rules" to keep abreast of it.

Today, in the 21st century, conventional war continues. However, there are other means of conducting war for which each nation must prepare. This type of war is described as N-B-C: nuclear war, biological war, and chemical war using these agents in place of (or in addition to) conventional arms. Nuclear war includes devices that produce explosions through fission or fusion, but now also uses conventional explosives to spread radioactive material with "dirty bombs." Biological war uses lethal viruses to spread disease and death in an enemy country. Chemical warfare uses agents that have progressed far beyond the mustard gas of World War I. These now include agents that can cause death to millions in a short time period after a brief exposure. Anthrax has been "weaponized" to create such a chemical weapon.

The Rules of War

The "rules" of war and codes of conduct in war have varied over time. In the sixth century, Sun Tzu wrote that "all war is based on deception." This is the one rule that may not have changed. In the 19th century, von Clausewitz wrote that moral principles were the most important element in war. He defined these moral principles as "everything that is created by intellectual and psychological influences." In the 20th century, while attempts were made to reduce armaments through the Washington Naval Conference and the agreements at the Hague and Geneva, wars took on the ability to end all life on the planet (see **Megadeath**). A question that follows from this is, can there be such a thing as a just war?

A "Just" War?

Ethicists and theologians have attempted to define what constitutes a just war. There is general agreement regarding several points that must be present for a war to be considered "just."

- *Cause:* The war must have a valid or just cause. Self-defense against an armed attack is always considered to be a just cause.
- *Last Resort:* War must be a last resort, used only after all other options are exhausted.
- *Waged by Legitimate Authority:* War must be waged by a legitimate authority and not by individuals or groups.
- *Proportionality:* The force used in the war must be a proportional response to the injury suffered.
- *Discrimination among Targets:* The tactics and weapons used must discriminate between combatants and noncombatants. Every effort must be taken to avoid killing civilians.

Even with all of those rules in place, as well as in practice, all levels of leadership, both military and civilian, must demonstrate actions and decisions that are oriented toward positive virtue before the individual soldier can be expected to act virtuously and to follow the rules of war.

The Cost of War

War exacts a cost for all parties, regardless of who wins and who loses. In addition to the financial burdens of war, recent studies suggest that many soldiers who in past years would have been said to be "fine" are, in fact, struggling with emotional and psychological scars that are a direct result of the aftermath of their participation in war. Traumatic brain injury (TBI) and posttraumatic stress disorder (PTSD) place a heavy toll on veterans and on their families.

The End Result

Wars are ultimately decided by a number of factors. The most obvious factor is by battles won or lost. After defeat at Waterloo, Napoleon and his army were finished. The French had lost their empire in Europe. After the defeat at Petersburg, the South had in effect lost the American Civil War. After their defeat at Yorktown, the British yielded to America its independence. The fall of the Maginot Line meant ultimate defeat for France in World War I.

Some military historians and strategists (such as British military historian B. H. Liddell Hart) believe that it is not the loss of lives or military battles that cause a war to be lost. Liddell Hart insisted that the real issues of a war were decided by hope. That is, defeat came to one side because of a "loss of hope" on the part of the vanquished. He describes a progression that starts with a feeling of *helplessness,* then moving to *hopelessness* and, finally, when hope had been lost, to the *capitulation* of one side. Those who believe wars are decided by a loss of hope can also look back to Yorktown to explain why the British, an empire with the most powerful fleets and armies in the world, agreed to withdraw and give independence to its former American colonies.

Perhaps the attraction of war lies in the possibility of a solution to some pressing issue. The flags, music, and comradeship of soldiers all seem romantic and can be a powerful attraction. However, a balanced view of war came from Confederate

General Robert E. Lee who, after seeing the slaughter that his men inflicted on attacking Union forces at Fredericksburg, Virginia, said, "It is good that war is so terrible, lest we grow too fond of it."

Robert G. Stevenson

See also: Megadeath; Terror Management Theory; Terrorism.

Further Reading

Chandler, David G. *The Campaigns of Napoleon: The Mind and Method of History's Greatest Soldier.* New York: Scribner, 1966.
Fisher, David. *Morality and War: Can War Be Just in the Twenty-First Century?* London: Oxford University Press, 2011.
Liddell Hart, B. H. *Strategy.* New York: Praeger Publishing, 1967.
Sun Tzu. *The Art of War.* Translated by Roger T. Ames. New York: Random House Publishing, 1993.
Von Clausewitz, Carl. *On War.* London, England: Penguin Books, 1982.

Z

ZOMBIES

Zombies, also known as "the living dead," are any of a number of types of reanimated corpses. They are a subset of the undead—creatures that formerly were alive, but are not presently dead or "at rest." Zombies can be further defined based on their type. Broadly speaking, zombies can be divided into two categories: supernatural and non-supernatural. There are also what are known in contemporary philosophical literature as "philosophical zombies."

Supernatural and Non-Supernatural Zombies

Supernatural zombies are those whose reanimation can be explained by supernatural or paranormal phenomena. Perhaps the most paradigmatic examples of supernatural zombies are corpses reanimated by Voodoo (both as seen in depictions within popular culture as well as actual Haitian religious rituals). Here, the corpses come under the control of a practitioner of Voodoo, by means of sorcery, magic, or witchcraft, much as would someone who has been hypnotized. Characteristic of such zombies is the complete loss of free will or independent cognitive activity. Other examples of supernatural zombies would be corpses who come to be possessed by other beings, in which case, nothing of the zombie's original personality remains; and corpses who are reanimated with some or all of the zombie's original cognitive traits and abilities intact. Supernatural zombies tend to pose a threat to nonzombie humans in the form of evil actions that they are being commanded to perform.

Non-supernatural zombies are those whose reanimation can be explained by natural phenomena. All known examples of non-supernatural zombies are provided by popular culture. Accordingly, the various cognitive abilities, varying degrees of cognitive ability, and presence or lack thereof of free will, vary on a case-by-case basis. This is in contrast with supernatural zombies, whose cognitive abilities, etc., are at least partially determined by the supernatural or paranormal phenomena that constitute their zombiedom. Examples of non-supernatural zombies include reanimated corpses who are reanimated by virtue of exposure to radioactive matter, chemicals, and viruses. Natural zombies tend to pose a threat to nonzombie humans in that a being bitten by a zombie or having one's bodily fluids exposed to zombie matter will result in death, followed by one becoming a zombie. For this reason, the threat of a zombie apocalypse is, typically, more closely associated with non-supernatural zombies than with supernatural zombies.

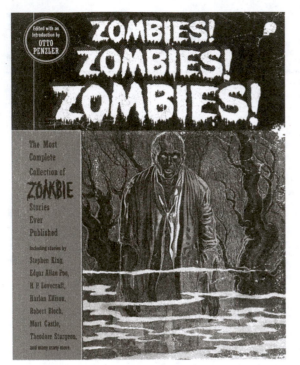

Due to their current cultural popularity, there are a variety of books, comics, and films featuring zombies being released. Shown is the book cover image released by Vintage Crime/Black Lizard, *Zombies! Zombies! Zombies!: The Most Complete Collection of Zombie Stories Ever Published*, edited by Otto Penzler. (AP Photo/Vintage Crime/Black Lizard)

Philosophical Zombies

Philosophical zombies are not reanimated corpses; rather, they are hypothetical creatures identical to human beings in every respect, except that they experience no mental phenomena. Philosophical zombies walk, talk, drive automobiles, and so on, but they don't have the corresponding inner experiences that humans have. They lack consciousness and the qualitative aspects of mental events. They are employed by philosophers in various thought experiments to challenge physicalism—the view that all worldly phenomena can be explained in purely physical terms. Philosophical zombies do not pose any threat to human beings that nonzombie human beings do not pose.

Richard Greene

Further Reading

Greene, Richard and K. Silem Mohammad (eds.). *Zombies, Vampires, and Philosophy.* Chicago IL: Open Court Publishing Company, 2010.

Stanford Encyclopedia of Philosophy. "Zombies." http://plato.stanford.edu/entries/zombies/

Index

Note: Page numbers in **boldface** reflect main entries in the book.

About the Editor

Michael Brennan was previously associate professor of sociology and director of the Center for Death Education and Bioethics at the University of Wisconsin–La Crosse, USA, and he currently teaches sociology in the faculty of business, school of government at Plymouth University, UK. He has written on a variety of topics of thanatological interest, including in his book *Mourning and Disaster* (2008), and has served as associate editor of the journal *Illness Crisis and Loss* and chair of the organizing committee for the International Conference on Death, Grief and Bereavement held annually at the University of Wisconsin–La Crosse, USA.